A Commemorative Issue in Honor of Professor Merlin G. Butler's Retirement: Unlocking Genetic Mysteries

A Commemorative Issue in Honor of Professor Merlin G. Butler's Retirement: Unlocking Genetic Mysteries

Guest Editors

David E. Godler
Olivia J. Veatch

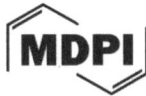

Basel • Beijing • Wuhan • Barcelona • Belgrade • Novi Sad • Cluj • Manchester

Guest Editors

David E. Godler
Genomic Medicine
Murdoch Children's
Research Institute
Melbourne
Australia

Olivia J. Veatch
Psychiatry and
Behavioral Sciences
University of Kansas
Medical Center
Kansas City, KS
United States

Editorial Office
MDPI AG
Grosspeteranlage 5
4052 Basel, Switzerland

This is a reprint of the Special Issue, published open access by the journal *International Journal of Molecular Sciences* (ISSN 1422-0067), freely accessible at: www.mdpi.com/journal/ijms/special_issues/Genetic_Mysteries.

For citation purposes, cite each article independently as indicated on the article page online and using the guide below:

Lastname, A.A.; Lastname, B.B. Article Title. *Journal Name* **Year**, *Volume Number*, Page Range.

ISBN 978-3-7258-3032-9 (Hbk)
ISBN 978-3-7258-3031-2 (PDF)
https://doi.org/10.3390/books978-3-7258-3031-2

© 2025 by the authors. Articles in this book are Open Access and distributed under the Creative Commons Attribution (CC BY) license. The book as a whole is distributed by MDPI under the terms and conditions of the Creative Commons Attribution-NonCommercial-NoDerivs (CC BY-NC-ND) license (https://creativecommons.org/licenses/by-nc-nd/4.0/).

Contents

About the Editors vii

Preface ix

Merlin G. Butler
Prader–Willi Syndrome and Chromosome 15q11.2 BP1-BP2 Region: A Review
Reprinted from: *Int. J. Mol. Sci.* **2023**, *24*, 4271, https://doi.org/10.3390/ijms24054271 1

Joyce Whittington and Anthony Holland
Next Steps in Prader-Willi Syndrome Research: On the Relationship between Genotype and Phenotype
Reprinted from: *Int. J. Mol. Sci.* **2022**, *23*, 12089, https://doi.org/10.3390/ijms232012089 14

Ranim Mahmoud, Virginia Kimonis and Merlin G. Butler
Clinical Trials in Prader–Willi Syndrome: A Review
Reprinted from: *Int. J. Mol. Sci.* **2023**, *24*, 2150, https://doi.org/10.3390/ijms24032150 19

Deepan Singh, Jennifer L. Miller, Edward Robert Wassman, Merlin G. Butler, Allison Foley Shenk and Monica Converse et al.
The Arduous Path to Drug Approval for the Management of Prader–Willi Syndrome: A Historical Perspective and Call to Action
Reprinted from: *Int. J. Mol. Sci.* **2023**, *24*, 11574, https://doi.org/10.3390/ijms241411574 34

Diana R. Mager, Krista MacDonald, Reena L. Duke, Hayford M. Avedzi, Edward C. Deehan and Jason Yap et al.
Comparison of Body Composition, Muscle Strength and Cardiometabolic Profile in Children with Prader-Willi Syndrome and Non-Alcoholic Fatty Liver Disease: A Pilot Study
Reprinted from: *Int. J. Mol. Sci.* **2022**, *23*, 15115, https://doi.org/10.3390/ijms232315115 37

Qiming Tan, Xiao Tian (Tim) He, Sabrina Kang, Andrea M. Haqq and Joanna E. MacLean
Preserved Sleep for the Same Level of Respiratory Disturbance in Children with Prader-Willi Syndrome
Reprinted from: *Int. J. Mol. Sci.* **2022**, *23*, 10580, https://doi.org/10.3390/ijms231810580 54

Lawrence P. Richer, Qiming Tan, Merlin G. Butler, Hayford M. Avedzi, Darren S. DeLorey and Ye Peng et al.
Evaluation of Autonomic Nervous System Dysfunction in Childhood Obesity and Prader–Willi Syndrome
Reprinted from: *Int. J. Mol. Sci.* **2023**, *24*, 8013, https://doi.org/10.3390/ijms24098013 65

Merlin G. Butler, Waheeda A. Hossain, Neil Cowen and Anish Bhatnagar
Chromosomal Microarray Study in Prader-Willi Syndrome
Reprinted from: *Int. J. Mol. Sci.* **2023**, *24*, 1220, https://doi.org/10.3390/ijms24021220 81

Caroline St. Peter, Waheeda A. Hossain, Scott Lovell, Syed K. Rafi and Merlin G. Butler
Mowat–Wilson Syndrome: Case Report and Review of *ZEB2* Gene Variant Types, Protein Defects and Molecular Interactions
Reprinted from: *Int. J. Mol. Sci.* **2024**, *25*, 2838, https://doi.org/10.3390/ijms25052838 96

Ranim Mahmoud, Virginia Kimonis and Merlin G. Butler
Genetics of Obesity in Humans: A Clinical Review
Reprinted from: *Int. J. Mol. Sci.* **2022**, *23*, 11005, https://doi.org/10.3390/ijms231911005 119

Merlin G. Butler, Waheeda A. Hossain, Jacob Steinle, Harry Gao, Eleina Cox and Yuxin Niu et al.
Connective Tissue Disorders and Fragile X Molecular Status in Females: A Case Series and Review
Reprinted from: *Int. J. Mol. Sci.* **2022**, *23*, 9090, https://doi.org/10.3390/ijms23169090 . . . . . . **134**

David E. Godler, Yoshimi Inaba, Minh Q. Bui, David Francis, Cindy Skinner and Charles E. Schwartz et al.
Defining the 3'Epigenetic Boundary of the *FMR1* Promoter and Its Loss in Individuals with Fragile X Syndrome
Reprinted from: *Int. J. Mol. Sci.* **2023**, *24*, 10712, https://doi.org/10.3390/ijms241310712 . . . . . **144**

Kathleen Rooney and Bekim Sadikovic
DNA Methylation Episignatures in Neurodevelopmental Disorders Associated with Large Structural Copy Number Variants: Clinical Implications
Reprinted from: *Int. J. Mol. Sci.* **2022**, *23*, 7862, https://doi.org/10.3390/ijms23147862 . . . . . . **161**

Valeria Orlando, Silvia Di Tommaso, Viola Alesi, Sara Loddo, Silvia Genovese and Giorgia Catino et al.
A Complex Genomic Rearrangement Resulting in Loss of Function of *SCN1A* and *SCN2A* in a Patient with Severe Developmental and Epileptic Encephalopathy
Reprinted from: *Int. J. Mol. Sci.* **2022**, *23*, 12900, https://doi.org/10.3390/ijms232112900 . . . . . **180**

About the Editors

David E. Godler

Dr. Godler is an Associate Professor at the University of Melbourne and a Group Leader of the Diagnosis and Development Laboratory at the Murdoch Children's Research Institute (MCRI). His research combines the power of omics technologies, population-scale cohort studies, and deep clinical phenotyping to improve outcomes for children and families with rare diseases.

Olivia J. Veatch

Dr. Veatch is an Assistant Professor in the Department of Psychiatry and Behavioral Sciences at the University of Kansas Medical Center. Her research combines innovative molecular and computational techniques for gene discovery and characterization to inform translational medicine for mental health conditions. Her research aims to help bridge the gap between basic science research endeavors and the clinical environment by finding efficient ways to translate biomedical data into clinically useful information.

Preface

This Special Issue of the *International Journal of Molecular Sciences* is dedicated to Professor Merlin G. Butler, in recognition of his retirement and to commemorate his substantial contributions to the field of genetics and genomics-driven medical care. Dr. Butler has been a pioneer in the expansion of our understanding of how genetics can help inform healthcare professionals regarding individuals with neurodevelopmental syndromes and conditions. For more than four decades, throughout his career as a physician scientist and laboratory and medical geneticist, he has cared for thousands of patients seeking genetic services in the clinical setting, also having performed extensive research, specifically regarding Prader–Willi, Angelman, Burnside–Butler, and fragile X syndromes, the genetics of autism and obesity, and the characterization, delineation, and natural history of rare genetic disorders using advanced genomic and pharmacogenetic methods. Rapid advancements in genomic technologies are continuing to improve the diagnosis, disease surveillance, counseling, research, and treatment of rare genetic diseases, chromosomal and neurodevelopmental disorders, autism, and congenital abnormalities. This commemorative Special Issue focuses on original research and review articles evaluating innovative molecular and computational approaches for studying the mechanisms underlying the expression and development of both common and rare genetic conditions.

David E. Godler and Olivia J. Veatch
Guest Editors

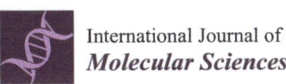 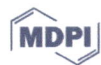

Review

Prader–Willi Syndrome and Chromosome 15q11.2 BP1-BP2 Region: A Review

Merlin G. Butler

Department of Psychiatry and Behavioral Sciences, University of Kansas Medical Center, 3901 Rainbow Blvd., MS 4015, Kansas City, MO 66160, USA; mbutler4@kumc.edu

Abstract: Prader–Willi syndrome (PWS) is a complex genetic disorder with three PWS molecular genetic classes and presents as severe hypotonia, failure to thrive, hypogonadism/hypogenitalism and developmental delay during infancy. Hyperphagia, obesity, learning and behavioral problems, short stature with growth and other hormone deficiencies are identified during childhood. Those with the larger 15q11-q13 Type I deletion with the absence of four non-imprinted genes (*NIPA1*, *NIPA2*, *CYFIP1*, *TUBGCP5*) from the 15q11.2 BP1-BP2 region are more severely affected compared with those with PWS having a smaller Type II deletion. *NIPA1* and *NIPA2* genes encode magnesium and cation transporters, supporting brain and muscle development and function, glucose and insulin metabolism and neurobehavioral outcomes. Lower magnesium levels are reported in those with Type I deletions. The *CYFIP1* gene encodes a protein associated with fragile X syndrome. The *TUBGCP5* gene is associated with attention-deficit hyperactivity disorder (ADHD) and compulsions, more commonly seen in PWS with the Type I deletion. When the 15q11.2 BP1-BP2 region alone is deleted, neurodevelopment, motor, learning and behavioral problems including seizures, ADHD, obsessive-compulsive disorder (OCD) and autism may occur with other clinical findings recognized as Burnside–Butler syndrome. The genes in the 15q11.2 BP1-BP2 region may contribute to more clinical involvement and comorbidities in those with PWS and Type I deletions.

Keywords: Prader–Willi syndrome (PWS); PWS molecular genetic classes; typical 15q11-q13 Type I; Type II deletions; 15q11.2 BP1-BP2 deletion; clinical findings

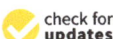

Citation: Butler, M.G. Prader–Willi Syndrome and Chromosome 15q11.2 BP1-BP2 Region: A Review. *Int. J. Mol. Sci.* **2023**, *24*, 4271. https://doi.org/10.3390/ijms24054271

Academic Editor: Lidia Larizza

Received: 12 January 2023
Revised: 13 February 2023
Accepted: 17 February 2023
Published: 21 February 2023

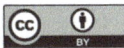

Copyright: © 2023 by the author. Licensee MDPI, Basel, Switzerland. This article is an open access article distributed under the terms and conditions of the Creative Commons Attribution (CC BY) license (https://creativecommons.org/licenses/by/4.0/).

1. Introduction

Prader–Willi syndrome (PWS) is caused by genomic imprinting errors with absence of expression of imprinted genes in the paternally derived PWS/Angelman syndrome (AS) region involving the chromosome 15q11.2-13 region by several genetic mechanisms. The most common cause is a paternal deletion followed by maternal disomy 15 where both 15s are from the mother, imprinting defects or chromosome 15 abnormalities (e.g., [1–5]). PWS affects about one in 15,000–20,000 individuals with an estimated 400,000 cases worldwide. This rare obesity-related genetic disorder has severe infantile hypotonia accompanied by poor suck with swallowing problems, sticky saliva and failure to thrive along with hypogonadism, hypogenitalism and development delay; many of these features compose the consensus diagnostic criteria triggering genetic testing for PWS [1,6–8]. Unique facial features are noted in PWS including bifrontal narrowing, almond-shaped eyes and a small chin with a high palate; additionally, small hands and feet with short stature due to growth and other hormone deficiencies involving the endocrine system and sex organs, pancreas, adrenal and thyroid glands occur [1,4,6–17]. Obesity, growth anomalies and hypogonadism are due to central and peripheral mechanisms involving the hypothalamus–pituitary–gonadal axis.

Nutritional phases previously described in PWS [7,18] display clinical stages of failure to thrive during infancy and excessive eating with hyperphagia in early childhood along with reduced physical activity and a lower metabolic rate leading to severe obesity, if not controlled externally [7,14]. Hyperphagia is an important health problem leading to both mortality and causes of death [19,20] with associated comorbidities typically lasting throughout life. The most common causes of death in a large survey of PWS patients studied were respiratory failure in 31%, followed by cardiac (16%), gastrointestinal (10%), infection (9%), obesity (7%) and pulmonary embolism (7%). Choking (6%) and accidents (6%) were reported more often in childhood or as young adults. The average age of death was 29.5 years [19,20]. The mortality rate for PWS is estimated at 3% per year across an age range of 0 to 47 years and 7% per year for patients aged >30 years. The most reported causes of death in children are respiratory infections and sudden deaths [21].

Mild intellectual disabilities in PWS are noted with an average IQ of 65 and about one-third having a normal IQ but often with delayed language and motor skills (e.g., [22]). Patients with PWS have unique symptoms and associated psychiatric or behavioral problems beginning in early childhood in greater than 70% of PWS patients, including emotional disturbances and obsessive-compulsive disorders, anxiety, depression, controlling and manipulative behavior, violent outbursts, stubbornness and skin picking [7,16,23]. The severity increases with age but diminishes in older patients. A high pain threshold is present along with eating nonfood or inedible items [1,6,7,11,14,16]. They also become easily frustrated with impulsivity, have a quick response to anger and lack of flexibility. Attention deficit hyperactivity with insistence to sameness is often observed in PWS and at an early age. Early diagnosis appears to lead to an improved prognosis and allows for potential treatment approaches to impact quality of life and life expectancy [24] (see Figure 1). An emerging disorder that shares genetic components with PWS is now recognized as the 15q11.2 BP1-BP2 deletion (Burnside–Butler) syndrome. The 15q11.2 BP1-BP2 region contains four genes in common with those with PWS having a typical chromosome 15q11-q13 deletion and will be discussed later in this review. Burnside–Butler syndrome is associated with motor and developmental delays, neurobehavioral problems including dyslexia, autism and psychosis with reported congenital anomalies [7,9]. Several of these findings are common in PWS, more so in those with the larger typical deletion.

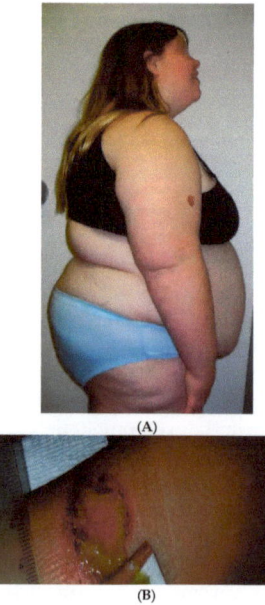

Figure 1. (**A**) A profile view from a 16-year-old female with Prader–Willi syndrome (PWS) showing central obesity as a major feature of this disorder. (**B**) A self-injury site noted in a separate patient with PWS, an abnormal clinical finding often seen in PWS.

2. Genetics of Prader–Willi Syndrome

The most recent studies using advanced genetic testing in the largest PWS cohort to date [2] showed that a 15q11-q13 paternal deletion is found in about 60% of PWS individuals, about 35% with maternal disomy 15, and the remaining individuals with imprinting defects, chromosome 15 translocations or inversions. The 15q11-13 proximal deletion breakpoint is located at two sites (i.e., breakpoint BP1 or breakpoint BP2) at the 15q11.2 band and located within either of two large duplicons predisposing for deletion hotspots at these sites (e.g., [25,26]). The larger Type I deletion at approximately 6 Mb in size involves the proximal BP1 breakpoint near the centromere and a distal 15q11-q13 breakpoint (BP3). The Type II deletion is smaller and involves proximal BP2 site located about 500 kilobases distal to breakpoint BP1 and the more distal breakpoint BP3, a breakpoint that is common in both the typical 15q11-q13 Type I or Type II deletion subtypes (e.g., [1,2,25,26], see Figure 2).

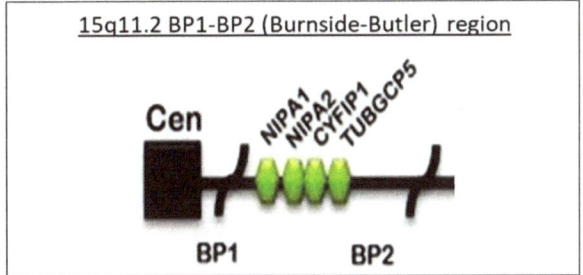

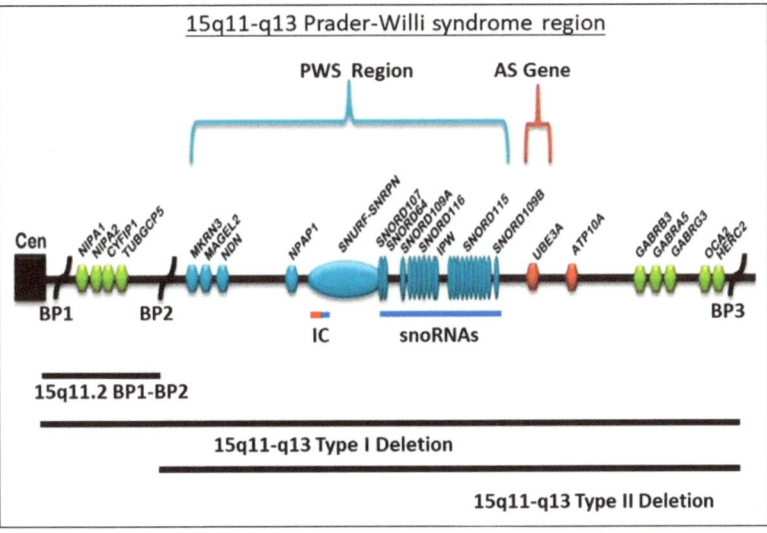

Figure 2. Chromosome 15q11-q13 region with gene and transcript symbols in blue and the location causing Prader–Willi syndrome (PWS) imprinted with paternal expression. Angelman syndrome (AS) and maternal expression is in red, including the causative AS gene (*UBE3A*). The non-imprinted genes are green. The three 15q11-q13 breakpoints (BP1, BP2 and BP3) are the sites for the three chromosome 15q deletions; the larger Type I at BP1 and BP3, smaller Type II at BP2 and BP3 and the 15q11.2 BP1-BP2 deletion alone designated as Burnside–Butler syndrome. IC designates the imprinting center that controls the activity of the imprinted genes in the region and dependent on the parent of origin. The 15q11.2 BP1-BP2 region is enlarged and illustrated at the top.

Prader–Willi syndrome is recognized as the first example of genomic imprinting in humans with dozens of genes and transcripts identified and located between chromosome 15q11-q13 breakpoints BP1 and BP3 flanked by low copy repeats prone to non-homologous recombination that leads to PWS. Genes in this 15q11-q13 region are both imprinted (*NDN, MAGEL2, MKRN3, SNURF-SNRPN, SNORDs, UBE3A, ATP10A*) and non-imprinted (*NIPA1, NIPA2, CYFIP1, TUBGCP5, GABA* receptors, *OCA2* albinism). There are 165 recognized human and 197 mouse genes currently known to be imprinted or active depending on the parent of origin. Several genes in the 15q11-q13 region have been implicated in neurodevelopment and function with a role in behavior and learning, ataxia, hyperphagia and obesity, magnesium transportation, hypogonadism and precocious puberty, circadian rhythm, autism and skin pigment production with albinism [1,2,7,17,24–28].

Information about the functional status of chromosome 15 genes, both imprinted and non-imprinted have been characterized. Specifically, the *NDN* (neurally differentiated EC cell-derived factor) gene which interacts with hundreds of encoded proteins such as brain-derived neurotrophic factor (BDNF) and ubiquitin E3 ligase has been studied which leads to degradation of the proapoptotic or cell cycle apoptosis regulatory protein. Additionally, *MAGEL2* or melanoma antigen-like 2 gene is imprinted in the brain and expressed from the paternal chromosome 15 allele. This gene is intron-less and associates with ubiquitin E3 ligase by altering activity, substrate specificity and subcellar location. Nonsense mutations of the *MAGEL2* gene are reported in Schaaf–Yang syndrome. At an early age, individuals with this syndrome have overlapping features including hyperphagia seen in PWS (e.g., [7,8]). The *MKRN3* or Makorin ring finger protein 3 gene is also imprinted and expressed on the paternal allele. The *MKRN3* gene plays a role in puberty and is expressed in the hypothalamus. It blocks transcription of *KISS* (KiSS-1 metastasis suppressor) and *TAC3* (tachykinin precursor 3), which are important for release of GnRH (gonadotrophin-releasing hormone) which initiates puberty [7,17]. *SNURF-SNRPN* (SNRPN upstream reading frame (SNURF)-small nuclear ribonucleoprotein polypeptide N (SNRPN)), a complex gene locus belonging to the *SNRPN* SmB/SmN family. The protein plays a role in pre-mRNA processing, tissue specific alternative splicing events and transcript production. *SNURF-SNRPN* is bi-cistronic in nature with over 100 exons that undergo alternative splicing and encodes two different proteins with exons 1–3 for SNURF producing a polypeptide and exons 4–10 generating a spliceosome protein (SmN) involved in mRNA splicing. The 5′ untranslated region component of this gene is identified as an imprinting center. This gene hosts six snoRNAs which are regulated or under the control by expression of the *SNURF-SNRPN* complex gene locus. SnoRNAs do not encode or generate protein but can impact the expression of genes and function of related proteins. Errors of paternally expressed genes/transcripts in this region do cause PWS and a second embedded imprinting center controls the maternally expressed *UBE3A* (ubiquitin-protein ligase E3A) gene causing Angelman syndrome when altered (deleted, mutated or by paternal disomy 15) (e.g., [7,16,17,29]).

SNORD116 is one of the snoRNAs in the chromosome 15q11-q13 region and is expressed in the hypothalamic region of the brain which regulates appetite, leading to obesity [17]. It appears to play a key role in the development of features seen in PWS as recognized in those with a deletion of this transcript [7]. In mice with a deletion of this transcript, postnatal growth retardation and increased food intake are noted in research studies. These mice also show dysregulation of diurnally expressed genes such as *Mtor* and circadian *Clock*, *Cry1* and *Per2* genes [7]. Sleep disturbances are also found in individuals with PWS [1,4,7,16].

Studies on prohormone convertase (PC1) are helping to further understand the clinical phenotype in PWS based on this protein involvement in several hormonal pathways and disturbances seen in PWS. These include hyperphagic obesity, hypogonadism, short stature, growth and other hormone deficiencies, hyperghrelinemia and relative hypoinsulinemia often due to impaired prohormone processing [30]. Rare microdeletions of the *SNORD116* in humans, *Snord116* knock-out mice models and induced pluripotent stem cell-derived neurons from PWS patients support the role of disturbed prohormone convertase (PC1) activity. Burnett et al. [30] in 2016 reported reduced levels and activity of prohormone convertase PC1 in their studies. They proposed and presented data that humans and mice who are deficient in PC1 display hyperphagic-related obesity. They also have high ghrelin levels (key appetite-inducing hormone produced by the stomach), hypogonadism, and decreased growth hormone and insulin levels. This leads to short stature with reduced growth and diabetes occurring as a result of impaired prohormone processing and lack of active or functional hormones required for normal response, affecting multiple organ systems as seen in PWS. For example, POMC (pro-opiomelanocortin) is a large prohormone that requires cleavage from inactive prohormone status to smaller active peptides for normal function, including for appetite regulation and normal eating behavior which is absent in PWS. Hence, PC1, which is the protein (enzyme) encoded by the *PCSK1* (proprotein convertase, subtilisin/kexin-type 1) gene located on chromosome 5q15 and is involved in post-translational modification or change of prohormone (inactive) to individual peptides (active) status, may be influential. It is suggested that several major neuroendocrine clinical findings seen in PWS could be due to PC1 deficiency requiring more investigations with the potential to lead to therapeutic agents [17,30].

3. Clinical Description of Prader–Willi Syndrome and 15q11.2 BP1-BP2 Deletion

Butler et al. [31] reported PWS patients and the chromosome 15q11-q13 deletion were more affected than patients with maternal disomy 15. Distinct differences were also reported in those with the two typical 15q11-q13 deletions compared with maternal disomy 15, particularly in phenotype, learning and psychiatric/behavioral parameters [31]. Specifically, Roof et al. [32] reported those with PWS and maternal disomy 15 had higher Verbal IQ scores than those with the 15q11-q13 deletion. Furthermore, PWS individuals with the deletion had more self-injury and severe behavior with lower intellectual ability than those with maternal disomy 15 [1,7,16]. The first clinical differences in individuals with PWS were described by Butler et al. [31] in 2004 when examining Type I or Type II deletions including assessments for intellectual, adaptive and aberrant behavior assessments, reading and math skills and visual-motor integration. Generally, poorer assessment scores were found in PWS individuals with Type I deletions compared to those with the smaller Type II deletions or maternal disomy 15. The larger typical Type I deletion accounts for about 40% of the typical 15q11-q13 deletions in PWS [2,31]. Specifically, those with the larger Type I deletions had more compulsions, poorer adaptive behavior and reduced cognition than those with the smaller Type II deletions. Those with the larger deletion had more severe compulsions related to grooming and bathing and compulsions that were more disruptive to daily living [1,31,33–35]. Intellectual ability and academic achievement skills were analyzed, and visual processing was poorer in those with the larger deletion [36,37]. Furthermore, self-injurious behaviors were more commonly observed in those with the larger Type I deletion. Hence, individuals with PWS and the larger 15q11-q13 Type I deletion including the four non-imprinted protein coding genes (*NIPA1*, *NIPA2*, *CYFIP1*, *TUBGCP5*) in the 15q11.2 BP1-BP2 region are more clinically impaired. Those individuals with 15q11.2 BP1-BP2 deletions are missing the four genes alone and do not have PWS but have Burnside–Butler syndrome (BBS) (e.g., [27,38,39]) with developmental motor and speech delays, congenital findings, behavioral problems including autism and brain imaging abnormalities (e.g., [27]).

Individuals with the larger typical 15q11–q13 Type I deletion were found to have more severe neurodevelopmental symptoms when compared to those with PWS or Angelman syndrome, a sister genomic imprinting disorder with loss of maternally expressed genes on the chromosome 15q11-q13 region with the smaller typical Type II deletions (e.g., [30,33–35,40–42]). Bittel et al. [43] reported on molecular gene expression (messenger-RNA) studies from lymphoblastoid cells obtained from PWS males and females from highly conserved *NIPA1*, *NIPA2*, *CYFIP1* and *TUBGCP5* genes. They found that 24–99% of the phenotypic variability seen in behavioral and academic measures in PWS subjects could be explained by individual gene expression patterns. Levels of messenger-RNA from *NIPA1*,

NIPA2, *CYFIP1* and *TUBGCP5* were reduced but detectable in individuals with PWS and the Type I deletion, supporting biallelic expression. Generally, messenger-RNA values were positively correlated with assessment measures, indicating a direct relationship between messenger-RNA levels and better assessment scores. The highest correlation was for *NIPA2*. Negative associations were found between age and behavior in the Type I deletion subtype only and implicating the four genes, specifically *CYFIP1* and *NIPA2*. Disturbed expression of *CYFIP1* is seen in other developmental disabilities including those with 15q disorders without PWS [44,45] and fragile X syndrome [46]. *NIPA1* and *NIPA2* are known to encode magnesium transporters and magnesium levels were recently reported to be lower in those with PWS and the Type I deletion compared to those with Type II deletions [28,47,48].

Clinical findings were reported in the literature from 200 patients with 15q11.2 BP1-BP2 deletion (Burnside–Butler) syndrome grouped into five categories [27]. These categories were (1) developmental (73% of cases), speech (67%) and motor delays (42%); (2) dysmorphic ear (46%) and palatal defects (46%); (3) writing (60%) and reading (57%) difficulties, memory problems (60%) and verbal IQ scores ≤ 75 (50%); (4) general behavioral problems, unspecified (55%); and (5) abnormal brain imaging including white matter disease (43%). Less often seen features were seizures/epilepsy (26%), autism spectrum disorder (ASD) (27%), attention-deficit hyperactivity disorder (ADHD) at 35% of cases and schizophrenia/paranoid psychosis (20%). Furthermore, Davis et al. [49] reported the parent of origin in dozens of families and found a maternal origin of the 15q11.2 BP1-BP2 deletion to be associated with a significantly higher risk for developmental, motor and speech delays, intellectual and learning problems, autism and behavioral/psychiatric diagnoses. Those with paternal chromosome 15q11.2 BP1-BP2 deletions were more prone to poor coordination/ataxia and congenital anomalies. The 15q11.2 BP1-BP2 region is deleted in PWS individuals having the larger Type I deletion. Butler [47] and Butler et al. [48] reported on the role of the four genes found in the 15q11.2 BP1-BP2 region involving magnesium transportation in the clinical presentation and potential treatment of those with Type I deletion. Figure 3 illustrates a frontal view of a non-dysmorphic mother and child having the 15q11.2 BP1-BP2 deletion (Burnside–Butler) syndrome.

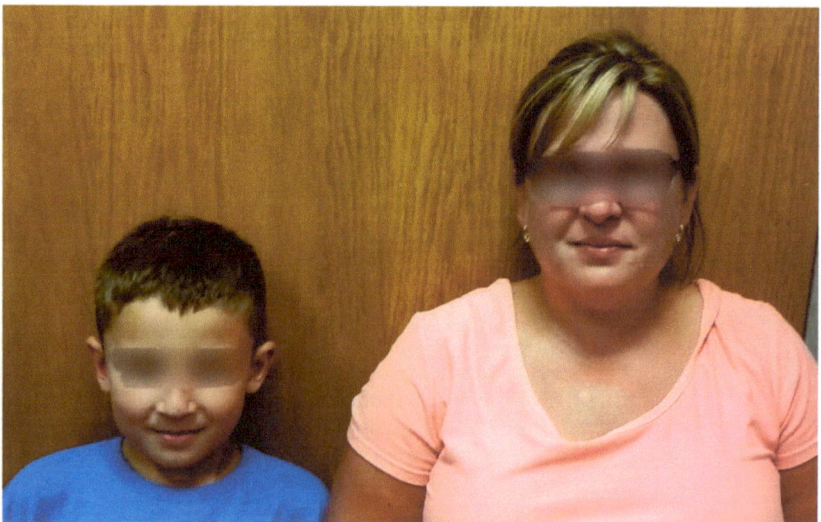

Figure 3. Frontal views of a mother and child with the 15q11.2 BP1-BP2 deletion (Burnside–Butler) syndrome.

4. Description, Evaluation and Gene Expression of Chromosome 15q11.2 BP1-BP2

4.1. Chromosome 15q11.2 BP1-BP2 Region Description

One allele is missing in each of the four genes (*NIPA1, NIPA2, CYFIP1, TUBGCP5*) in the 15q11.2 BP1-BP2 region due to a deletion designated as Burnside–Butler syndrome, emerging with variable clinical findings including a neurodevelopmental-autism non-dysmorphic phenotype with low penetrance. This phenotype presents with features including language and/or motor delay, cognitive impairment, aberrant behavior and autism, poor coordination with ataxia, seizures and congenital anomalies [50–57]. This small proximal 15q11.2 deletion characterized by Burnside et al. [39] in 2011 is now recognized as the most common chromosome finding in large cohorts of those presenting with neurodevelopmental problems and/or autism [50].

Ho et al. [50] in 2016 used 2.8 million DNA markers including single nucleotide polymorphic (SNP) and copy number variant (CNV) probes optimized for detection of regions of homozygosity and CNVs associated with neurodevelopmental disorders with high-resolution chromosomal microarrays. Neurodevelopmental disorders include developmental delay and intellectual disabilities with ASD, which affect up to 15% of all children. About 40% of those with ASD also have learning disabilities and approximately 30% show other comorbidities including seizures (e.g., [58,59]). Genetic testing may allow pinpointing the causes critical for clinical management and genetic counseling of at-risk family members.

Ho et al. [50] summarized results in a total of 10,351 custom microarrays performed on patients over a period of four years with a male to female ratio of 2.5:1 and a mean age of 7.0 years. This neurodevelopmental patient cohort comprised 55% of cases with a diagnosis of ASD with or without other features (ASD+ and ASD only). Neurologists were the most common referring physician group at 36%, followed by developmental pediatricians at 31%, pediatricians at 16% and medical geneticists at 14%. Psychiatrists referred only 2% of the total cases but had the highest indication of ASD at 72% with or without features. In the study, 74% of ASD cases were referred by pediatric neurologists or developmental/behavioral pediatricians. Potentially abnormal CNVs were observed in 28% of cases with an average 1.2 reportable CNVs per individual. Overall detection rate for individuals with ASD was significant at 24.4%. The detection rate for a pathogenic cause using chromosome microarray analysis varied by indication for testing, age and gender as well as specialty of the ordering physician.

The most common genetic defect identified in the combined ASD group (N = 5694 patients) was the 15q11.2 BP1-BP2 deletion, and the 22q11.2 deletion was seen most often in the non-ASD group (N = 4657). The most common cytogenetic finding seen in both the ASD+ group (N = 2844) and ASD only group (N = 2850) was also the 15q11.2 BP1-BP2 deletion. This chromosome 15 defect was the most common finding in both females and males. Of the 85 genetic findings reported by Ho et al. [50], 9% of the patients had the 15q11.2 BP1-BP2 deletion, followed by the 16p11.2 deletion at 5% and 16p11.2 duplication at 5%. Other findings included the 15q13.3 deletion, 16p13.1 duplication and *NRXN1* gene deletion all at 4%. Hence, a greater understanding of the 15q11.2 BP1-BP2 deletion may further impact the role in the context of PWS, the most classical chromosome 15 disorder in humans.

4.2. Chromosome 15q11.2 BP1-BP2 Genes, Functions and Pathway Analysis

To further investigate biological pathways involving the 15q11.2 BP1-BP2 region, Rafi and Butler [28] examined STRING protein–protein interactions that encompass the four 15q11.2 BP1-BP2 genes with predicted Gene Ontology (GO) functions and processes. They found a role in magnesium ion transport, regulation of cellular growth and development with production of bone morphogenetic protein (BMP) and signaling pathways, regulation of axonogenesis and axon extension, cellular growth and development, and plasma membrane bounded cell projection and mitotic spindle organization. Using searchable genomic disease websites and tabulating disease data, they found the top ten overlapping significant neurodevelopmental disorders to be Prader–Willi Syndrome (PWS); Angelman

Syndrome (AS); 15q11.2 Deletion Syndrome with Attention Deficit Hyperactive Disorder and Learning Disability; Autism Spectrum Disorder (ASD); Schizophrenia; Epilepsy; Down Syndrome; Microcephaly; Developmental Disorder; and Peripheral Nervous System Disease. These were also individually associated with PWS, ASD, ataxia, intellectual disability, schizophrenia, epilepsy and Down syndrome.

Of the four non-imprinted biallelic genes and their encoded proteins, NIPA1 protein interacts with 11 other proteins, of which five (45%) are bone morphogenic protein (BMP) superfamily members, three (27%) are BMP receptors and one is the TGFB1 (9%) protein [28]. Therefore, three-fourths of NIPA1 interacting proteins are important for developmental bone morphogenesis or involved in multifunctional proteins controlling proliferation, differentiation and other cellular functions. The *NIPA2* gene and protein interact with 19 other proteins and of these three (16%) are involved with the BMP protein superfamily, three (16%) proteins interact with BMP receptors ACVR1 and TGFBR1, and six are members of the SMAD superfamily of proteins (42%). These genes are important as intracellular signal transducers and transcriptional modulators activated by TGFB [28]. *NIPA1* and *NIPA2* genes also encode magnesium transporter proteins (e.g., [28,54]). Picinelli et al. [55] reported on a small number of patients with 15q11.2 BP1–BP2 deletions or duplications and found an inverse relationship for the NIPA2 gene encoding a magnesium transporter in both central nervous system (CNS) and renal tubules to be directly associated with urinary magnesium levels. Those with this gene deletion had higher urinary magnesium and those with this gene duplicated showed lower urinary levels. PWS patients with the larger Type I deletion had lower plasma magnesium levels [48]. In addition, Xie et al. [56] reported *NIPA2* gene mutations that showed incorrect localization of the NIPA2 transporter protein in neurons. This resulted in decreased intracellular magnesium levels apparently due to reduced cross-membrane transport involving renal tubules. Furthermore, Mg^{2+} is involved in gating and activation of channels and receptors including NMDARs, playing a role in memory processing and altered neural extracellular Mg2+ concentrations caused by *NIPA2* deletions in neuronal cells.

NIPA1 (non-imprinted in PWS/AS 1) gene defects cause autosomal dominant hereditary spastic paraplegia and postural disturbance [60,61]. *NIPA1* is known to mediate Mg^{2+} transport and is highly expressed in the brain [28]. The NIPA1 protein can also transport other divalent cations such as Fe^{2+}, Sr^{2+}, Ba^{2+}, Mn^{2+} and Co^{2+} and possibly impacting their levels. The *NIPA2* (non-imprinted in PWS/AS 2) gene encodes a protein acting as a renal Mg^{2+} transporter. Three reported *NIPA2* mutations (p.I178F, p.N244S and p.N334_E335insD) are found in childhood absence epilepsy [54,56]. *NIPA2* gene variants and functional studies have shown decreased intracellular magnesium concentrations in neurons, suggesting lower intracellular magnesium levels may enhance N-methyl-d-aspartate receptor (NMDAR) currents impacting neuron excitability and brain function.

CYFIP1 (cytoplasmic fragile X mental retardation 1 FMR1 interacting protein 1) is reported to interact with other proteins with functions related to actin filament binding with cell-matrix adhesion, cytoskeleton organization, MAP kinase signal transduction of cell growth, survival and differentiation with stimulation of glucose uptake, intracellular protein breakdown and tissue remodeling and mediation of translational repression. These interactions may impact brain morphology associated with learning and memory impairment. The *CYFIP1* gene encodes a protein that also interacts with FMRP, the protein coded by the *FMR1* gene. It is associated with fragile X syndrome, the most common cause of intellectual disabilities and autism found in families [45,62].

The *TUBGCP5* (tubulin gamma complex associated protein 5) generates an interaction with proteins involved with mitotic spindle formation and assembly along with microtubule organization and production of centrosomal proteins. These are involved in centriole duplication and regulation during cell division. They are also associated with chorioretinopathy and microcephaly (e.g., [28,44,55]) as well as ADHD and obsessive-compulsive disorder (OCD) [28].

Seven genes interact directly with the non-imprinted 15q11.2 BP1-BP2 genes including *CFHR1* or complement factor H-related protein 1 interacting with complement regulation;

SPAST or Spastin, an ATP-dependent microtubule-severing protein involved in movement; *SPG20* or Spartin implicated in endosomal trafficking participating in cytokinesis; *CFHR3* or complement factor H-related protein involved with complement regulation; *MNS1* or meiosis-specific nuclear structural protein 1 controlling meiotic division and germ cell differentiation; *IGFBF2* or insulin-like growth factor-binding protein 2 inhibiting IGF-mediated growth and developmental rates with *BMPR2* or bone morphogenetic protein receptor 2 [26].

4.3. Clinical Evaluation and Findings in 15q11.2 BP1-BP2 Deletion

Clinical and brain imaging data support brain disturbances with global morphology and subcortical volume differences in those with the 15q11.2 BP1-BP2 deletion [63]. Significantly lower nucleus accumbens volume and total surface brain area were found along with thicker cortices reported in those with the deletion when compared to individuals without the deletion, typically across the frontal lobe, anterior cingulate and precentral and postcentral gyri regions using brain magnetic resonance imaging. The investigators also measured cognitive function and found lower performance on all tasks in those with the 15q11.2 BP1-BP2 deletion and larger intracranial volume and total surface area were associated with higher performance on nearly all cognitive tasks. Generally, frontal cortex surface regions were found to be associated with task performance, particularly for fluid intelligence and trail-making tasks.

In addition, onset of adverse perinatal events and early life outcomes have been examined in pregnancies with 15q11.2 BP1-BP2 anomalies [64,65]. For example, Chu et al. [64] analyzed 1,337 pregnancies with genetic amniocentesis and found that 0.7% of cases had the 15q11.2 BP1-BP2 deletion and 0.8% had a duplication of the same region. They compared the pregnancies with normal microarray results to those with the 15q11.2 BP1-BP2 deletion and more cases with the deletion received neonatal intensive care, Apgar scores less than 7 (at 1 min) and recorded neonatal deaths. Perinatal findings noted in other studies included development delays and more infantile deaths in the deletion group, specifically related to congenital heart disease [66]. Other birth defects reported at birth in those with this deletion include congenital arthrogryposis [67] and tracheoesophageal fistula with congenital cataracts [68].

The published abnormal results associated with the 15q11.2 BP1-BP2 deletion do not fit one molecular dysfunction, but multiple altered functions of the four genes, suggesting involvement in neuro-plasticity, development and function. One important interactive gene involved in this cytogenetic region and is associated with learning and motor delays, autism and schizophrenia is *CYFIP1*, which encodes a protein involved with actin cytoskeletal dynamics. It interacts with the fragile X mental retardation protein and when disturbed causes fragile X syndrome with abnormal white matter microstructure and postnatal hippocampal neurogenesis microglial disturbances [69–71]. For example, Silva et al. [69] applied a brain-wide voxel-based approach and analyzed diffusion tensor imaging data from healthy individuals and those with 15q11.2 BP1-BP2 deletions or duplications. A reciprocal effect was found for 15q11.2 BP1-BP2 on white matter microstructure suggesting reciprocal chromosomal imbalances may lead to opposite changes in brain structure. For example, findings in the deletion group overlapped with more white matter differences previously reported in the fragile X syndrome suggesting common pathogenic mechanisms derived from disruptions of the cytoplasmic CYFIP1–fragile X mental retardation protein complexes. In addition, other interactive genes including solute carrier (SLC) family composed of at least 43 gene families and hundreds of transporters may impact features seen in PWS and Burnside–Butler syndrome [28,52]. This collection of gene interactions may contribute to comorbidities seen in PWS, particularly those with the larger Type I deletion including glucose and insulin metabolic alterations [48]. Identified components of the 15q11.2 BP1-BP2 phenotype and neurobiological mechanisms should stimulate more studies to test similarities between the 15q11.2 BP1-BP2 disorder and in those with PWS having the larger typical 15q11-q13 Type I deletion with these four genes deleted.

5. Conclusions

Bi-allelic *NIPA1*, *NIPA2*, *TUBGCP5* and *CYFIP1* genes located in the proximal 15q11 chromosomal region between breakpoints BP1 and BP2 are implicated in compulsivity, aberrant behavior and lower intellectual ability in individuals with Prader–Willi syndrome with Type I versus Type II deletions. For example, the coefficient of determination for the deletion type alone explained 5 to 50% of the variation in the clinical parameters that were assessed when examining expression of the four genes [43].

In summary, this chromosome deletion has been unequivocally associated with congenital defects, neurobehavior disturbances including autism, schizophrenia, dyslexia or dyscalculia in the vast majority of individuals studied related to these four genes. Additional studies are needed to identify the function of the four genes and their interaction with gene networks to clarify their potential role and include brain gene expression patterns with involved pathways. Parent of origin and gender-based differences should be studied. These may impact fetal phenotype, prognosis and development/behavior/psychiatry with the need for follow-up and long-term care, including echocardiography due to the higher risk of congenital anomalies and heart defects with developmental assessments from disturbances seen in those with the 15q11.2 BP1-BP2 deletion.

The clinical presentation and findings seen in Burnside–Butler syndrome (BBS) are also seen in individuals with PWS, particularly those with the larger Type I deletion coined PWS and BBS, with mounting evidence of more severity than is observed in other genetic defects in PWS such as the smaller Type II deletion or maternal disomy 15. The description and explanation of the clinical findings focused on this report and associations could be recognized as a separate category of PWS, particularly in the 25 to 30% of all PWS patients who have the larger Type I deletion with loss of the four described genes and their interactions. These observations could lead to the potential for earlier intervention, treatment and surveillance when applied at a young age, particularly magnesium surveillance and supplementation, if low, with close medical care. More research is requested to pursue and confirm these potentially associated findings with impact on prognosis, longevity and quality of life.

Funding: This research was supported by the National Institute of Child Health and Human Development (NICHD) and U54 grant number HD06122.

Acknowledgments: I thank all patients and families with PWS or Burnside–Butler syndrome as information learned is based on their participation in clinical and genetics studies. I thank Corina Fryman and Waheeda Hossain, MD for their assistance in manuscript preparation and submission.

Conflicts of Interest: There are no conflict of interest from the author.

References

1. Butler, M.G. Single Gene and Syndromic Causes of Obesity: Illustrative Examples. *Prog. Mol. Biol. Transl. Sci.* **2016**, *140*, 1–45. [CrossRef]
2. Butler, M.G.; Hartin, S.N.; Hossain, W.A.; Manzardo, A.M.; Kimonis, V.; Dykens, E.; Gold, J.A.; Kim, S.J.; Weisensel, N.; Tamura, R.; et al. Molecular genetic classification in Prader-Willi syndrome: A multisite cohort study. *J. Med. Genet.* **2019**, *56*, 149–153. [CrossRef]
3. Strom, S.P.; Hossain, W.A.; Grigorian, M.; Li, M.; Fierro, J.; Scaringe, W.; Yen, H.Y.; Teguh, M.; Liu, J.; Gao, H.; et al. A Streamlined Approach to Prader-Willi and Angelman Syndrome Molecular Diagnostics. *Front Genet.* **2021**, *12*, 608889. [CrossRef]
4. Duis, J.; Butler, M.G. Syndromic and Nonsyndromic Obesity: Underlying Genetic Causes in Humans. *Adv. Biol.* **2022**, *6*, e2101154. [CrossRef]
5. Butler, M.G.; Duis, J. Chromosome 15 Imprinting Disorders: Genetic Laboratory Methodology and Approaches. *Front Pediatr.* **2020**, *8*, 154. [CrossRef]
6. Cassidy, S.B.; Schwartz, S.; Miller, J.L.; Driscoll, D.J. Prader-Willi syndrome. *Genet. Med.* **2012**, *14*, 10–26. [CrossRef]
7. Butler, M.G.; Lee, P.; Whitman, B. *Management of Prader-Willi Syndrome*, 4th ed.; Springer Publishers: New York, NY, USA, 2022.
8. Butler, M.G. Imprinting disorders in humans: A review. *Curr. Opin. Pediatr.* **2020**, *32*, 719–729. [CrossRef]
9. Butler, M.G.; Miller, B.S.; Romano, A.; Ross, J.; Abuzzahab, M.J.; Backeljauw, P.; Bamba, V.; Bhangoo, A.; Mauras, N.; Geffner, M. Genetic conditions of short stature: A review of three classic examples. *Front Endocrinol.* **2022**, *13*, 1011960. [CrossRef]

10. Alves, C.; Franco, R.R. Prader-Willi syndrome: Endocrine manifestations and management. *Arch. Endocrinol. Metab.* **2020**, *64*, 223–234. [CrossRef]
11. Butler, M.G. Prader-Willi syndrome: Current understanding of cause and diagnosis. *Am. J. Med. Genet.* **1990**, *35*, 319–332. [CrossRef]
12. Angulo, M.A.; Butler, M.G.; Hossain, W.A.; Castro-Magana, M.; Corletto, J. Central adrenal insufficiency screening with morning plasma cortisol and ACTH levels in Prader-Willi syndrome. *J. Pediatr. Endocrinol. Metab.* **2022**, *35*, 733–740. [CrossRef]
13. Mahmoud, R.; Kimonis, V.; Butler, M.G. Genetics of Obesity in Humans: A Clinical Review. *Int. J. Mol. Sci.* **2022**, *23*, 11005. [CrossRef]
14. Butler, M.G.; Miller, J.L.; Forster, J.L. Prader-Willi Syndrome—Clinical Genetics, Diagnosis and Treatment Approaches: An Update. *Curr. Pediatr. Rev.* **2019**, *15*, 207–244. [CrossRef] [PubMed]
15. Butler, M.G.; Kimonis, V.; Dykens, E.; Gold, J.A.; Miller, J.; Tamura, R.; Driscoll, D.J. Prader-Willi syndrome and early-onset morbid obesity NIH rare disease consortium: A review of natural history study. *Am. J. Med. Genet A* **2018**, *176*, 368–375. [CrossRef] [PubMed]
16. Driscoll, D.J.; Miller, J.L.; Schwartz, S.; Cassidy, S.B. Prader-Willi Syndrome. In *GeneReviews®*; Adam, M.P., Everman, D.B., Mirzaa, G.M., Pagon, R.A., Wallace, S.E., Bean, L.J.H., Gripp, K.W., Amemiya, A., Eds.; University of Washington: Seattle, WA, USA, 1998; pp. 1993–2022.
17. Napolitano, L.; Barone, B.; Morra, S.; Celentano, G.; La Rocca, R.; Capece, M.; Morgera, V.; Turco, C.; Caputo, V.F.; Spena, G.; et al. Hypogonadism in Patients with Prader Willi Syndrome: A Narrative Review. *Int. J. Mol. Sci.* **2021**, *22*, 1993. [CrossRef]
18. Miller, J.L.; Lynn, C.H.; Driscoll, D.C.; Goldstone, A.P.; Gold, J.A.; Kimonis, V.; Dykens, E.; Butler, M.G.; Shuster, J.J.; Driscoll, D.J. Nutritional phases in Prader-Willi syndrome. *Am. J. Med. Genet. A* **2011**, *155A*, 1040–1049. [CrossRef] [PubMed]
19. Butler, M.G.; Manzardo, A.M.; Heinemann, J.; Loker, C.; Loker, J. Causes of death in Prader-Willi syndrome: Prader-Willi Syndrome Association (USA) 40-year mortality survey. *Genet. Med.* **2017**, *19*, 635–642. [CrossRef]
20. Manzardo, A.M.; Loker, J.; Heinemann, J.; Loker, C.; Butler, M.G. Survival trends from the Prader-Willi Syndrome Association (USA) 40-year mortality survey. *Genet. Med.* **2018**, *20*, 24–30. [CrossRef] [PubMed]
21. Whittington, J.E.; Holland, A.J.; Webb, T.; Butler, J.; Clarke, D.; Boer, H. Population prevalence and estimated birth incidence and mortality rate for people with Prader-Willi syndrome in one UK Health Region. *J. Med. Genet.* **2001**, *38*, 792–798. [CrossRef]
22. Butler, M.G.; Matthews, N.A.; Patel, N.; Surampalli, A.; Gold, J.A.; Khare, M.; Thompson, T.; Cassidy, S.B.; Kimonis, V.E. Impact of genetic subtypes of Prader-Willi syndrome with growth hormone therapy on intelligence and body mass index. *Am. J. Med. Genet. A* **2019**, *179*, 1826–1835. [CrossRef]
23. Huisman, S.; Mulder, P.; Kuijk, J.; Kerstholt, M.; van Eeghen, A.; Leenders, A.; van Balkom, I.; Oliver, C.; Piening, S.; Hennekam, R. Self-injurious behavior. *Neurosci. Biobehav. Rev.* **2018**, *84*, 483–491. [CrossRef]
24. Kimonis, V.E.; Tamura, R.; Gold, J.A.; Patel, N.; Surampalli, A.; Manazir, J.; Miller, J.L.; Roof, E.; Dykens, E.; Butler, M.G.; et al. Early Diagnosis in Prader-Willi Syndrome Reduces Obesity and Associated Co-Morbidities. *Genes* **2019**, *10*, 898. [CrossRef]
25. Nicholls, R.D.; Knepper, J.L. Genome organization, function, and imprinting in Prader-Willi and Angelman syndromes. *Annu. Rev. Genomics. Hum. Genet.* **2001**, *2*, 153–175. [CrossRef]
26. Bittel, D.C.; Butler, M.G. Prader-Willi syndrome: Clinical genetics, cytogenetics and molecular biology. *Expert Rev. Mol. Med.* **2005**, *7*, 1–20. [CrossRef] [PubMed]
27. Butler, M.G. Clinical and genetic aspects of the 15q11.2 BP1-BP2 microdeletion disorder. *J. Intellect. Disabil. Res.* **2017**, *61*, 568–579. [CrossRef] [PubMed]
28. Rafi, S.K.; Butler, M.G. The 15q11.2 BP1-BP2 Microdeletion (*Burnside-Butler*) Syndrome: In Silico Analyses of the Four Coding Genes Reveal Functional Associations with Neurodevelopmental Phenotypes. *Int. J. Mol. Sci.* **2020**, *21*, 3296. [CrossRef]
29. Kalsner, L.; Chamberlain, S.J. Prader-Willi, Angelman, and 15q11-q13 Duplication Syndromes. *Pediatr. Clin. North. Am.* **2015**, *62*, 587–606. [CrossRef] [PubMed]
30. Burnett, L.C.; LeDuc, C.A.; Sulsona, C.R.; Paull, D.; Rausch, R.; Eddiry, S.; Carli, J.F.; Morabito, M.V.; Skowronski, A.A.; Hubner, G.; et al. Deficiency in prohormone convertase PC1 impairs prohormone processing in Prader-Willi syndrome. *J. Clin. Investig.* **2017**, *127*, 293–305. [CrossRef] [PubMed]
31. Butler, M.G.; Bittel, D.C.; Kibiryeva, N.; Talebizadeh, Z.; Thompson, T. Behavioral differences among subjects with Prader-Willi syndrome and type I or type II deletion and maternal disomy. *Pediatrics* **2004**, *113*, 565–573. [CrossRef]
32. Roof, E.; Stone, W.; MacLean, W.; Feurer, I.D.; Thompson, T.; Butler, M.G. Intellectual characteristics of Prader-Willi syndrome: Comparison of genetic subtypes. *J. Intellect. Disabil. Res.* **2000**, *44*, 25–30. [CrossRef] [PubMed]
33. Hartley, S.L.; Maclean, W.E., Jr.; Butler, M.G.; Zarcone, J.; Thompson, T. Maladaptive behaviors and risk factors among the genetic subtypes of Prader-Willi syndrome. *Am. J. Med. Genet A* **2005**, *136*, 140–145. [CrossRef]
34. Zarcone, J.; Napolitano, D.; Peterson, C.; Breidbord, J.; Ferraioli, S.; Caruso-Anderson, M.; Holsen, L.; Butler, M.G.; Thompson, T. The relationship between compulsive behaviour and academic achievement across the three genetic subtypes of Prader-Willi syndrome. *J. Intellect. Disabil. Res.* **2007**, *51*, 478–487. [CrossRef]
35. Holsen, L.M.; Zarcone, J.R.; Chambers, R.; Butler, M.G.; Bittel, D.C.; Brooks, W.M.; Thompson, T.I.; Savage, C.R. Genetic subtype differences in neural circuitry of food motivation in Prader-Willi syndrome. *Int. J. Obes.* **2009**, *33*, 273–283. [CrossRef] [PubMed]
36. Fox, R.; Sinatra, R.B.; Mooney, M.A.; Feurer, I.D.; Butler, M.G. Visual capacity and Prader-Willi syndrome. *J. Pediatr. Ophthalmol. Strabismus.* **1999**, *36*, 331–336. [CrossRef]

37. Fox, R.; Yang, G.S.; Feurer, I.D.; Butler, M.G.; Thompson, T. Kinetic form discrimination in Prader-Willi syndrome. *J. Intellect. Disabil. Res.* **2001**, *45*, 317–325. [CrossRef]
38. Cox, D.M.; Butler, M.G. The 15q11.2 BP1-BP2 microdeletion syndrome: A review. *Int. J. Mol. Sci.* **2015**, *16*, 4068–4082. [CrossRef]
39. Burnside, R.D.; Pasion, R.; Mikhail, F.M.; Carroll, A.J.; Robin, N.H.; Youngs, E.L.; Gadi, I.K.; Keitges, E.; Jaswaney, V.L.; Papenhausen, P.R.; et al. Microdeletion/microduplication of proximal 15q11.2 between BP1 and BP2: A susceptibility region for neurological dysfunction including developmental and language delay. *Hum. Genet.* **2011**, *130*, 517–528. [CrossRef]
40. Chai, J.H.; Locke, D.P.; Greally, J.M.; Knoll, J.H.; Ohta, T.; Dunai, J.; Yavor, A.; Eichler, E.E.; Nicholls, R.D. Identification of four highly conserved genes between breakpoint hotspots BP1 and BP2 of the Prader-Willi/Angelman syndromes deletion region that have undergone evolutionary transposition mediated by flanking duplicons. *Am. J. Hum. Genet.* **2003**, *73*, 898–925. [CrossRef]
41. Dagli, A.; Buiting, K.; Williams, C.A. Molecular and Clinical Aspects of Angelman Syndrome. *Mol. Syndromol.* **2012**, *2*, 100–112. [CrossRef]
42. Bonello, D.; Camilleri, F.; Calleja-Agius, J. Angelman Syndrome: Identification and Management. *Neonatal. Netw.* **2017**, *36*, 142–151. [CrossRef]
43. Bittel, D.C.; Kibiryeva, N.; Butler, M.G. Expression of 4 genes between chromosome 15 breakpoints 1 and 2 and behavioral outcomes in Prader-Willi syndrome. *Pediatrics* **2006**, *118*, e1276–e1283. [CrossRef]
44. Chen, C.P.; Lin, S.P.; Lee, C.L.; Chern, S.R.; Wu, P.S.; Chen, Y.N.; Chen, S.W.; Wang, W. Familial transmission of recurrent 15q11.2 (BP1-BP2) microdeletion encompassing NIPA1, NIPA2, CYFIP1, and TUBGCP5 associated with phenotypic variability in developmental, speech, and motor delay. *Taiwan J. Obstet. Gynecol.* **2017**, *56*, 93–97. [CrossRef]
45. Clifton, N.E.; Thomas, K.L.; Wilkinson, L.S.; Hall, J.; Trent, S. FMRP and CYFIP1 at the Synapse and Their Role in Psychiatric Vulnerability. *Complex Psychiatry* **2020**, *6*, 5–19. [CrossRef]
46. Salcedo-Arellano, M.J.; Dufour, B.; McLennan, Y.; Martinez-Cerdeno, V.; Hagerman, R. Fragile X syndrome and associated disorders: Clinical aspects and pathology. *Neurobiol. Dis.* **2020**, *136*, 104740. [CrossRef]
47. Butler, M.G. Magnesium Supplement and the 15q11.2 BP1-BP2 Microdeletion (Burnside-Butler) Syndrome: A Potential Treatment? *Int. J. Mol. Sci.* **2019**, *20*, 2914. [CrossRef]
48. Butler, M.G.; Cowen, N.; Bhatnagar, A. Prader-Willi syndrome, deletion subtypes, and magnesium: Potential impact on clinical findings. *Am. J. Med. Genet A* **2022**, *188*, 3278–3286. [CrossRef] [PubMed]
49. Davis, K.W.; Serrano, M.; Loddo, S.; Robinson, C.; Alesi, V.; Dallapiccola, B.; Novelli, A.; Butler, M.G. Parent-of-Origin Effects in 15q11.2 BP1-BP2 Microdeletion (Burnside-Butler) Syndrome. *Int. J. Mol. Sci.* **2019**, *20*, 1459. [CrossRef] [PubMed]
50. Ho, K.S.; Wassman, E.R.; Baxter, A.L.; Hensel, C.H.; Martin, M.M.; Prasad, A.; Twede, H.; Vanzo, R.J.; Butler, M.G. Chromosomal Microarray Analysis of Consecutive Individuals with Autism Spectrum Disorders Using an Ultra-High Resolution Chromosomal Microarray Optimized for Neurodevelopmental Disorders. *Int. J. Mol. Sci.* **2016**, *17*, 2070. [CrossRef]
51. Baldwin, I.; Shafer, R.L.; Hossain, W.A.; Gunewardena, S.; Veatch, O.J.; Mosconi, M.W.; Butler, M.G. Genomic, Clinical, and Behavioral Characterization of 15q11.2 BP1-BP2 Deletion (Burnside-Butler) Syndrome in Five Families. *Int. J. Mol. Sci.* **2021**, *22*, 1660. [CrossRef] [PubMed]
52. Vanlerberghe, C.; Petit, F.; Malan, V.; Vincent-Delorme, C.; Bouquillon, S.; Boute, O.; Holder-Espinasse, M.; Delobel, B.; Duban, B.; Vallee, L.; et al. 15q11.2 microdeletion (BP1-BP2) and developmental delay, behaviour issues, epilepsy and congenital heart disease: A series of 52 patients. *Eur. J. Med. Genet.* **2015**, *58*, 140–147. [CrossRef] [PubMed]
53. Farrell, M.; Lichtenstein, M.; Harner, M.K.; Crowley, J.J.; Filmyer, D.M.; Lázaro-Muñoz, G.; Dietterich, T.E.; Bruno, L.M.; Shaughnessy, R.A.; Biondi, T.F.; et al. Treatment-resistant psychotic symptoms and the 15q11.2 BP1-BP2 (Burnside-Butler) deletion syndrome: Case report and review of the literature. *Transl. Psychiatry.* **2020**, *10*, 42. [CrossRef]
54. Jiang, Y.; Zhang, Y.; Zhang, P.; Sang, T.; Zhang, F.; Ji, T.; Huang, Q.; Xie, H.; Du, R.; Cai, B.; et al. NIPA2 located in 15q11.2 is mutated in patients with childhood absence epilepsy. *Hum. Genet.* **2012**, *131*, 1217–1224. [CrossRef]
55. Picinelli, C.; Lintas, C.; Piras, I.S.; Gabriele, S.; Sacco, R.; Brogna, C.; Persico, A.M. Recurrent 15q11.2 BP1-BP2 microdeletions and microduplications in the etiology of neurodevelopmental disorders. *Am. J. Med. Genet. B Neuropsychiatr. Genet.* **2016**, *171*, 1088–1098. [CrossRef]
56. Xie, H.; Zhang, Y.; Zhang, P.; Wang, J.; Wu, Y.; Wu, X.; Netoff, T.; Jiang, Y. Functional study of NIPA2 mutations identified from the patients with childhood absence epilepsy. *PLoS ONE* **2014**, *9*, e109749. [CrossRef]
57. Stefanski, A.; Calle-López, Y.; Leu, C.; Pérez-Palma, E.; Pestana-Knight, E.; Lal, D. Clinical sequencing yield in epilepsy, autism spectrum disorder, and intellectual disability: A systematic review and meta-analysis. *Epilepsia* **2021**, *62*, 143–151. [CrossRef]
58. Genovese, A.; Butler, M.G. Clinical Assessment, Genetics, and Treatment Approaches in Autism Spectrum Disorder (ASD). *Int. J. Mol. Sci.* **2020**, *21*, 4726. [CrossRef]
59. Lord, C.; Brugha, T.S.; Charman, T.; Cusack, J.; Dumas, G.; Frazier, T.; Jones, E.J.H.; Jones, R.M.; Pickles, A.; State, M.W.; et al. Autism spectrum disorder. *Nat. Rev. Dis. Primers* **2020**, *6*, 5. [CrossRef]
60. Rainier, S.; Chai, J.H.; Tokarz, D.; Nicholls, R.D.; Fink, J.K. NIPA1 gene mutations cause autosomal dominant hereditary spastic paraplegia (SPG6). *Am. J. Hum. Genet.* **2003**, *73*, 967–971. [CrossRef]
61. Spagnoli, C.; Schiavoni, S.; Rizzi, S.; Salerno, G.G.; Frattini, D.; Koskenvuo, J.; Fusco, C. SPG6 (NIPA1 variant): A report of a case with early-onset complex hereditary spastic paraplegia and brief literature review. *J. Clin. Neurosci.* **2021**, *94*, 281–285. [CrossRef]
62. Hagerman, R.J.; Berry-Kravis, E.; Hazlett, H.C.; Bailey, D.B., Jr.; Moine, H.; Kooy, R.F.; Tassone, F.; Gantois, I.; Sonenberg, N.; Mandel, J.L.; et al. Fragile X syndrome. *Nat. Rev. Dis. Primers* **2017**, *3*, 17065. [CrossRef]

63. van der Meer, D.; Sønderby, I.E.; Kaufmann, T.; Walters, G.B.; Abdellaoui, A.; Ames, D.; Amunts, K.; Andersson, M.; Armstrong, N.J.; Bernard, M.; et al. Association of Copy Number Variation of the 15q11.2 BP1-BP2 Region With Cortical and Subcortical Morphology and Cognition. *JAMA Psychiatry* **2020**, *77*, 420–430. [PubMed]
64. Chu, F.C.; Shaw, S.W.; Lee, C.H.; Lo, L.M.; Hsu, J.J.; Hung, T.H. Adverse Perinatal and Early Life Outcomes following 15q11.2 CNV Diagnosis. *Genes* **2021**, *12*, 1480. [CrossRef] [PubMed]
65. Huang, X.; Chen, J.; Hu, W.; Li, L.; He, H.; Guo, H.; Liao, Q.; Ye, M.; Tang, D.; Dai, Y. A report on seven fetal cases associated with 15q11-q13 microdeletion and microduplication. *Mol. Genet. Genomic. Med.* **2021**, *9*, e160. [CrossRef] [PubMed]
66. Williams, S.G.; Nakev, A.; Guo, H.; Frain, S.; Tenin, G.; Liakhovitskaia, A.; Saha, P.; Priest, J.R.; Hentges, K.E.; Keavney, B.D. Association of congenital cardiovascular malformation and neuropsychiatric phenotypes with 15q11.2 (BP1-BP2) deletion in the UK Biobank. *Eur. J. Hum. Genet.* **2020**, *28*, 1265–1273. [CrossRef] [PubMed]
67. Usrey, K.M.; Williams, C.A.; Dasouki, M.; Fairbrother, L.C.; Butler, M.G. Congenital Arthrogryposis: An Extension of the 15q11.2 BP1-BP2 Microdeletion Syndrome? *Case Rep. Genet.* **2014**, *2014*, 127258. [CrossRef] [PubMed]
68. Wong, D.; Johnson, S.M.; Young, D.; Iwamoto, L.; Sood, S.; Slavin, T.P. Expanding the BP1-BP2 15q11.2 Microdeletion Phenotype: Tracheoesophageal Fistula and Congenital Cataracts. *Case Rep. Genet.* **2013**, *2013*, 801094. [CrossRef] [PubMed]
69. Silva, A.I.; Ulfarsson, M.O.; Stefansson, H.; Gustafsson, O.; Walters, G.B.; Linden, D.E.J.; Wilkinson, L.S.; Drakesmith, M.; Owen, M.J.; Hall, J.; et al. Reciprocal White Matter Changes Associated With Copy Number Variation at 15q11.2 BP1-BP2: A Diffusion Tensor Imaging Study. *Biol. Psychiatry* **2019**, *85*, 563–572. [CrossRef] [PubMed]
70. Silva, A.I.; Haddon, J.E.; Ahmed Syed, Y.; Trent, S.; Lin, T.E.; Patel, Y.; Carter, J.; Haan, N.; Honey, R.C.; Humby, T.; et al. Cyfip1 haploinsufficient rats show white matter changes, myelin thinning, abnormal oligodendrocytes and behavioural inflexibility. *Nat. Commun.* **2019**, *10*, 3455. [CrossRef]
71. Haan, N.; Westacott, L.J.; Carter, J.; Owen, M.J.; Gray, W.P.; Hall, J.; Wilkinson, L.S. Haploinsufficiency of the schizophrenia and autism risk gene Cyfip1 causes abnormal postnatal hippocampal neurogenesis through microglial and Arp2/3 mediated actin dependent mechanisms. *Transl. Psychiatry* **2021**, *11*, 313. [CrossRef]

Disclaimer/Publisher's Note: The statements, opinions and data contained in all publications are solely those of the individual author(s) and contributor(s) and not of MDPI and/or the editor(s). MDPI and/or the editor(s) disclaim responsibility for any injury to people or property resulting from any ideas, methods, instructions or products referred to in the content.

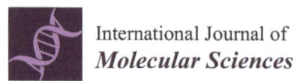 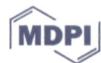

Hypothesis

Next Steps in Prader-Willi Syndrome Research: On the Relationship between Genotype and Phenotype

Joyce Whittington * and Anthony Holland

Department of Psychiatry, University of Cambridge, Douglas House, 18b Trumpington Road, Cambridge CB2 8AH, UK
* Correspondence: jew1000@cam.ac.uk; Tel.: +41 (0)1223 465255; Fax: +41 (0) 1223 465270

Abstract: This article reviews what we know of the phenotype and genotype of Prader-Willi syndrome and hypothesizes two possible paths from phenotype to genotype. It then suggests research that may strengthen the case for one or other of these hypotheses.

Keywords: Prader-Willi syndrome; genotype; phenotype; hypothalamus; brain development

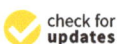

Citation: Whittington, J.; Holland, A. Next Steps in Prader-Willi Syndrome Research: On the Relationship between Genotype and Phenotype. *Int. J. Mol. Sci.* **2022**, *23*, 12089. https://doi.org/10.3390/ijms232012089

Academic Editors: David E. Godler and Olivia J. Veatch

Received: 17 September 2022
Accepted: 6 October 2022
Published: 11 October 2022

Publisher's Note: MDPI stays neutral with regard to jurisdictional claims in published maps and institutional affiliations.

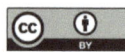

Copyright: © 2022 by the authors. Licensee MDPI, Basel, Switzerland. This article is an open access article distributed under the terms and conditions of the Creative Commons Attribution (CC BY) license (https://creativecommons.org/licenses/by/4.0/).

1. Introduction

In the short-term, research in Prader-Willi syndrome (PWS) aimed at alleviating symptoms is more likely to achieve quick results and provide some benefit to people with the syndrome and their families. However, in the long term, research needs to concentrate on elucidating the mechanisms whereby the absence of the expression of specific gene(s) gives rise to the particular symptoms associated with PWS so that interventions can be more precisely targeted. Our aim in this article is not to stifle the search for treatments to alleviate symptoms, indeed in [1] we made various suggestions for such research. Rather, it is to suggest ways that research on how the phenotype arises from the genotype may be carried forward.

In this article, we first describe the PWS phenotypes before continuing to what is known of the gene(s) whose absence of expression results in PWS and, in particular, the single gene now thought most likely to lie at the heart of the syndrome. We identify what we consider to be particular key questions that need to be addressed and suggest hypotheses as to how the absence of expression of this gene gives rise to the phenotype. We propose that this is either due to a direct effect on brain development, particularly affecting the hypothalamus [2] by impacting on foetal nutrition or by failing to modify the expression levels of a cascade of other (as yet unidentified) genes, which in turn affect brain development. The ultimate effect of the pattern of atypical brain development specific to PWS is to alter the response thresholds for particular networks in the brain thereby impairing the ability to maintain homeostasis, such as ensuring energy balance or responding to environmental change. Finally, based on these hypotheses we suggest new areas for research.

2. PWS

PWS arises from the loss of maternally imprinted genes from the paternal chromosome 15 in the region q11-q13. There are two main subtypes, resulting respectively from a deletion in the region q11-q13 (deletion subtype) or from the inheritance of two maternally marked chromosome 15s and no paternally marked chromosome 15 (maternal disomy subtype, (mUPD) or imprinting centre deficit (IC)). The early phenotype is characterised by restricted foetal movement, evidence of foetal growth retardation, severe hypotonia and failure to thrive. The infant with PWS is described as then passing through a period of normal growth and feeding, to a gain in weight not obviously related to an increase in food intake, to an obsessive interest in food in which restriction of food access is necessary to prevent obesity [3]. Later developmental delay, cognitive impairments, short stature due to low growth hormone (GH) levels, and impaired sexual development (undescended testes in males and small labia in females apparent at birth) as well as continued propensity to obesity in the absence of intervention are recognised as part of the PWS phenotype. Ritualistic behaviours, severe emotional outbursts, skin picking, an abnormal sleep pattern, poor temperature regulation and a high pain threshold are also frequently seen. Those with PWS due to the maternal disomy subtype are also more prone to develop a psychotic illness from teenage years on (very high lifetime risk) and more likely to be diagnosed with autism [4,5]. While the diagnostic criteria listed by [6] are extensive, some signs and symptom cluster together and can be explained by a single abnormality. For example, children with PWS who have been on growth hormone since early childhood not only have a normal height they also have normal sized hands and feet and the facial characteristics associated with PWS are much less marked [7]. It is the changing core phenotype, from a foetus and infant that is undernourished, fails to thrive, and is sexually immature to a child who develops hyperphagia, has relative sex and growth hormone deficiencies and developmental delay and intellectual impairments, that ultimately has to be explained by the genetics. We note that the foetus appears to develop normally up to the point where brain development is predominant, in that internal organs are not impaired and it is in the second half of pregnancy that the first symptoms (eg reduced foetal movement) appear.

3. PWS Gene

The genes involved in PWS are imprinted, but we do not know for certain how many such genes exist in the PWS region. Much progress on the functions of these genes has been made using mouse models. Mouse chromosome 7 is similar to human chromosome 15, but there is not a perfect match, as shown by the Cl5orf2 gene, which has no mouse counterpart [8]. Knock-out mouse models and studies of people with mutations in the MAGEL2 (i.e., Schaaf-Yang syndrome) and/or NECDIN genes suggest that these genes are involved in hypotonia, respiratory problems, sleep abnormalities, adiposity, developmental and cognitive delay, socialisation difficulties, and skin picking [9–12]. MAGEL2 knock-out mice show the poor suck/failure to thrive characteristic of PWS and the demonstration that in these mice, oxytocin administration in the first five hours after birth restored normal suckling [13] raised hopes of a treatment in humans. However, reviews of trials of oxytocin administration in humans reported mixed results [14,15]. Moreover, two people have been described lacking expression of the genes MKRN3, MAGEL2, and NECDIN but showing only developmental and cognitive delay from the major PWS criteria (see [6] for consensus diagnostic criteria) and a high pain threshold from minor criteria [16,17]. Furthermore, accounts in the literature of people with very small deletions, not involving MKRN3, MAGEL2, or NECDIN, but with most or all PWS characteristics also support the non-involvement of these genes in the PWS core characteristics in humans [18–20]. Core characteristics in these cases were: hypotonia, feeding difficulties, hyperphagia/obesity, hypogonadism, intellectual disability, and behaviour problems. The most likely single candidate gene, from studies of people with PWS, is now considered to be SNORD116 but mouse models are inconsistent: [21] support this hypothesis, [22] question it, and others suggest that IPW is also involved [23]. Summarising this evidence, it seems that findings in humans and mice differ, and that, in humans, the gene(s) responsible for the core characteristics of PWS is, or lies in the vicinity of, SNORD116. Further support for this hypothesis comes from the observation that the brain is the only major organ involved in the syndrome. Organs that develop earlier in gestation, such as the heart and lungs, are normal, suggesting that the gene, whose absence of expression results in PWS, is expressed in the brain and not in these other organs.

4. The SNORD116 Gene

The gene cluster SNORD116 encoding small nucleolar RNAs is considered to be a cluster of orphan C/D box snoRNAs since it does not target rRNAs or snRNAs. It is expressed prevalently in the brain and lacks any significant complementarity with ribosomal RNA. Due to its affinity with the brain, most studies are performed in mice. Although SNORD116 contains major sequences that are conserved across a number of species, there are some nucleotide differences between human and mouse [24] SNORD116 changes the expression levels of multiple genes [25], which may explain why, in PWS, its absence can affect so many areas. In mouse models selective deletion of SNORD116 from NPY expressing neurons resulted in upregulation of NPY mRNA and low birth weight, increased weight gain in early adulthood, increased energy expenditure, and hyperphagia [26].

5. Genotype to Phenotype

As noted above, in PWS threshold levels for several characteristics are changed; this means that the distribution of the particular characteristic in people with PWS is shifted relative to the distribution of that characteristic in the typically developing population towards the more deleterious end. However, significantly, no characteristic is entirely absent or 100% dominant. This might be explained by the relevant gene-controlled threshold levels for these characteristics being changed, exactly what we would expect of a gene that altered expression levels in a number of other genes but did not entirely eliminate expression in these genes.

One possible version of our single gene hypothesis follows from our earlier observations: SNORD116 changes the expression levels of genes involved in several different regulatory processes (satiation, pain, sleep, temperature) and its absence, as in the case of NPY (related to satiation), causes an increase in the threshold level at which satiety is reached. As [27,28] noted in the case of satiety, the threshold for reaching satiety is increased but satiation is not completely absent in PWS. The persistence of satiation has been demonstrated recently [29]. Thus, SNORD116 appears to be a regulatory gene that regulates other genes by changing their expression levels and its absence therefore changes expression levels from those observed in the non-PWS population in the opposite direction. With this model PWS can therefore be regarded as fundamentally a single gene disorder but it may also be considered to be a polygenic disorder, involving respectively a single gene from the PWS region and multiple genes not yet identified from other areas of the genome.

Another possible explanation of the genotype to phenotype transition is outlined in [1]. Prader-Willi syndrome arises as a consequence of absent paternal copies of maternally imprinted genes at 15q11-13. Such gender-of-origin imprinted genes are expressed in the brain and also in mammalian placenta where paternally expressed imprinted genes drive foetal nutritional demand. We hypothesise that the PWS phenotype is the result of the genotype impacting two pathways: firstly, directly on brain development and secondly, on placental nutritional pathways that results in its down-regulation and relative foetal starvation. The early PWS phenotype establishes the basis for the later characteristic phenotype. Hyperphagia and other phenotypic characteristics arise as a consequence of impaired hypothalamic development. Hypothalamic feeding pathways become set in a state indicative of starvation, with a high satiety threshold and a dysfunctional neurophysiological state due to incorrect representations of reward needs, based on inputs that indicate a false requirement for food. In this model PWS might be considered to be a single gene disorder in which the phenotype arises as a consequence of abnormal brain development driven by the absence of expression of SNORD 116. A paper by [2] reported on recent neuroimaging findings showing significantly smaller hypothalamic nuclei in people with PWS compared to an aged-matched typically developing control group and also an obese group. The authors argue that the hypothalamus fails to develop in PWS and this would explain the varied phenotypic characteristics of hypothalamic origin.

6. Research Directions

The above hypotheses give rise to possible fruitful research directions: firstly, investigation of genes whose expression levels are changed by SNORD116 including investigation of

PWS placental genes, especially those whose expression levels are changed by SNORD116. Secondly, using mouse models, the investigation of placental foetal nutritional pathways to see if these are down-regulated, and thirdly; from a phenotypic perspective, to take a symptom such as high pain threshold, whose extreme would be a complete inability to feel pain, as in Congenital Insensitivity to Pain (CIPA), for example, whose cause is the inheritance of two copies of the NTRK1 gene [30]. Then ask the questions: Would over-expression of a single copy lead to a higher pain threshold and does SNORD116 alter the expression level of this gene? FOURTHLY, from the observation that the motor cortex and hypothalamus are involved in PWS symptoms, are there any genes specific to these areas? Are the expression levels of any such genes changed by the absence of SNORD116 expression?

The genotype to phenotype pathways in PWS remain an enigma. Fundamental to understanding the syndrome and to the development of new treatments is understanding how the genotype leads to the initial failure to thrive phenotype and then how this then results in the characteristic PWS phenotype. We challenge the accepted wisdom on this proposing two contrasting perspectives. We hope that this article will help to stimulate research.

Author Contributions: Concept and writing, J.W. and A.H. All authors have read and agreed to the published version of the manuscript.

Funding: This research received no external funding.

Institutional Review Board Statement: Not applicable.

Informed Consent Statement: Not applicable.

Conflicts of Interest: The authors declare no conflict of interest.

References

1. Holland, A.; Manning, K.; Whittington, J.E. The paradox of Prader-Willi syndrome revisited: Making sense of the phenotype. *BioMedicine* **2022**, *78*, 103952. [CrossRef] [PubMed]
2. Brown, S.S.G.; Manning, K.E.; Fletcher, P.; Holland, A. In-vivo neuroimaging evidence of hypothalamic alteration in Prader-Willi syndrome. *Brain Commun.* **2022**, *4*, fcac229. [CrossRef] [PubMed]
3. Miller, J.L.; Lynn, C.H.; Driscoll, D.C.; Goldstone, A.P.; Gold, J.A.; Kimonis, V.; Dykens, E.; Butler, M.G.; Shuster, J.J.; Driscoll, D.J. Nutritional phases in Prader-Willi syndrome. *Am. J. Med. Genet. A.* **2011**, *155A*, 1040–1049. [CrossRef]
4. Boer, H.; Holland, A.J.; Whittington, J.E.; Butler, J.V.; Webb, T.; Clarke, D.J. Psychotic illness in people with Prader-Willi syndrome due to chromosome 15 maternal uniparental disomy. *Lancet* **2002**, *359*, 135–136. [CrossRef]
5. Bennett, J.A.; Germani, T.; Haqq, A.M.; Zwaigenbaum, L. Autism spectrum disorder in Prader-Willi syndrome: A systematic review. *Am. J. Med. Genet. A.* **2015**, *167A*, 2936–2944. [CrossRef] [PubMed]
6. Holm, V.A.; Cassidy, S.B.; Butler, M.G.; Hanchett, J.M.; Greenswag, L.R.; Whitman, B.Y.; Greenberg, F. Prader-Willi syndrome: Consensus Diagnostic Criteria. *Pediatrics* **1993**, *91*, 398–402. [CrossRef]
7. De Souza, M.A.; McAllister, C.; Suttie, M.; Perrotta, C.; Mattina, T.; Faravelli, F.; Forzano, F.; Holland, A.; Hammond, P. Growth hormone, gender and face shape in Prader-Willi syndrome. *Am. J. Med. Genet. A.* **2013**, *161A*, 2453–2463. [CrossRef]
8. Wawrzik, M.; Unmehopa, U.A.; Swaab, D.F.; van de Nes, J.; Buiting, K.; Horsthemke, B. The C15orf2 gene in the Prader-Willi syndrome region is subject to genomic imprinting and positive selection. *Neurogenetics* **2010**, *11*, 153–156. [CrossRef]
9. Fountain, M.D.; Tao, H.; Chen, C.A.; Yin, J.; Schaaf, C.P. Magel2 knockout mice manifest altered social phenotypes and a deficit in preference for social novelty. *Genes Brain Behav.* **2017**, *16*, 592–600. [CrossRef]
10. Fountain, M.D.; Schaaf, C.P. Prader-Willi Syndrome and Schaaf-Yang Syndrome: Neurodevelopmental Diseases Intersecting at the *MAGEL2* Gene. *Diseases* **2016**, *4*, 2. [CrossRef]
11. Matarazzo, V.; Caccialupi, L.; Schaller, F.; Shvarev, Y.; Kourdougli, N.; Bertoni, A.; Menuet, C.; Voituron, N.; Deneris, E.; Gaspar, P.; et al. Necdin shapes serotonergic development and SERT activity modulating breathing in a mouse model for Prader-Willi syndrome. *eLife* **2017**, *31*, e32640. [CrossRef] [PubMed]
12. Muscatelli, F.; Abrous, D.N.; Massacrier, A.; Boccaccio, I.; Le Moal, M.; Cau, P.; Cremer, H. Disruption of the mouse Necdin gene results in hypothalamic and behavioral alterations reminiscent of the human Prader-Willi syndrome. *Hum. Mol. Genet.* **2000**, *9*, 3101–3110. [CrossRef] [PubMed]
13. Schaller, F.; Watrin, F.; Sturny, R.; Massacrier, A.; Szepetowski, P.; Muscatelli, F. A single postnatal injection of oxytocin rescues the lethal feeding behaviour in mouse newborns deficient for the imprinted *Magel2* gene. *Hum. Mol. Genet.* **2010**, *15*, 4895–4905. [CrossRef] [PubMed]

14. Rice, L.J.; Einfeld, S.L.; Hu, N.; Carter, C.S. A review of clinical trials of oxytocin in Prader-Willi syndrome. *Curr. Opin. Psychiatry* **2018**, *31*, 123–127. [CrossRef] [PubMed]
15. Althammer, F.; Muscatelli, F.; Grinevich, V.; Schaaf, C.P. Oxytocin-based therapies for treatment of Prader-Willi and Schaaf-Yang syndromes: Evidence, disappointments, and future research strategies. *Transl. Psychiatry* **2022**, *12*, 318. [CrossRef] [PubMed]
16. Kanber, D.; Giltay, J.; Wieczorek, D.; Zogel, C.; Hochstenbach, R.; Caliebe, A.; Kuechler, A.; Horsthemke, B.; Buiting, K. A paternal deletion of MKRN3, MAGEL2 and NDN does not result in Prader-Willi syndrome. *Eur. J. Hum. Genet.* **2009**, *17*, 582–590. [CrossRef]
17. Buiting, K.; Di Donato, N.; Beygo, J.; Bens, S.; von der Hagen, M.; Hackmann, K.; Horsthemke, B. Clinical phenotypes of *MAGEL2* mutations and deletions. *Orphanet J. Rare Dis.* **2014**, *9*, 40. [CrossRef]
18. Sahoo, T.; del Gaudio, D.; German, J.R.; Shinawi, M.; Peters, S.U.; Person, R.; Garnica, A.; Cheung, S.W.; Beaudet, A.L. Prader-Willi phenotype caused by paternal deficiency for the HBII-85 C/D box small nucleolar RNA cluster. *Nat. Genet.* **2008**, *40*, 719–721. [CrossRef]
19. De Smith, A.J.; Purmann, C.; Walters, R.G.; Ellis, R.J.; Holder, S.E.; Van Haelst, M.M.; Brady, A.F.; Fairbrother, U.L.; Dattani, M.; Keogh, J.M.; et al. A deletion of the HBII-85 class of small nucleolar RNAs (snoRNAs) is associated with hyperphagia, obesity and hypogonadism. *Hum. Mol. Genet.* **2009**, *18*, 3257–3265. [CrossRef]
20. Duker, A.L.; Ballif, B.C.; Bawle, E.V.; Person, R.E.; Mahadevan, S.; Alliman, S.; Thompson, R.; Traylor, R.; Bejjani, B.A.; Shaffer, L.G.; et al. Paternally inherited microdeletion at 15q11.2 confirms a significant role for the SNORD116 C/D box snoRNA cluster in Prader-Willi syndrome. *Eur. J. Hum. Genet.* **2010**, *18*, 1196–1201. [CrossRef]
21. Zhang, Q.; Bouma, G.J.; McClellan, K.; Tobet, S. Hypothalamic expression of snoRNA Snord116 is consistent with a link to the hyperphagia and obesity symptoms of Prader-Willi syndrome. *Int. J. Dev. Neurosci.* **2012**, *30*, 479–485. [CrossRef] [PubMed]
22. Rodriguez, J.A.; Zigman, J.M. Hypothalamic loss of Snord116 and Prader-Willi syndrome hyperphagia: The buck stops here? *J. Clin. Investig.* **2018**, *128*, 900–902. [CrossRef] [PubMed]
23. Davies, J.R.; Dent, C.L.; McNamara, G.I.; Isles, A.R. Behavioural effects of imprinted genes. *Curr. Opin. Behav. Sci.* **2015**, *2*, 28–33. [CrossRef]
24. Good, D.J.; Kocher, M.A. Phylogenetic Analysis of the SNORD116 Locus. *Genes* **2017**, *8*, 358.
25. Falaleeva, M.; Surface, J.; de la Grange, P.; Stamm, S. SNORD116 and SNORD115 change expression of multiple genes and modify each other's activity. *Gene* **2015**, *72*, 266–273. [CrossRef]
26. Qi, Y.; Purtell, L.; Fu, M.; Zhang, L.; Zolotukhin, S.; Campbell, L.; Herzog, H.J. Hypothalamus Specific Re-Introduction of SNORD116 into Otherwise Snord116 Deficient Mice Increased Energy Expenditure. *J. Neuroendocrinol.* **2017**, *29*, e12457. [CrossRef]
27. Hinton, E.C.; Holland, A.J.; Gellatly, M.S.N.; Soni, S.; Ghatei, M.A.; Owen, A.M. Neural Representations of hunger and satiety in Prader-Willi syndrome. *Int. J. Obes.* **2006**, *30*, 313–321. [CrossRef]
28. Hinton, E.C.; Holland, A.J.; Gellatly, M.S.; Soni, S.; Owen, A.M. An investigation into food preferences and the neural basis of food-related incentive motivation in Prader-Willi syndrome. *J. Intellect Disabil. Res.* **2006**, *50*, 633–642. [CrossRef]
29. Rigamonti, A.E.; Bini, S.; Grugni, G.; Agosti, F.; DeCol, A.; Mallone, M.; Cella, S.G.; Sartorio, A. Unexpectedly increasedanorexigenic postprandial responses of PYY and GLP-1 to fast ice cream consumption in adult patients with Prader-Willi syndrome. *Clin. Endoccrinol.* **2014**, *81*, 542–550. [CrossRef]
30. Franco, M.L.; Melero, C.; Sarasola, E.; Acebo, P.; Luque, A.; Calatayud-Baselga, I.; García-Barcina, M.; Vilar, M. Mutations in TrkA causing congenital insensitivity to pain with anhidrosis (CIPA) induce misfolding, aggregation, and mutation-dependent neurodegeneration by dysfunction of the autophagic flux. *J. Biol Chem.* **2016**, *291*, 21363–21374. [CrossRef]

Review

Clinical Trials in Prader–Willi Syndrome: A Review

Ranim Mahmoud [1,2], Virginia Kimonis [1,3,4] and Merlin G. Butler [5,*]

1. Department of Pediatrics, University of California, Irvine, CA 92697, USA
2. Department of Pediatrics, Faculty of Medicine, Mansoura University, Mansoura, 35516, Egypt
3. Departments of Neurology and Pathology, University of California, Irvine, CA 92697, USA
4. Children's Hospital of Orange County, Orange, CA 92868, USA
5. Departments of Psychiatry & Behavioral Sciences and Pediatrics, University of Kansas Medical Center, Kansas City, KS 66160, USA
* Correspondence: mbutler4@kumc.edu

Abstract: Prader–Willi syndrome (PWS) is a complex, genetic, neurodevelopmental disorder. PWS has three molecular genetic classes. The most common defect is due to a paternal 15q11-q13 deletion observed in about 60% of individuals. This is followed by maternal disomy 15 (both 15 s from the mother), found in approximately 35% of cases. the remaining individuals have a defect of the imprinting center that controls the activity of imprinted genes on chromosome 15. Mild cognitive impairment and behavior problems in PWS include self-injury, anxiety, compulsions, and outbursts in childhood, impacted by genetic subtypes. Food seeking and hyperphagia can lead to morbid obesity and contribute to diabetes and cardiovascular or orthopedic problems. The control of hyperphagia and improving food-related behaviors are the most important unmet needs in PWS and could be addressed with the development of a new therapeutic agent, as currently no approved therapeutics exist for PWS treatment. The status of clinical trials with existing results for the management of obesity and hyperphagia in PWS will be discussed in this review, including treatments such as beloranib, setmelanotide, a diazoxide choline controlled-release tablet (DCCR), an unacylated ghrelin analogue, oxytocin and related compounds, glucagon-like peptide 1 receptor agonists, surgical intervention, and transcranial direct-current stimulation.

Keywords: Prader–Willi syndrome; obesity; hyperphagia; clinical trials; genetics

1. Introduction

Prader–Willi syndrome (PWS) is a rare, genetic, neurodevelopmental disorder caused by errors in a complex genomic mechanism, referred to as genomic imprinting, comprised of three PWS molecular genetic classes. PWS is characterized by severe hypotonia with a poor suck and feeding difficulties causing failure to thrive during infancy, hypogenitalism/hypogonadism in both sexes, motor and cognitive delays, low muscle tone, slow metabolism, behavior disturbances, and endocrine findings involving growth and other hormone deficiencies with short stature, infertility, and small hands and feet (e.g., [1–6]). Mild cognitive impairment and behavior problems, including self-injury, anxiety, compulsions, and outbursts, can occur in childhood along with food seeking and hyperphagia, leading to morbid obesity and a shortened life expectancy if not controlled (e.g., [7]). PWS is considered the most commonly known cause of life-threatening obesity in humans, affecting approximately 400,000 people worldwide and one in every 20,000 live births [8]. Occurrences of this rare disorder are sporadic, but the cause is due to errors in the genomic imprinting of the chromosome 15q11-q13 region in humans. The most common defect is due to a paternal 15q11-q13 deletion observed in about 60% of individuals. This is followed by maternal disomy 15 (both 15 s from the mother), found in approximately 35% of cases. The remaining individuals have a defect of the imprinting center that controls the activity of imprinted genes on chromosome 15 or have chromosome 15 translocations or inversions (e.g., [4]). Individuals with the different PWS molecular classes present with varying clinical findings. Those with the typical 15q11-q13 deletion, specifically the larger 15q11-q13 type I deletion, have a more severe phenotype with self-injuries, compulsions, and lower cognition than those with the typical, smaller 15q11-q13 Type II deletion or maternal disomy 15 (e.g., [9–11]). A typical patient with Prader–Willi syndrome is shown in Figure 1.

If not externally controlled, significant hyperphagia leads to morbid obesity in PWS and contributes to diabetes, cardiovascular or orthopedic problems, and even death [12]. The most common cause of death in PWS is respiratory failure followed by cardiac failure, gastrointestinal failure, and infection [7,13]. According to a 2014 survey of parents and caregivers of PWS patients, reducing hunger and improving food-related behaviors were the most important unmet needs in PWS. These needs could be addressed with the development of a new therapeutic agent, as currently no approved therapeutics exist for the treatment of hyperphagia in PWS.

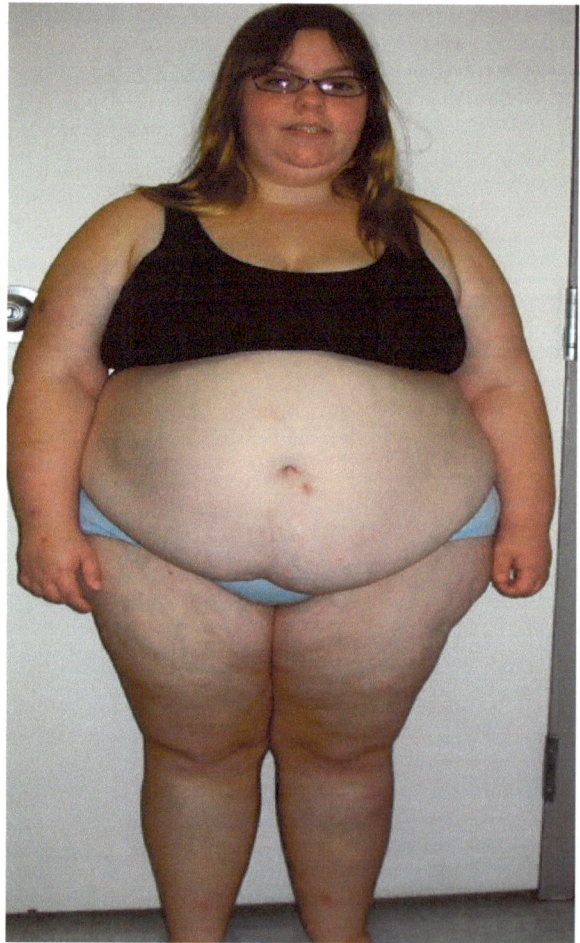

Figure 1. Frontal view of a 16-year-old female with Prader–Willi syndrome due to maternal disomy 15. (Modified from Mahmoud et al. [14]).

2. Beloranib Clinical Trial in Prader–Willi Syndrome

Beloranib treatment was undertaken in a large cohort of individuals with genetic confirmation of PWS in a clinical trial sponsored by Zafgen, Inc. (Boston, MA, USA). The goal was to investigate the efficacy of beloranib treatment for hyperphagia and obesity, as well as to determine its safety with tolerability over 26 weeks of treatment in both PWS adolescent and adult participants. The study was stimulated by early reported data indicating a clinically significant and sustained weight loss with decreased hunger in obese subjects using beloranib [15]. Beloranib inhibits methionine aminopeptidase 2 (MetAP2) by removing methionine residue from proteins, impacting fat metabolism. Inhibitors of MetAP2 were found to reduce food intake, body weight, fat content and adipocyte size in animal models [15]. Hence, a Phase Three, randomized, placebo-controlled, double-blind trial was conducted in 15 states in the United States between 2014 and 2015. Those with genetically confirmed PWS were enrolled between the ages of 12 to 65 years. Participants had an elevated body mass index (BMI) (ages 12 to 17 years: BMI $\geq$ 95th percentile for age and sex; ages 18 to 65 years: BMI 27–60 kg/m^2), with a total score $\geq$ 13 on the Hyperphagia Questionnaire for Clinical Trials (HQ-CT), and a stable weight for at least three months, but otherwise demonstrated health-related findings, such as blood pressure readings, within the normal range. Those with type II diabetes were accepted, if stable. Growth hormone treatment was allowed if a stable dose was prescribed for at least three months before entry into the trial. Participants living in a group home for less than 50% of the time were excluded. All participants were randomized via computer access using a centralized interactive system with a 1:1:2:2 ratio of lower dose placebo: higher dose placebo: lower dose beloranib (1.8 mg): higher dose beloranib (2.4 mg) per participant.

Following a two-week single-blind placebo lead-in, participants were randomized to study treatment with doses selected based on previous experience, with the study drug administered twice weekly. The study included an optional twenty-six-week, open-label extension trial in which all participants received four weeks of 1.8 mg beloranib, followed by 2.4 mg beloranib use for 22 weeks. The prespecified co-primary endpoints were a change in hyperphagia-related behaviors, captured via a questionnaire form, and a percent change in body weight from baseline to week 26. The HQ-CT form consisted of nine question items with responses ranging from 0 to 4 units each, with a possible total score range of 0 to 36 designed to measure symptoms of food-related preoccupations and behaviors. The form was completed by the caregiver for each participant. It was estimated that a sample size of 20 participants per group would provide 94% power to detect the between-group difference in each of the co-primary endpoints. Out of 126 screened individuals, 108 participants were randomized and 107 received the study drug. Demographic and baseline characteristics were well-matched across the treatment groups for age, sex, growth hormone use, weight, BMI, fat mass, and genetic subtype. The participants were primarily Caucasian. A significant reduction in fat mass was found in both the low- and high-dosage beloranib-treated groups when compared with the placebo, with participants having a weight loss greater than or equal to 5%. A change in HQ-CT individual question scores indicating improvement were found for eight out of the nine measures in the beloranib-treated participants. The questionnaire measures were classified as: upset when denied food, bargain to get more food, forage through trash for food, up at night to seek food, persistent asking for food, time spent talking about food, distress when stopped from asking about food, and interferes with activities. Unfortunately, the randomized, double-blind portion of the trial was stopped early due to venous thromboembolic events, including two participant deaths in the beloranib-treated group.

3. Oxytocin Clinical Trials in PWS

Oxytocin is a neuropeptide hormone which plays an important role in social interactions, social skills, food intake, anxiety, energy expenditure, maternal behaviors, and body weight regulation [16,17]. All of these parameters are severely affected in patients with PWS. They have a decreased number of oxytocin-producing neurons in the hypothalamic periventricular nuclei and a small number of observed periventricular nuclei [18]. The deficiency of these neurons could be related to PWS patients' poor social judgement and their inability to control their emotions. Two mouse models deficient for PWS genes, including necdin and Magel2, also showed decreased oxytocin levels [19]. Additionally, postnatal treatment with oxytocin has been reported to normalize suckling and feeding behavior in the Magel2-knockout mouse [20]. Approximately one half of the surviving mice showed an improvement in social recognition skills, which would suggest that oxytocin could be helpful in managing behavioral problems in PWS [21].

To date, there have been seven clinical trials on the use of oxytocin in PWS. The first study was a double-blind, randomized, placebo-controlled trial undertaken by Tauber et al. [22] in 2011. Twenty-four patients were included, with a median age of 28.5 years, and grouped based on gender and intelligence quotient (IQ). Every patient received a single dose (24 IU) of either oxytocin or a placebo. The behavior of the patients was assessed three times: the first at two days before drug administration, the second at one half-day after administration (early effects), and for the last time at two days after drug administration (late effects). A behavior grid was developed to assess ten social and emotional behaviors. There was also as a separate set of four questions relating to eating behavior. There was no difference between the two groups before intranasal administration, but a significant increase in trust in others, less sadness tendencies, and disruptive behavior were observed in the two days after intranasal drug administration. While no statistical difference was observed in the eating behavior scores between both groups, there was improvement in social skills in the oxytocin-treated group. The limitations of this study were the use of only one dose of oxytocin and a placebo with the effect of treatment appearing only in the behavior grid.

The second study was a double-blind, randomized, controlled trial with intranasal use of oxytocin in patients with PWS to examine its effect on physical, behavioral, and cognitive function. Thirty patients with PWS were included in this study, and two different doses of oxytocin were used according to the age of patients: a 24 IU dosage for patients aged 16 years and more, and an 18 IU dosage for patients aged between 12 and 15 years. The dose was increased to 40 IU for patients older than 16 years and 32 IU for patients between 12 and 15 years. The oxytocin and placebo were given for eight weeks; this was followed by a two-week washout period. The Developmental Behavior Checklist (DBC), the Yale–Brown Obsessive Compulsive Scale (Y-BOCS), the Dykens Hyperphagia Questionnaire, the Reading the Mind in the Eyes Test (RMET), and the Epworth Sleepiness Scale (ESS) were used to assess behavioral and related problems. No improvement was found in any of the behavioral problems or in hyperphagia in response to the oxytocin treatment [23].

The third trial was applied only to children with PWS [24]. The randomized, double-blind, placebo-controlled, cross-over study was conducted on 25 children with the aim of investigating the effect of oxytocin on social and eating behavior in PWS. Children received either oxytocin or a placebo for four weeks. They then crossed over to the alternative treatment for another four weeks. The Dykens Hyperphagia Questionnaire was used to evaluate changes in eating behavior and hyperphagia and the Oxytocin Study Questionnaire, designed by PWS experts, was used for the evaluation of social behavior. When the participants were divided into two groups, <11 years and >11 years, there was no significant effect between either oxytocin or the placebo in the whole group. The younger children showed beneficial effects of oxytocin on social behavior and hyperphagia. Less anger and sadness and an improvement in social behavior were noted during oxytocin treatment when compared with the placebo, as was documented by the participants' parents. The lack of response in the older group could be related to the small number of older children, a miscalculation of the oxytocin dose, the wrong administration of oxytocin, or that the behavior of older children may be more fixed in their personality and may need a longer duration of treatment to generate a significant effect [24].

The fourth study was a double-blinded, placebo-controlled, crossover trial performed on 24 children with PWS, reported by Miller et al. [25] in 2017. The participants received

16 IU of intranasal oxytocin or placebo for five days, followed by a four-week washout period, and finally an adjustment to the alternative treatment for another five days. The Aberrant Behavior Checklist, Social Responsiveness Scale (SRS-P), Repetitive Behavior Scale- Revised (RBS-R), Hyperphagia Questionnaire, and the Clinical Global Impression (CGI) scale were used to evaluate hyperphagia and other behaviors. The authors reported that the use of oxytocin in children over five days was safe, and a significant improvement was noted in anxiety and self-injurious behavior when compared to the placebo [25].

The fifth study was performed to examine the safety and efficacy of a single dose of oxytocin in infants less than six months of age with PWS. Oxytocin was well-tolerated in infants, with no side effects noted during the seven days of treatment. The effects of oxytocin on oral feeding and social skills in human infants were first reported in this study. Sucking and swallowing were also evaluated before and after oxytocin administration by using the Neonatal Oral–Motor Assessment Scale (NOMAS), video fluoroscopy of swallowing, and the Clinical Global Impression (CGI) scale. The authors reported positive treatment effects on social and feeding behaviors [26].

Damen et al. [27] in 2021 conducted a randomized, double-blind, placebo-controlled cross-over study on the effects of oxytocin versus placebo treatment for three months in children with PWS. The primary outcomes were changes in social behavior and hyperphagia, with differences between males and females and between PWS molecular genetic classes [4]. Forty-six children with PWS were blindly assigned to receive twice-daily intranasal doses of either oxytocin or a placebo during four visits in an outpatient clinic setting. The parents completed questionnaires at all visits. The completed questionnaire forms (e.g., Oxytocin Questionnaire and Dykens Hyperphagia Questionnaire) measured changes in eating or repetitive behaviors using the Repetitive Behavior Scale-Revised (RBS-R) form. According to the Dykens Hyperphagia Questionnaire form, patients who received oxytocin showed a trend of being less hyperphagic. RBS-R scores showed that patients receiving oxytocin had less repetitive behavior. The Oxytocin Questionnaire and Dykens Hyperphagia Questionnaire scores were significantly improved during oxytocin treatment in comparison with placebo treatment in patients with the 15q11-q13 deletion, while patients with maternal disomy 15 showed no differences between oxytocin and placebo treatment. In addition, there were positive effects of oxytocin treatment in PWS males compared to females. The cause for this was not known, but it could be explained by differences in the oxytocin biological system between males and females. Males may be more sensitive to the effect of oxytocin than females; however, more studies are needed. The limitations of this study included the small sample size and the insufficient number of questionnaires used for the assessment of changes in both eating and social behavior [27].

The final study conducted by Hollander et al. [28] in 2021 on children and adolescents with PWS investigated the effect of intranasal oxytocin on hyperphagia and repetitive behaviors. Their double-blind, placebo-controlled, randomized trial was conducted over eight weeks on 23 patients with PWS. The participants received 16 IU/per day and had evaluation visits every two weeks for an eight-week period. The primary outcome measure of food-seeking behavior was assessed by using the Dykens Hyperphagia Questionnaire form. The secondary outcomes were repetitive behaviors, assessed using the Repetitive Behavior Scale-Revised (RBS-R). Significant reductions in hyperphagia and repetitive behaviors were noted across time for the placebo group. There was no reduction for the group that received oxytocin treatment, which could be due to subjective expectation bias from caregivers and clinicians [28]. Overall, the reported studies demonstrated the beneficial effects of oxytocin treatment in PWS, except for the two study trials described. The absence of a positive effect of oxytocin treatment in all studies may reflect the dosage and administration differences and may not indicate that oxytocin does not have a role in treating the PWS phenotype, particularly hyperphagia and behavioral problems. More studies are needed to further understand the role of oxytocin in treating those with PWS.

4. Setmelanotide Clinical Trial in PWS

A clinical trial on 40 participants diagnosed with PWS was sponsored by Rhythm Pharmaceuticals (Boston, MA, USA) to treat hyperphagia and obesity. The preliminary results were reported in abstract format at the 2017 PWSA Scientific Conference (Orlando, FL, USA) and are available online [29–31]. Studies on Setmelanotide, a melanocortin (MC)-4 receptor agonist that impacts satiety and feeding centers to decrease eating, were undertaken with a once-per-day administration via subcutaneous injection in those with PWS. The proof-of-concept trial included 40 participants diagnosed with PWS (19 males and 21 females) with a mean age of 26.4 years, with an age range of 16 to 25 years; a mean body mass index (BMI) of 39.4 kg/m^2, with a BMI range of 26.1 to 74.1; and a mean Dykens Hyperphagia Questionnaire (HQ) score of 23.9, with a range of 12 to 45.

The results of this phase-two study using the MC-4 receptor (MC4R) agonist (Setmelanotide) were obtained in a four-week trial at five centers in the U.S.A. A primary study was randomized as a double-blind comparison of a placebo to three daily doses of Setmelanotide (0.5, 1.5, and 2.5 mg) preceded by a two-week, single-blind placebo run-in time interval. A percent bodyweight change was the primary endpoint, with secondary endpoints including HQ scores; dual-energy x-ray absorptiometry (DEXA) measures of body composition for fat, muscle, and bone; metabolic and laboratory parameters; and safety with tolerability assessments. The mean weight changes at four weeks showed no difference when comparing the Setmelanotide versus the placebo. The mean hyperphagia questionnaire scores demonstrated a small, not-statistically-significant reduction from baseline at the two highest Setmelanotide doses. No changes were observed in the DEXA measurements or laboratory findings. Adverse events included occasional, mild-to-moderate injection-site reactions reported in approximately two-thirds of the participants for both active and placebo administration. Skin and nevi darkening was noted, along with intermittent, spontaneous penile erections. There were no serious adverse events, but one patient discontinued the trial due to injection site reactions. Although the results in PWS were not promising, later studies in other rare, monogenic obesity disorders, such as those with POMC gene mutations or Bardet–Biedel syndrome—a ciliary protein group of genetic disorders—have met with success using this MC4R agonist [32].

5. Diazoxide Choline Controlled-Release Clinical Trial in PWS

Diazoxide choline, a new chemical entity, is a benzothiadiazine that acts by stimulating an ion flux through ATP-sensitive K+ channels (KATP). It is the choline salt of diazoxide, and is currently used to treat infants, children, and adults with hyperinsulinemia hypoglycemia. Diazoxide choline controlled-release (DCCR) is diazoxide choline formulated as an oral, once-a-day, extended-release tablet.

The hyperphagia signal in PWS likely occurs due to the dysregulation of neuropeptide Y/Agouti Related Protein/Gamma-aminobutyric Acid (NAG) neurons, which are regulated by leptin via reduction in their excitability [33]. This dysregulation results in marked elevations in the synthesis and secretion of NPY, the most potent endogenous neuropeptide. Leptin's activation of adenosine triphosphate (ATP)-sensitive potassium channels (K_{ATP}) via phosphoinositide-3-kinase (PI3-K) [34–36] serves to hyperpolarize the resting membrane potential, which results in a limitation in the release of NPY by these neurons. Depolarizing the resting membrane potential of neurons in the arcuate nucleus (including the NAG neurons) via perfusion with potassium chloride results in the doubling of the NPY release rate, which returns to normal following perfusion [37]. There is strong evidence that the activation of NAG neurons results in insulin resistance and impaired glucose tolerance [38]. Inhibiting these neurons by agonizing the K_{ATP} channel has the potential to improve insulin sensitivity and improve glucose tolerance. Agonizing the K_{ATP} channel in NAG neurons using diazoxide choline is expected to result in reduced NPY secretion. Diazoxide readily crosses the blood–brain barrier [39], and diazoxide choline can be orally administered and can effectively agonize the K_{ATP} channels in the hypothalamic NAG neurons. Therefore, agonizing the K_{ATP} channel in these neurons amplifies the regulatory effects of leptin, reducing the secretion of NPY and likely AgRP and GABA, blunting hyperphagia and impacting obesity.

This preliminary trial consisted of a single-center, Phase II clinical study including a 1ten-week open-label treatment period followed by a four-week double-blind, placebo-controlled, randomized-withdrawal treatment period conducted at the University of California, Irvine. Patients were initiated on a once-daily oral DCCR dose of approximately 1.5 mg/kg (maximum starting dose of 145 mg) and titrated every two weeks to approximately 2.4 mg/kg, 3.3 mg/kg, 4.2 mg/kg, and 5.1 mg/kg (or to a maximum dose of 507.5 mg, whichever was less) at the discretion of the investigator. Any patient who showed any increase in resting energy expenditure and/or any reduction in hyperphagia from baseline through week six or week eight was designated a responder and was eligible to be randomized in the double-blind treatment period. During the double-blind treatment period, all individuals designated as responders were to be randomized in a 1:1 ratio to either continue active treatment at the dose they were treated at during week eight or to the placebo equivalent of that dose for an additional four weeks. Non-responder patients continued open-label treatment for an additional four weeks. Screening began in June 2014, and the last subject's visit took place in April 2015. The trial was registered on www.clinicaltrials.gov, identifier NCT02034071. Hyperphagia was measured in the study using a nine-question Modified Dykens Hyperphagia questionnaire, posed to the parent or caregiver, which utilized a two-week recall period. Changes in body fat and lean body mass were measured using dual-energy x-ray absorptiometry (DEXA) at baseline and at the end of the open-label treatment period. Behavioral assessments were also conducted using a questionnaire to assess the presence or absence of 23 PWS-associated behaviors (grouped into four categories) at baseline and at the end of the open-label treatment period. Resting energy expenditure (REE) and respiratory quotient (RQ) were measured by indirect calorimetry.

The patients enrolled included both males and females and consisted of overweight and obese patients between the ages of 10 and 22 years with genetically confirmed PWS. Fifteen patients were screened, and thirteen subjects were enrolled in the study. Patients treated with growth hormone for at least one year prior to the start of study could be enrolled.

The open-label treatment period was completed on 11 of the 13 enrolled patients (84.6%). All 11 patients who completed the open-label treatment period were designated as responders and showed improvements in hyperphagia. Most had also shown improvements in REE and were randomized into the double-blind treatment period. All 11 patients who were randomized into the double-blind treatment period completed the period [40]. After two weeks of treatment, there was a significant reduction in the hyperphagia score, and comments by parents were supportive of a marked improvement in hyperphagia. Treatment with DCCR for ten weeks had a significant impact on body composition, including reductions in body fat, increases in lean body mass, and a marked increase in the lean-body-mass to body-fat ratio. However, there was no significant change in weight from baseline to the end of the study. Waist circumference was significantly reduced during the open-label treatment period, suggesting the loss of visceral fat.

6. Livoletide Clinical Trial in PWS

Livoletide is an unacylated or inactive ghrelin analogue which works by decreasing the amount of active ghrelin in the brain. Ghrelin is a neuropeptide, produced by the stomach, which directly stimulates eating behavior in the hypothalamus in humans and is reportedly elevated in PWS (e.g., [41]). The ZEPHYR study sponsored by Millendo (Ann Arbor, MI, USA) was a randomized, double-blind, placebo-controlled, pivotal Phase 2b/3 study [42]. The therapy showed promising results in the phase 2a trial, in which daily Livoletide treatment or a placebo were administered via subcutaneous injection for 12 weeks. The Phase 2b study included 158 patients with PWS who were randomized to either (60 µg/kg or 120 µg/kg) receive the Livoletide dosage or the placebo. Livoletide was well-tolerated during this time, and the most-reported side effect was an injection site reaction of mild severity. However, no significant change was found in the Hyperphagia Questionnaire for Clinical Trials (HQ-CT) scores, which measured hunger and food-related behaviors, when compared with placebo. Hence, Livoletide also did not significantly improve hyperphagia and food-related behaviors and had no effect on fat mass, body weight, or waist circumference via DEXA data. As this drug was rigorously studied and the results were negative, it has been suggested that ghrelin may not be a driving force for the hyperphagia observed in PWS patients via this therapeutic route. However, this study may stimulate other gene–protein interactions or pathway analysis to study therapeutic options for treating hyperphagia and obesity in PWS. The company announced that it would discontinue this therapeutic development as a potential treatment model for PWS.

7. Cannabinoid Use in PWS

The cannabinoid-1 receptor (CB1R) plays an important role in the regulation of appetitive behavior. CB1Rs are important elements, encoded by genes located on chromosome 6 at bands q14-q15. The receptors are expressed most densely in the brain in areas involved in appetite regulation in the hypothalamus, but they also present in many peripheral tissues such as the liver, adrenal and pituitary glands, adipose tissue, and gonads. Research has shown that the activation of CB1R increases appetite, and the blockade of peripheral CB1R can decrease obesity and metabolic complications. Cannabidiol (CBD) is one of the common, non-psychotropic constituents of the Cannabis plant. It has an antagonist effect on CB1R, and thereby an anti-obesity effect [43]. Its use in PWS to treat hyperphagia progressed to an initial clinical-trial development with subject recruitment; however, the trial did not progress due to unforeseen problems.

8. Exenatide Use in PWS

Glucagon-like peptide-1 (GLP-1) is a hormone synthesized from the L- cells of the ileum and colon. It is released in response to food intake, contributing to postprandial glucose regulation. It also augments meal-related insulin secretion from the pancreas. The effect of GLP-1 receptor agonists on weight loss has been studied, with delays in gastric emptying and decreased appetite noted [44]. Exenatide is a GLP-1 receptor agonist, and its use has resulted in persistent weight loss in animals and obese adults [43]. In 2016, Salehi et al. [45] investigated the effect of exenatide treatment in a six-month trial in ten obese, adult patients with PWS. Body weight, body mass index (BMI), truncal fat, appetite measures, and plasma-acylated ghrelin and leptin levels were analyzed. They found no significant effect on body weight, BMI, or truncal adiposity, but did note a significant decrease in appetite scores and eating behavior [45], requiring more testing.

9. Transcranial Direct-Current Stimulation (tDCS) Clinical Trial and Startle Response in PWS

Transcranial direct-current stimulation (tDCS) is a safe, painless, and non-invasive technique to modify neuronal and cognitive function in areas of the brain (e.g., [46]). This technique has been undertaken in multiple studies in humans and can stimulate targeted brain regions and networks to increase or decrease cortical excitability in children or adults. In addition, the dorsolateral prefrontal cortex (DLPFC) is involved in the regulation and processing of food craving and motivation accessible by tDCS [46–48].

In 2015, Bravo et al. [46] investigated the efficacy of tDCS on the right DLPFC to modulate food craving and hyperphagia in patients with PWS by undertaking a double-blind, sham-controlled multicenter study of tDCS in ten adults with genetically confirmed PWS, eleven adult, obese subjects, and eleven adult, healthy-weight controls. The PWS and obese subjects received five consecutive daily sessions of active or sham tDCS over the right DLPFC, while healthy-weight subjects received a single sham and active tDCS in a crossover design. Standardized assessments for food cravings, drive, and hyperphagia from self-reporting and caregiver information were obtained over 30 days. The observed baseline differences were robust for severity scores for the Three Factor Eating Questionnaire (TFEQ) and the Dyken's Hyperphagia Questionnaire (DHQ) for PWS subjects when compared to healthy-weight controls, while the obese subjects were more similar to the healthy-weight controls. Active tDCS sessions in PWS were associated with a significant change from baseline in the TFEQ disinhibition component and for total scores. The participant ratings for the DHQ severity category and total scores were also significant. The reports of food craving using the Food Craving Analogue Scale, provided through self-reporting or by caregivers, supported the hypothesis of primary disturbances in cognitive and emotional aspects and food preoccupation in PWS [46].

In 2021, Poje et al. [48] further investigated the effect of tDCS on the DLPFC and hyperphagia in patients with PWS by reporting on the positive effects of brief tDCS sessions on the Go/NoGo task performance involving food and non-food stimuli images. Alterations in N2-brainwave-amplitude were recorded utilizing a skull-cap electroencephalogram apparatus, and PWS molecular genetic class differences before and after tDCS were assessed by event-related potentials (ERPs) in ten adults with PWS. The results indicated a group effect on baseline NoGo N2 amplitude in PWS patients with the 15q11-q13 deletion versus maternal disomy 15, a decrease in NoGo N2 brain amplitude in PWS adults with the deletion versus maternal disomy 15, and a decrease in NoGo N2 amplitude following tDCS. The tDCS approach demonstrated a trend towards a decreased response time. It collectively replicated and expanded prior work, highlighting neurophysiological differences in patients with PWS according to their genetic subtype and demonstrating the feasibility of examining neuromodulatory effects on information processing in individuals with PWS. The study supported the positive effect of tDCS on hyperphagic behavior in patients with PWS [46], requiring more testing.

In 2018, Gabrielli et al. [49] reported on the emotional processing of food and eating behavior in PWS by using startle-response modulation. The startle-eyeblink response is an involuntary reflex activated by the autonomic nervous system in response to sudden or disturbing auditory/visual stimuli. It may be modulated by the emotional valence of concurrently viewed visual stimuli. Gabrielli et al. studied thirteen individuals with PWS and eight healthy controls while viewing standard neutral, negative, positive, and food-derived images. Electromyogram (EMG) recordings of the orbicularis oculi muscle were measured in response to binaural white noise before and after the consumption of a standard 500 kcal meal. Participants reported their pre- and post-meal perceived emotional valence for each image using a one to ten Likert rating scale. Subjective ratings of food images and the urge to eat were significantly higher in PWS than found in controls and did not significantly decline post-meal. Acoustic startle responses detected in PWS were significantly lower than observed in controls under all conditions. Startle responses to food images in PWS were attenuated relative to other picture types, with a potentially abnormal emotional modulation of responses to non-food images, which contrasted with self-reported picture ratings. A stable, positive emotional valence to food images was observed pre-and post-feeding with a sustained urge to consume food in the PWS participants. Researchers concluded that the emotional processing measured using startle-modulation-responsive, non-food images was abnormal in PWS, which may reflect their unique features, such as hypotonia or increased fat mass and distribution, possibly impacting skin conductivity. It may also reflect an autonomic-nervous-system derangement in PWS that requires more testing [49].

10. Surgical Management of Obesity in PWS

The role of bariatric surgery in patients with PWS is controversial. Alqahtani et al. [50] and Fong et al. [51] reported decreased food seeking and a reduction in body weight and comorbidities such as obstructive sleep apnea, hypertension, and diabetes mellitus in PWS patients after laparoscopic sleeve gastrectomy. By contrast, Liu et al. [52] reported the rebound of symptoms and the development of obesity complications four to five years following bariatric surgery, which was described as ineffective in producing sustainable weight loss.

Scheimann et al. [53] reported a retrospective review on 60 published cases of PWS patients who underwent bariatric surgery. They found a variety of postoperative complications in PWS patients after bariatric surgery. Patients with PWS have special medical problems, such as a higher degree of insulin sensitivity, growth-hormone deficiency, hyperlipidemia, a decreased ability to vomit, and abnormal eating behavior with hyperphagia; therefore, a high potential for the development of gastric dilation/necrosis exists. These factors suggest that patients with PWS may have a higher potential risk of bariatric surgical complications than those seen in obese individuals without PWS. After jejunoileal bypass, one patient died. Another experienced wound infection and deep vein thrombosis. Furthermore, the patients who underwent gastric bypass with PWS found that one patient died, and two patients underwent splenectomy at the time of bariatric surgery. Most of the PWS patients who underwent gastroplasty reported a loss of weight, but this was followed by rebound weight gain. However, one PWS patient underwent laparoscopic, silicone gastric banding and died 45 days post-operatively [53]. Additionally, DePeppo et al. [54] reported a significant improvement in BMI after endoscopic intragastric balloon (BIB) placements in 12 patients with PWS, but two patients died from gastric perforation. Two other PWS patients developed severe, symptomatic gastric distension associated with food consumption. Although there are a small number of reported case series in PWS, there appears to be little justification for subjecting PWS patients to the potential high risk of complications from bariatric surgery (e.g., [53]).

11. Conclusions

As most individuals with PWS begin marked food seeking and hyperphagia during early childhood and often develop extreme obesity over time if uncontrolled, a safe and effective treatment is warranted to control both hyperphagia and obesity in PWS. Hence, several agents are currently in the clinical-trial stage or have been studied for treating hyperphagia and obesity in PWS patients as described. No specific differences were noted in drug responses in the individual clinical trials related to the PWS molecular genetic classes identified in the enrolled participants. Other drugs which impact features seen in PWS includes the antiepileptic drug topiramate, which showed a potential effect on disordered eating in several small studies in PWS patients [55,56]. It is also recommended for the treatment of skin-picking, a common obsessive-compulsive manifestation observed in individuals with PWS [57]. Furthermore, Holland et al. [58] recently investigated the efficacy of transcutaneous vagus nerve stimulation (t-VNS) for the treatment of temper outbursts and related behavioral findings in PWS, including hyperphagia; five individuals were studied. They found a significant decrease in temper outbursts in four out of the five PWS participants, with an improvement in emotional control, responses to interventions, and an increased ability to control and manage outburst-stimulating situations. However, they did not observe any reduction in hyperphagia [58].

Various drugs and devices investigated in clinical trials are discussed in this review and are summarized in Table 1, including beloranib, setmelanotide, DCCR, unacylated ghrelin analogue, oxytocin or related compounds, glucagon-like peptide 1 receptor agonists, transcranial direct-current stimulation, and transcutaneous vagus nerve stimulation. Other agents have been used, proposed, or are under development such as tesofensine/metoprolol, cannabinoids, topiramate, and histamine-related agents for the treatment of PWS findings that include hyperphagia and obesity [28,55,56,59–61]. Medical devices for treating hyperphagia and modulating eating behavior in PWS have shown promise. These include transcranial direct-current stimulation and transcutaneous vagus nerve stimulation in individuals with PWS, as well as generated information relating to brain regions and function impacted by the PWS diagnosis which require more testing. No specific differences were noted in response to the individual clinical-trial protocols or therapeutic agents related to the PWS molecular genetic classes identified in the PWS participants enrolled in the clinical trials [23,40,46–49,58].

Two of the trials that we reviewed hold promise for impacting hyperphagia and obesity in PWS. The reported success for the use of beloranib for weight loss and decreased appetite would have been of interest for continued testing; however, this trial was discontinued due to reported deaths. The second trial used DCCR tablets to treat hyperphagia and obesity and reported changes in both body composition measures and hyperphagia in a small number of subjects with PWS. More detailed studies are currently under study and review. Oxytocin trials have shown mixed results in treating PWS; this may be related to identifying the correct dose needed for use and may depend on the age of participants. Additionally, more research is needed to identify more objective measures for determining the level of hyperphagia. For example, the startle response and food-image processing in Prader–Willi syndrome reported by Gabrielli et al. [49] before and after consuming a standard meal may prove useful as an objective measure of hyperphagia and food-driven responses. More research is needed to identify objective measures of hyperphagia instead of using the subjective questionnaire forms that current exist for clinical trial use. Body composition measures using DEXA, weight, circumference, and body mass index (BMI) are the currently available objective data for studying obesity in clinical trials.

New pharmacotherapies aimed at controlling hyperphagia and appetite behavior in PWS patients are of interest for this patient population, with potential direct applications in the treatment of non-syndromic or exogenous obesity, which is on a significant rise worldwide and contributes to growing morbidity and mortality and healthcare costs. The identification of new mechanisms of the cause of hyperphagia and weight gain in patients with PWS, based on advances in genetic technology, bioinformatics, and gene variant testing, will be important. Computational biology to identify gene–gene–protein interactions and biological–molecular processes with pathways will lead to a better understanding of the cause and mechanism of other rare, obesity-related disorders (e.g., [62]). The recently reviewed research regarding the genetics of obesity and the newly acquired information about the role of genes [14,62,63] will yield promising new molecular targets for potentially novel pharmaceutical agents.

Table 1. Summary of drugs and medical devices used in PWS clinical trials.

Mechanism of Action	Studies Reviewed	Age Range	Reason Chosen for Treatment
Beloranib Beloranib inhibits methionine aminopeptidase 2 (MetAP2) by removing methionine residue from proteins, impacting fat metabolism and adipocyte size in animal models.	McCandless et al. [15]	12–65 years	Inhibitors of MetAP2 were found to reduce food intake, affect adipose tissue, and reduce fat synthesis with weight loss in humans.
Oxytocin Oxytocin is a neuropeptide hormone produced in the brain that plays an important role in social interactions and skills, food intake, anxiety, energy expenditure, and body-weight regulation.	Tauber et al. [22] Einfeld et al. [23] Kuppens et al. [24] Miller et al. [25] Tauber et al. [26] Damen at al. [27] Hollander et al. [28]	18.7–43.6 years >12 years 6–14 years 5–11 years <6 months 3–11 years 5–18 years	Patients with PWS have been reported to have decreased oxytocin-producing neurons. This deficiency could be related to their inability to control their emotions, with poor social adjustment and food intake.
Setmelanotide Setmelanotide is a melanocortin (MC)-4 receptor agonist that impacts satiety and feeding to decrease eating.	Rhythm Pharmaceuticals [29–31]	16–25 years	Patients with PWS begin marked food seeking and hyperphagia during early childhood and develop extreme obesity over time if not externally controlled.

Table 1. *Cont.*

Mechanism of Action	Studies Reviewed	Age Range	Reason Chosen for Treatment
Diazoxide choline controlled release (DCCR) DCCR is a benzothiadiazine that acts by stimulating ion flux through ATP-sensitive K+ channels used to treat infants, children, and adults with hyperinsulinemia hypoglycemia.	Kimonis et al. [40]	10–22 years	Hyperphagia in PWS relates to dysregulation of neuropeptide Y/Agouti Related Protein/Gamma-aminobutyric Acid (NAG) neurons, which are regulated by leptin via the reduction of their excitability. This dysregulation results in marked elevations in the synthesis and secretion of NPY, the most potent endogenous neuropeptide. Leptin's activation of adenosine triphosphate (ATP)-sensitive potassium channels (K_{ATP}) via phosphoinositide-3-kinase (PI3-K) serves to hyperpolarize the resting membrane potential, resulting in a limitation of the release of NPY by these neurons, thus blunting the hyperphagia signal.
Livoletide Livoletide is an inactive ghrelin analogue which works by decreasing the amount of the active form of ghrelin in the brain. Ghrelin is a neuropeptide produced by the stomach which directly stimulates eating behavior in the hypothalamus in humans.	Millendo Therapeutics SAS [42]	8–65 years	Patients with PWS have elevated ghrelin levels.
Exenatide Glucagon-like peptide-1 (GLP-1) is a hormone synthesized from L-cells of the ileum and colon and released in response to food intake. GLP-1 receptor agonists such as Exenatide affect weight loss in the form of a delay in gastric emptying and decreased appetite.	Salehi et al. [45]	13–25 years	Exenatide is a GLP-1 receptor agonist and its use has resulted in persistent weight loss in animals and obese adults.
Transcranial direct-current stimulation (tDCS) Transcranial direct-current stimulation (tDCS) is a safe, painless, and non-invasive technique to modify neuronal and cognitive function in areas of the brain to help modulate food craving.	Bravo et al. [46] Poje et al. [48] Gabrielli et al. [49]	18–64 years 19–44 years 16–65 years	The dorsolateral prefrontal cortex (DLPFC) is involved in the regulation and processing of food craving and motivation in humans.

Author Contributions: Writing—original draft preparation, R.M.; writing—review and editing, M.G.B. and V.K.; visualization, V.K. and M.G.B.; supervision, V.K. and M.G.B. All authors have read and agreed to the published version of the manuscript.

Funding: This research was funded by National Institute of Health (NIH) U54 Grant HD061222 and support from Prader-Willi Syndrome Association (PWSA)-USA.

Informed Consent Statement: No consent is required for the discussion of clinical trial data that is available to the public as no identifying information related to the individual participants is shared.

Data Availability Statement: The data supporting the reported material can be obtained upon request.

Acknowledgments: We thank all the patients and families with PWS for their participation in clinical trials to help identify an agent to treat hyperphagia and obesity.

Conflicts of Interest: The authors declare no conflict of interest.

References

1. Butler, M.G. Prader-Willi Syndrome: Current Understanding of Cause and Diagnosis. *Am. J. Med. Genet.* **1990**, *35*, 319–332. [CrossRef] [PubMed]
2. Butler, M.G. Prader-Willi Syndrome: Obesity due to Genomic Imprinting. *Curr. Genom.* **2011**, *12*, 204–215. [CrossRef] [PubMed]
3. Butler, M.G.; Manzardo, A.M.; Forster, J.L. Prader-Willi Syndrome: Clinical Genetics and Diagnostic Aspects with Treatment Approaches. *Curr. Pediatr. Rev.* **2016**, *12*, 136–166. [CrossRef]
4. Butler, M.G.; Hartin, S.N.; Hossain, W.A.; Manzardo, A.M.; Kimonis, V.; Dykens, E.; Gold, J.A.; Kim, S.-J.; Weisensel, N.; Tamura, R.; et al. Molecular Genetic Classification in Prader-Willi Syndrome: A Multisite Cohort Study. *J. Med. Genet.* **2018**, *56*, 149–153. [CrossRef]
5. Cassidy, S.B.; Schwartz, S.; Miller, J.L.; Driscoll, D.J. Prader-Willi syndrome. *Genet. Med.* **2012**, *14*, 10–26. [CrossRef] [PubMed]
6. Butler, M.G.; Kimonis, V.; Dykens, E.; Gold, J.A.; Miller, J.; Tamura, R.; Driscoll, D.J. Prader-Willi syndrome and early-onset morbid obesity NIH rare disease consortium: A review of natural history study. *Am. J. Med. Genet. A* **2018**, *176*, 368–375. [CrossRef] [PubMed]
7. Butler, M.G.; Manzardo, A.M.; Heinemann, J.; Loker, C.; Loker, J. Causes of death in Prader-Willi syndrome: Prader-Willi Syndrome Association (USA) 40-year mortality survey. *Genet. Med.* **2017**, *19*, 635–642. [CrossRef] [PubMed]
8. Butler, M.G.; Thompson, T. Prader-Willi Syndrome. *Endocrinologist.* **2000**, *10* (Suppl. S1), 3S16S. [CrossRef] [PubMed]
9. Roof, E.; Stone, W.; MacLean, W.; Feurer, I.D.; Thompson, T.; Butler, M.G. Intellectual characteristics of Prader-Willi syndrome: Comparison of genetic subtypes. *J. Intellect. Disabil. Res.* **2000**, *44 Pt 1*, 25–30. [CrossRef] [PubMed]
10. Butler, M.G.; Bittel, D.C.; Kibiryeva, N.; Talebizadeh, Z.; Thompson, T. Behavioral differences among subjects with Prader-Willi syndrome and type I or type II deletion and maternal disomy. *Pediatrics* **2004**, *113 Pt 1*, 565–573. [CrossRef]
11. Zarcone, J.; Napolitano, D.; Peterson, C.; Breidbord, J.; Ferraioli, S.; Caruso-Anderson, M.; Holsen, L.; Butler, M.G.; Thompson, T. The relationship between compulsive behaviour and academic achievement across the three genetic subtypes of Prader-Willi syndrome. *J. Intellect. Disabil. Res.* **2007**, *51 Pt 6*, 478–487. [CrossRef]
12. Hedgeman, E.; Ulrichsen, S.P.; Carter, S.; Kreher, N.C.; Malobisky, K.P.; Braun, M.M.; Fryzek, J.; Olsen, M.S. Long-term health outcomes in patients with Prader-Willi Syndrome: A nationwide cohort study in Denmark. *Int. J. Obes.* **2017**, *41*, 1531–1538. [CrossRef]
13. Manzardo, A.M.; Loker, J.; Heinemann, J.; Loker, C.; Butler, M.G. Survival Trends from the Prader–Willi Syndrome Association (USA) 40-Year Mortality Survey. *Genet. Med.* **2017**, *20*, 24–30. [CrossRef] [PubMed]
14. Mahmoud, R.; Kimonis, V.; Butler, M.G. Genetics of Obesity in Humans: A Clinical Review. *Int. J. Mol. Sci.* **2022**, *23*, 11005. [CrossRef] [PubMed]
15. McCandless, S.E.; Yanovski, J.A.; Miller, J.; Fu, C.; Bird, L.M.; Salehi, P.; Chan, C.L.; Stafford, D.; Abuzzahab, M.J.; Viskochil, D.; et al. Effects of MetAP2 Inhibition on Hyperphagia and Body Weight in Prader-Willi Syndrome: A Randomized, Double-Blind, Placebo-Controlled Trial. *Diabetes Obes. Metab.* **2017**, *19*, 1751–1761. [CrossRef]
16. Johnson, L.; Manzardo, A.M.; Miller, J.L.; Driscoll, D.J.; Butler, M.G. Elevated Plasma Oxytocin Levels in Children with Prader-Willi Syndrome Compared with Healthy Unrelated Siblings. *Am. J. Med. Genet. Part A* **2015**, *170*, 594–601. [CrossRef] [PubMed]
17. Love, T.M. Oxytocin, Motivation and the Role of Dopamine. *Pharmacol. Biochem. Behav.* **2014**, *119*, 49–60. [CrossRef] [PubMed]
18. Swaab, D.F.; Purba, J.S.; Hofman, M.A. Alterations in the hypothalamic paraventricular nucleus and its oxytocin neurons (putative satiety cells) in Prader-Willi syndrome: A study of five cases. *J. Clin. Endocrinol. Metab.* **1995**, *80*, 573–579. [PubMed]
19. Muscatelli, F.; Abrous, D.N.; Massacrier, A.; Boccaccio, I.; Le Moal, M.; Cau, P.; Cremer, H. Disruption of the mouse Necdin gene results in hypothalamic and behavioral alterations reminiscent of the human Prader-Willi syndrome. *Hum. Mol. Genet.* **2000**, *9*, 3101–3110. [CrossRef] [PubMed]
20. Schaller, F.; Watrin, F.; Sturny, R.; Massacrier, A.; Szepetowski, P.; Muscatelli, F. A single postnatal injection of oxytocin rescues the lethal feeding behaviour in mouse newborns deficient for the imprinted Magel2 gene. *Hum. Mol. Genet.* **2010**, *19*, 4895–4905. [CrossRef] [PubMed]
21. Meziane, H.; Schaller, F.; Bauer, S.; Villard, C.; Matarazzo, V.; Riet, F.; Guillon, G.; Lafitte, D.; Desarmenien, M.G.; Tauber, M.; et al. An Early Postnatal Oxytocin Treatment Prevents Social and Learning Deficits in Adult Mice Deficient for Magel2, a Gene Involved in Prader-Willi Syndrome and Autism. *Biol. Psychiatry* **2015**, *78*, 85–94. [CrossRef]
22. Tauber, M.; Mantoulan, C.; Copet, P.; Jauregui, J.; Demeer, G.; Diene, G.; Roge, B.; Laurier, V.; Ehlinger, V.; Arnaud, C.; et al. Oxytocin may be useful to increase trust in others and decrease disruptive behaviours in patients with Prader-Willi syndrome: A randomised placebo-controlled trial in 24 patients. *Orphanet J. Rare Dis.* **2011**, *6*, 47. [CrossRef] [PubMed]
23. Einfeld, S.L.; Smith, E.; McGregor, I.S.; Steinbeck, K.; Taffe, J.; Rice, L.J.; Horstead, S.K.; Rogers, N.; Hodge, M.A.; Guastella, A.J. A double-blind randomized controlled trial of oxytocin nasal spray in Prader Willi syndrome. *Am. J. Med. Genetics. Part A* **2014**, *164A*, 2232–2239. [CrossRef] [PubMed]

24. Kuppens, R.J.; Donze, S.H.; Hokken-Koelega, A.C. Promising effects of oxytocin on social and food-related behaviour in young children with Prader-Willi syndrome: A randomized, double-blind, controlled crossover trial. *Clin. Endocrinol.* **2016**, *85*, 979–987. [CrossRef] [PubMed]
25. Miller, J.L.; Tamura, R.; Butler, M.G.; Kimonis, V.; Sulsona, C.; Gold, J.A.; Driscoll, D.J. Oxytocin treatment in children with Prader-Willi syndrome: A double-blind, placebo-controlled, crossover study. *Am. J. Med. Genetics. Part A* **2017**, *173*, 1243–1250. [CrossRef]
26. Tauber, M.; Boulanouar, K.; Diene, G.; Cabal-Berthoumieu, S.; Ehlinger, V.; Fichaux-Bourin, P.; Molinas, C.; Faye, S.; Valette, M.; Pourrinet, J.; et al. The Use of Oxytocin to Improve Feeding and Social Skills in Infants with Prader-Willi Syndrome. *Pediatrics* **2017**, *139*, e20162976. [CrossRef] [PubMed]
27. Damen, L.; Grootjen, L.N.; Juriaans, A.F.; Donze, S.H.; Huisman, T.M.; Visser, J.A.; Delhanty, P.J.D.; Hokken-Koelega, A.C.S. Oxytocin in young children with Prader-Willi syndrome: Results of a randomized, double-blind, placebo-controlled, crossover trial investigating 3 months of oxytocin. *Clin. Endocrinol.* **2021**, *94*, 774–785. [CrossRef] [PubMed]
28. Hollander, E.; Levine, K.G.; Ferretti, C.J.; Freeman, K.; Doernberg, E.; Desilva, N.; Taylor, B.P. Intranasal oxytocin versus placebo for hyperphagia and repetitive behaviors in children with Prader-Willi Syndrome: A randomized controlled pilot trial. *J. Psychiatr. Res.* **2021**, *137*, 643–651. [CrossRef]
29. Rhythm Pharmaceuticals, Inc. A Ph 2, Randomized, Double-Blind, Placebo-Controlled Pilot Study to Assess the Effects of RM-493, a Melanocortin 4 Receptor (MC4R) Agonist, in Obese Subjects with Prader-Willi Syndrome (PWS) on Safety, Weight Reduction, and Food-Related Behaviors. Available online: https://clinicaltrials.gov/ct2/show/NCT02311673 (accessed on 2 November 2022).
30. Duis, J.; van Wattum, P.J.; Scheimann, A.; Salehi, P.; Brokamp, E.; Fairbrother, L.; Childers, A.; Shelton, A.R.; Bingham, N.C.; Shoemaker, A.H.; et al. A Multidisciplinary Approach to the Clinical Management of Prader–Willi Syndrome. *Mol. Genet. Genom. Med.* **2019**, *7*, e514. [CrossRef]
31. Miller, J.; Roof, E.; Butler, M.G.; Kimonis, V.; Angulo, M.; Folster, C.; Hylan, M.; Fred, T.; Fiedorek, F.T. Results of a Phase 2 Study of the Melanocortin (MC)-4 Receptor (R) Agonist Setmelanotide (SET) in Prader-Willi Syndrome (PWS). In Proceedings of the 2017 PWSA 34th Scientific Day National Convention, Orlando, FL, USA, 15–18 November 2017.
32. Markham, A. Setmelanotide: First Approval. *Drugs* **2021**, *81*, 397–403. [CrossRef]
33. Baver, S.B.; Hope, K.; Guyot, S.; Bjorbaek, C.; Kaczorowski, C.; O'Connell, K.M. Leptin modulates the intrinsic excitability of AgRP/NPY neurons in the arcuate nucleus of the hypothalamus. *J. Neurosci.* **2014**, *34*, 5486–5496. [CrossRef] [PubMed]
34. Baquero, A.F.; de Solis, A.J.; Lindsley, S.R.; Kirigiti, M.A.; Smith, M.S.; Cowley, M.A.; Zeltser, L.M.; Grove, K.L. Developmental switch of leptin signaling in arcuate nucleus neurons. *J. Neurosci.* **2014**, *34*, 9982–9994. [CrossRef]
35. Spanswick, D.; Smith, M.A.; Groppi, V.E.; Logan, S.D.; Ashford, M.L. Leptin inhibits hypothalamic neurons by activation of ATP-sensitive potassium channels. *Nature* **1997**, *390*, 521–525. [CrossRef] [PubMed]
36. van den Top, M.; Lee, K.; Whyment, A.D.; Blanks, A.M.; Spanswick, D. Orexigen-sensitive NPY/AgRP pacemaker neurons in the hypothalamic arcuate nucleus. *Nat. Neurosci.* **2004**, *7*, 493–494. [CrossRef] [PubMed]
37. Stricker-Krongrad, A.; Barbanel, G.; Beck, B.; Burlet, A.; Nicolas, J.P.; Burlet, C. K(+)-stimulated neuropeptide Y release into the paraventricular nucleus and relation to feeding behavior in free-moving rats. *Neuropeptides* **1993**, *24*, 307–312. [CrossRef] [PubMed]
38. Ruud, J.; Steculorum, S.M.; Bruning, J.C. Neuronal control of peripheral insulin sensitivity and glucose metabolism. *Nat. Commun.* **2017**, *8*, 15259. [CrossRef]
39. Kishore, P.; Boucai, L.; Zhang, K.; Li, W.; Koppaka, S.; Kehlenbrink, S.; Schiwek, A.; Esterson, Y.B.; Mehta, D.; Bursheh, S.; et al. Activation of K(ATP) channels suppresses glucose production in humans. *J. Clin. Investig.* **2011**, *121*, 4916–4920. [CrossRef] [PubMed]
40. Kimonis, V.; Surampalli, A.; Wencel, M.; Gold, J.-A.; Cowen, N.M. A Randomized Pilot Efficacy and Safety Trial of Diazoxide Choline Controlled-Release in Patients with Prader-Willi Syndrome. *PLoS ONE* **2019**, *14*, e0221615. [CrossRef] [PubMed]
41. Butler, M.G.; Bittel, D.C. Plasma Obestatin and Ghrelin Levels in Subjects with Prader–Willi Syndrome. *Am. J. Med. Genet. Part A* **2007**, *143A*, 415–421. [CrossRef] [PubMed]
42. Millendo Therapeutics SAS. A Phase 2b/3 Study to Evaluate the Safety, Tolerability, and Effects of Livoletide (AZP-531), an Unacylated Ghrelin Analogue, on Food-Related Behaviors in Patients with Prader-Willi Syndrome. Available online: https://clinicaltrials.gov/ct2/show/NCT03790865 (accessed on 1 November 2022).
43. Thomas, A.; Baillie, G.L.; Phillips, A.M.; Razdan, R.K.; Ross, R.A.; Pertwee, R.G. Cannabidiol Displays Unexpectedly High Potency as an Antagonist of CB1 and CB2 Receptor Agonists in Vitro. *Br. J. Pharmacol.* **2009**, *150*, 613–623. [CrossRef] [PubMed]
44. Van Bloemendaal, L.; ten Kulve, J.S.; la Fleur, S.E.; Ijzerman, R.G.; Diamant, M. Effects of Glucagon-like Peptide 1 on Appetite and Body Weight: Focus on the CNS. *J. Endocrinol.* **2013**, *221*, T1–T16. [CrossRef] [PubMed]
45. Salehi, P.; Hsu, I.; Azen, C.G.; Mittelman, S.D.; Geffner, M.E.; Jeandron, D. Effects of Exenatide on Weight and Appetite in Overweight Adolescents and Young Adults with Prader-Willi Syndrome. *Pediatr. Obes.* **2016**, *12*, 221–228. [CrossRef]
46. Bravo, G.L.; Poje, A.B.; Perissinotti, I.; Marcondes, B.F.; Villamar, M.F.; Manzardo, A.M.; Luque, L.; LePage, J.F.; Stafford, D.; Fregni, F.; et al. Transcranial Direct Current Stimulation Reduces Food-Craving and Measures of Hyperphagia Behavior in Participants with Prader-Willi Syndrome. *Am. J. Med. Genet. Part B Neuropsychiatr. Genet.* **2015**, *171*, 266–275. [CrossRef] [PubMed]

47. Azevedo, C.C.; Trevizol, A.P.; Gomes, J.S.; Akiba, H.; Franco, R.R.; Simurro, P.B.; Ianni, R.M.; Grigolon, R.B.; Blumberger, D.M.; Dias, A.M. Transcranial Direct Current Stimulation for Prader-Willi Syndrome. *J. ECT* **2020**, *37*, 58–63. [CrossRef]
48. Poje, A.B.; Manzardo, A.; Gustafson, K.M.; Liao, K.; Martin, L.E.; Butler, M.G. Effects of Transcranial Direct Current Stimulation (TDCS) on Go/NoGo Performance Using Food and Non-Food Stimuli in Patients with Prader–Willi Syndrome. *Brain Sci.* **2021**, *11*, 250. [CrossRef] [PubMed]
49. Gabrielli, A.; Poje, A.B.; Manzardo, A.; Butler, M.G. Startle response analysis of food-image processing in Prader-Willi Syndrome. *J. Rare Disord.* **2018**, *6*, 18–27.
50. Alqahtani, A.R.; Elahmedi, M.O.; Al Qahtani, A.R.; Lee, J.; Butler, M.G. Laparoscopic Sleeve Gastrectomy in Children and Adolescents with Prader-Willi Syndrome: A Matched-Control Study. *Surg. Obes. Relat. Dis.* **2016**, *12*, 100–110. [CrossRef] [PubMed]
51. Fong, A.K.W.; Wong, S.K.H.; Lam, C.C.H.; Ng, E.K.W. Ghrelin Level and Weight Loss after Laparoscopic Sleeve Gastrectomy and Gastric Mini-Bypass for Prader–Willi Syndrome in Chinese. *Obes. Surg.* **2012**, *22*, 1742–1745. [CrossRef] [PubMed]
52. Liu, S.Y.; Wong, S.K.; Lam, C.C.; Ng, E.K. Bariatric Surgery for Prader-Willi Syndrome Was Ineffective in Producing Sustainable Weight Loss: Long Term Results for up to 10 Years. *Pediatr. Obes.* **2019**, *15*, e12575. [CrossRef] [PubMed]
53. Scheimann, A.; Butler, M.; Gourash, L.; Cuffari, C.; Klish, W. Critical Analysis of Bariatric Procedures in Prader-Willi Syndrome. *J. Pediatr. Gastroenterol. Nutr.* **2008**, *46*, 80–83. [CrossRef] [PubMed]
54. De Peppo, F.; Di Giorgio, G.; Germani, M.; Ceriati, E.; Marchetti, P.; Galli, C.; Ubertini, M.G.; Spera, S.; Ferrante, G.; Cuttini, M.; et al. BioEnterics Intragastric Balloon for Treatment of Morbid Obesity in Prader–Willi Syndrome: Specific Risks and Benefits. *Obes. Surg.* **2008**, *18*, 1443–1449. [CrossRef] [PubMed]
55. Smathers, S.A.; Wilson, J.G.; Nigro, M.A. Topiramate Effectiveness in Prader-Willi Syndrome. *Pediatr. Neurol.* **2003**, *28*, 130–133. [CrossRef] [PubMed]
56. Consoli, A.; Çabal Berthoumieu, S.; Raffin, M.; Thuilleaux, D.; Poitou, C.; Coupaye, M.; Pinto, G.; Lebbah, S.; Zahr, N.; Tauber, M.; et al. Effect of Topiramate on Eating Behaviours in Prader-Willi Syndrome: TOPRADER Double-Blind Randomised Placebo-Controlled Study. *Transl. Psychiatry* **2019**, *9*, 274. [CrossRef]
57. Symons, F.J.; Butler, M.G.; Sanders, M.D.; Feurer, I.D.; Thompson, T. Self-Injurious Behavior and Prader-Willi Syndrome: Behavioral Forms and Body Locations. *Am. J. Ment. Retard.* **1999**, *104*, 260–269. [CrossRef]
58. Holland, A.; Manning, K. T-VNS to Treat Disorders of Behaviour in Prader-Willi Syndrome and in People with Other Neurodevelopmental Conditions. *Auton. Neurosci.* **2022**, *239*, 102955. [CrossRef] [PubMed]
59. Dykens, E.M.; Miller, J.; Angulo, M.; Roof, E.; Reidy, M.; Hatoum, H.T.; Willey, R.; Bolton, G.; Korner, P. Intranasal Carbetocin Reduces Hyperphagia in Individuals with Prader-Willi Syndrome. *JCI Insight* **2018**, *3*, e98333. [CrossRef]
60. Tan, Q.; Orsso, C.E.; Deehan, E.C.; Triador, L.; Field, C.J.; Tun, H.M.; Han, J.C.; Müller, T.D.; Haqq, A.M. Current and Emerging Therapies for Managing Hyperphagia and Obesity in Prader-Willi Syndrome: A Narrative Review. *Obes. Rev.* **2020**, *21*, e12992. [CrossRef] [PubMed]
61. Muscogiuri, G.; Barrea, L.; Faggiano, F.; Maiorino, M.I.; Parrillo, M.; Pugliese, G.; Ruggeri, R.M.; Scarano, E.; Savastano, S.; Colao, A. Obesity in Prader–Willi Syndrome: Physiopathological Mechanisms, Nutritional and Pharmacological Approaches. *J. Endocrinol. Investig.* **2021**, *44*, 2057–2070. [CrossRef]
62. Butler, M.G. Single Gene and Syndromic Causes of Obesity: Illustrative Examples. *Prog. Mol. Biol. Transl. Sci.* **2016**, *140*, 1–45. [CrossRef]
63. Duis, J.; Butler, M.G. Syndromic and Nonsyndromic Obesity: Underlying Genetic Causes in Humans. *Adv. Biol.* **2022**, *6*, e2101154. [CrossRef]

Disclaimer/Publisher's Note: The statements, opinions and data contained in all publications are solely those of the individual author(s) and contributor(s) and not of MDPI and/or the editor(s). MDPI and/or the editor(s) disclaim responsibility for any injury to people or property resulting from any ideas, methods, instructions or products referred to in the content.

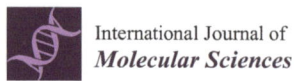

Editorial

The Arduous Path to Drug Approval for the Management of Prader–Willi Syndrome: A Historical Perspective and Call to Action

Deepan Singh [1,*], Jennifer L. Miller [2], Edward Robert Wassman [3], Merlin G. Butler [4], Allison Foley Shenk [3], Monica Converse [3] and Maria Picone [3]

1. Department of Psychiatry, Maimonides Medical Center, Brooklyn, New York, NY 11219, USA
2. Department of Pediatrics, Division of Pediatric Endocrinology, University of Florida, Gainesville, FL 32611, USA; millejl@peds.ufl.edu
3. TREND Community, Philadelphia, PA 19103, USA; drbobwassman@gmail.com (E.R.W.); alifoleyshenk.trend@gmail.com (A.F.S.); maria@trend.community (M.P.)
4. Departments of Psychiatry & Behavioral Sciences and Pediatrics, University of Kansas Medical Center, Kansas City, KS 66160, USA; mbutler4@kumc.edu
* Correspondence: desingh@maimonidesmed.org

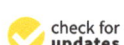

Citation: Singh, D.; Miller, J.L.; Wassman, E.R.; Butler, M.G.; Foley Shenk, A.; Converse, M.; Picone, M. The Arduous Path to Drug Approval for the Management of Prader–Willi Syndrome: A Historical Perspective and Call to Action. *Int. J. Mol. Sci.* **2023**, *24*, 11574. https://doi.org/10.3390/ijms241411574

Received: 25 May 2023
Accepted: 19 June 2023
Published: 18 July 2023

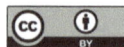

Copyright: © 2023 by the authors. Licensee MDPI, Basel, Switzerland. This article is an open access article distributed under the terms and conditions of the Creative Commons Attribution (CC BY) license (https://creativecommons.org/licenses/by/4.0/).

Prader–Willi syndrome (PWS) is a neuroendocrine genetic disorder resulting from the loss of paternally expressed imprinted genes in chromosome 15q11-q13 [1,2]. Although characterized most prominently by life-threatening hyperphagia and obesity, PWS can also be accompanied by a multitude of other issues, including growth and other hormone deficiencies, behavioral problems, skin picking, abnormal body composition [3,4], and sleep disruption [5,6]. Despite the well-established burden of illness and the social costs of PWS, the only medication that has been approved by the Food and Drug Administration (FDA) for the management of this disorder is recombinant human growth hormone (rhGH), which was approved in 2000 [7,8]. However, since then, every PWS clinical trial that has reached phase 3 has failed to achieve final approval. Here, we discuss some insights into the challenges associated with the approval of drugs to treat PWS.

The increased awareness of PWS has led to earlier diagnosis and resultant intervention and treatment [9]. With the approval and introduction of rhGH during early development and the implementation of individualized dietary and exercise plans [10], progress has been made in improving stature and body composition associated with PWS; however, limited progress has been made regarding neurobehavioral manifestations of the disease. Although PWS was once considered a disorder marked by cognitive impairment, some individuals with PWS now attend mainstream school classrooms and have a wealth of options for attending college, demonstrating the potential for more independent living for those with this disorder.

Despite these incremental advances, hyperphagia, its repercussions, and behavioral dysregulation in PWS remain severe and life-threatening. Hence, the importance of novel drug development and approval cannot be overstated. A recent review by Mahmoud et al. [11] detailed clinical trials of multiple proposed therapeutics for PWS and highlighted other potential prospects for evaluation. Thus far, these therapies and others have mostly been discontinued or failed to receive approval from the FDA.

The challenges inherent in rare disease clinical trials are well known. Notably, the intrinsic limitation in sample size is exponentially compounded by the geographical scale needed for recruitment and enrollment for studies to attain sufficient power to reach statistical significance.

To address these challenges, the FDA has used its regulatory flexibility to its advantage, ultimately approving drugs to treat many illnesses, predominantly hematological–oncological diseases and, more recently, neurodegenerative disorders such as Alzheimer's disease and amyotrophic lateral sclerosis (ALS). Such regulatory discretion applies when a disease is serious, life-threatening, and has few or no therapies available. All of these factors apply to PWS, and any therapeutic approval pathway for this syndrome should therefore be eligible for "flexibility". This would allow for the acceptance of greater-than-usual uncertainty about the effi-cacy of a treatment modality for an unmet medical need. However, the FDA has yet to apply its regulatory flexibility regarding medications developed for this population.

Arguments posed by the FDA include a lack of sufficiently well-described mechanisms of action for agents and inadequate direct or surrogate study endpoints. The lack of established biomarkers in PWS that serve as potentiating surrogate endpoints remains a barrier to successful studies, which historically have been heavily influenced by subjective caregiver questionnaires. The result is an inherent rigidity to the regulatory flexibility process and no path forward to address the unmet needs of PWS.

Under the current regulatory construct, in which reliance on biomarkers and the requirement of prestated narrow goals cannot be changed to include other relevant clinical improvements, the approval of new treatments for PWS remains scarce. We contend that recent clinical trials that failed to meet primary endpoints still had significant off-target benefits for participants, often with minimal to no adverse effects. A recent example is carbetocin and its effects on PWS-related anxiousness and hyperphagia [12]. Additionally, diazoxide choline controlled-release (DCCR) recently demonstrated significant improvements in hyperphagia, as well as in anxiety, depression, and compulsive and self-injurious behavior; however, the top-line analysis was negatively affected by the COVID-19 pandemic, which caused the overall analysis to miss its primary endpoint. Long-term data continue to show improvements in hyperphagia as well as several behavioral parameters, and comparisons with a contemporaneous natural history study have shown the significant benefits of DCCR treatment [13]. The fact that the significant beneficial effects of this agent are disastrously overshadowed by the rigid analytical process in this setting is a major concern of the patient–caregiver–clinical community.

Many manifestations of PWS have multidimensional and complex etiologies, including genetic factors that remain poorly understood or characterized. Some therapeutic agents or approaches may focus on physical findings or comorbidities such as obesity and abnormal body composition, but not on behavioral manifestations, which also impair quality of life across many domains [3]. The complexity of PWS and history of failed trials are leading to the further marginalization of patients with PWS and risk causing a feeling of disinterest among the scientific and pharmaceutical communities; the barriers to treatment might seem insurmountable and not worth pursuing.

The future envisioned by the patient–caregiver–clinician community is one in which people with PWS can make meaningful contributions to society and have purposeful lives of their own without having to face as-yet-unaddressed biological and psychological challenges. This is within reach in the near future if the scientific, clinical, industry, and regulatory communities work toward this common goal. For this to happen, we must remove obstacles to the approval of reasonable and effective treatments for people with PWS. We strongly recommend that the FDA apply the broadest regulatory flexibility to the statutory standards and use clinically grounded scientific judgment, as we discussed, paired with an understanding that patients and their families are willing to accept greater risk and uncertainty for the opportunity to ameliorate the severely disabling, life-threatening symptoms of PWS.

Author Contributions: D.S., M.C. and A.F.S. contributed to drafting the editorial. All authors were involved in critical revision of the manuscript. All authors have read and agreed to the published version of the manuscript.

Conflicts of Interest: Merlin Butler and Allison Foley Shenk have no conflict of interest to declare. Deepan Singh received grants from the Foundation for Prader-Willi Research and has served as a consultant for Soleno Therapeutics, Acadia, and ConSynance. Jennifer Miller received research funding from Soleno Therapeutics, Rhythm Therapeutics, TRYP Pharmaceuticals, and Harmony Biosciences. E. Robert Wassman, Monica Converse, and Maria Picone are employees of TREND Community. TREND Community's clients are pharmaceutical and biotechnology companies including, but not limited to Horizon Therapeutics, Chiesi Global Rare Disease, Novartis, Harmony Biosciences, and Avadel.

References

1. Irizarry, K.A.; Miller, M.; Freemark, M.; Haqq, A.M. Prader Willi syndrome: Genetics, metabolomics, hormonal function, and new approaches to therapy. *Adv. Pediatr.* **2016**, *63*, 47–77. [CrossRef]
2. Butler, M.G.; Hartin, S.N.; Hossain, W.A.; Manzardo, A.M.; Kimonis, V.; Dykens, E.; Gold, J.A.; Kim, S.J.; Weisensel, N.; Tamura, R.; et al. Molecular genetic classification in Prader-Willi syndrome: A multisite cohort study. *J. Med. Genet.* **2019**, *56*, 149–153. [CrossRef]
3. Cassidy, S.B.; Schwartz, S.; Miller, J.L.; Driscoll, D.J. Prader-Willi syndrome. *Genet. Med.* **2012**, *14*, 10–26. [CrossRef]
4. Butler, M.G.; Miller, J.L.; Forster, J.L. Prader-Willi syndrome—Clinical genetics, diagnosis and treatment approaches: An update. *Curr. Pediatr. Rev.* **2019**, *15*, 207–244. [CrossRef] [PubMed]
5. Veatch, O.J.; Malow, B.A.; Lee, H.S.; Knight, A.; Barrish, J.O.; Neul, J.L.; Lane, J.B.; Skinner, S.A.; Kaufmann, W.E.; Miller, J.L.; et al. Evaluating sleep disturbances in children with rare genetic neurodevelopmental syndromes. *Pediatr. Neurol.* **2021**, *123*, 30–37. [CrossRef] [PubMed]
6. Duis, J.; Pullen, L.C.; Picone, M.; Friedman, N.; Hawkins, S.; Sannar, E.; Pfalzer, A.C.; Shelton, A.R.; Singh, D.; Zee, P.C.; et al. Diagnosis and management of sleep disorders in Prader-Willi syndrome. *J. Clin. Sleep Med.* **2022**, *18*, 1687–1696. [CrossRef] [PubMed]
7. Butler, M.G.; Miller, B.S.; Romano, A.; Ross, J.; Abuzzahab, M.J.; Backeljauw, P.; Bamba, V.; Bhangoo, A.; Mauras, N.; Geffner, M. Genetic conditions of short stature: A review of three classic examples. *Front. Endocrinol.* **2022**, *13*, 1011960. [CrossRef] [PubMed]
8. Food and Drug Administration (FDA). Treatment of Short Stature with Prader-Willi Syndrome. Orphan Drug Designations and Approvals. Available online: https://www.accessdata.fda.gov/scripts/opdlisting/oopd/detailedIndex.cfm?cfgridkey=124799 (accessed on 21 March 2023).
9. Kimonis, V.E.; Tamura, R.; Gold, J.A.; Patel, N.; Surampalli, A.; Manazir, J.; Miller, J.L.; Roof, E.; Dykens, E.; Butler, M.G.; et al. Early diagnosis in Prader-Willi syndrome reduces obesity and associated co-morbidities. *Genes* **2019**, *10*, 898. [CrossRef] [PubMed]
10. Woods, S.G.; Knehans, A.; Arnold, S.; Dionne, C.; Hoffman, L.; Turner, P.; Baldwin, J. The associations between diet and physical activity with body composition and walking a timed distance in adults with Prader-Willi syndrome. *Food Nutr. Res.* **2018**, *62*. [CrossRef] [PubMed]
11. Mahmoud, R.; Kimonis, V.; Butler, M.G. Clinical trials in Prader-Willi syndrome: A review. *Int. J. Mol. Sci.* **2023**, *24*, 2150. [CrossRef] [PubMed]
12. Roof, E.; Deal, C.L.; McCandless, S.E.; Cowan, R.L.; Miller, J.L.; Hamilton, J.K.; Roeder, E.R.; McCormack, S.E.; Roshan Lal, T.R.; Abdul-Latif, H.D.; et al. Intranasal carbetocin reduces hyperphagia, anxiousness and distress in Prader-Willi syndrome: CARE-PWS phase 3 trial. *J. Clin. Endocr. Metab.* **2023**, *108*, 1696–1708. [CrossRef]
13. Miller, J.L.; Gevers, E.; Bridges, N.; Yanovski, J.A.; Salehi, P.; Obrynba, K.S.; Felner, E.I.; Bird, L.M.; Shoemaker, A.H.; Angulo, M.; et al. Diazoxide choline extended-release tablet in people with Prader-Willi syndrome: A double-blind, placebo-controlled trial. *J. Clin. Endocr. Metab.* **2023**, *108*, 1676–1685. [CrossRef] [PubMed]

Disclaimer/Publisher's Note: The statements, opinions and data contained in all publications are solely those of the individual author(s) and contributor(s) and not of MDPI and/or the editor(s). MDPI and/or the editor(s) disclaim responsibility for any injury to people or property resulting from any ideas, methods, instructions or products referred to in the content.

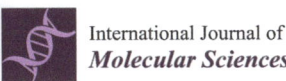

Article

Comparison of Body Composition, Muscle Strength and Cardiometabolic Profile in Children with Prader-Willi Syndrome and Non-Alcoholic Fatty Liver Disease: A Pilot Study

Diana R. Mager [1,2], Krista MacDonald [1], Reena L. Duke [2], Hayford M. Avedzi [2], Edward C. Deehan [2], Jason Yap [3], Kerry Siminoski [4] and Andrea M. Haqq [2,*]

[1] Department of Agricultural Food and Nutritional Science, University of Alberta, Edmonton, AB T6G 2R3, Canada
[2] Department of Pediatrics, University of Alberta, Edmonton, AB T6G 2R3, Canada
[3] Department of Paediatrics, University of Melbourne, Melbourne, VIC 3010, Australia
[4] Faculty of Medicine and Dentistry, Radiology, University of Alberta, Edmonton, AB T6G 2R3, Canada
* Correspondence: haqq@ualberta.ca; Tel.: +1-780-492-0015

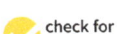

Citation: Mager, D.R.; MacDonald, K.; Duke, R.L.; Avedzi, H.M.; Deehan, E.C.; Yap, J.; Siminoski, K.; Haqq, A.M. Comparison of Body Composition, Muscle Strength and Cardiometabolic Profile in Children with Prader-Willi Syndrome and Non-Alcoholic Fatty Liver Disease: A Pilot Study. *Int. J. Mol. Sci.* **2022**, *23*, 15115. https://doi.org/10.3390/ijms232315115

Academic Editor: Gil Atzmon

Received: 1 November 2022
Accepted: 28 November 2022
Published: 1 December 2022

Publisher's Note: MDPI stays neutral with regard to jurisdictional claims in published maps and institutional affiliations.

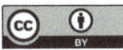

Copyright: © 2022 by the authors. Licensee MDPI, Basel, Switzerland. This article is an open access article distributed under the terms and conditions of the Creative Commons Attribution (CC BY) license (https://creativecommons.org/licenses/by/4.0/).

Abstract: Syndromic and non-syndromic obesity conditions in children, such as Prader-Willi syndrome (PWS) and non-alcoholic fatty liver disease (NAFLD), both lower quality of life and increase risk for chronic health complications, which further increase health service utilization and cost. In a pilot observational study, we compared body composition and muscle strength in children aged 7–18 years with either PWS ($n = 9$), NAFLD ($n = 14$), or healthy controls ($n = 16$). Anthropometric and body composition measures (e.g., body weight, circumferences, skinfolds, total/segmental composition, and somatotype), handgrip strength, six minute-walk-test (6MWT), physical activity, and markers of liver and cardiometabolic dysfunction (e.g., ALT, AST, blood pressure, glucose, insulin, and lipid profile) were measured using standard procedures and validated tools. Genotyping was determined for children with PWS. Children with PWS had reduced lean body mass (total/lower limb mass), lower handgrip strength, 6MWT and increased sedentary activity compared to healthy children or those with NAFLD ($p < 0.05$). Children with PWS, including those of normal body weight, had somatotypes consistent with relative increased adiposity (endomorphic) and reduced skeletal muscle robustness (mesomorphic) when compared to healthy children and those with NAFLD. Somatotype characterizations were independent of serum markers of cardiometabolic dysregulation but were associated with increased prevalence of abnormal systolic and diastolic blood pressure Z-scores ($p < 0.05$). Reduced lean body mass and endomorphic somatotypes were associated with lower muscle strength/functionality and sedentary lifestyles, particularly in children with PWS. These findings are relevant as early detection of deficits in muscle strength and functionality can ensure effective targeted treatments that optimize physical activity and prevent complications into adulthood.

Keywords: body composition; muscle strength; non-alcoholic fatty liver disease; Prader-Willi syndrome; children

1. Introduction

Obesity is defined as excessive adiposity, with a body mass index (BMI) above 30 kg/m^2, that increases potential health risks for the individual [1]. More than 340 million children 5–19 years worldwide had obesity in 2016, reflecting almost a fivefold increase from 1975 [1]. Factors such as high birth weight, parental overweight and obesity, and parental education and income may increase risk for childhood obesity [2,3]. Rare genetic conditions, such as Prader-Willi syndrome (PWS), predispose children to increased adiposity, which may lead to obesity when triggered by environmental factors [3–6]. In contrast, the childhood obesity epidemic has been attributed mostly to unhealthy diets high in saturated fat and simple sugars and living environments that promote sedentary lifestyles and positive energy balance [7]. The increasing prevalence of obesity among children poses a significant public health challenge as it increases risk for adverse cardiometabolic disorders such as non-alcoholic fatty liver disease (NAFLD) and early onset insulin resistance [8–11], reduced quality of life, and higher mortality [12–14]. Childhood obesity increases long-term health service utilization and expenditure, placing significant burdens on healthcare systems and governments worldwide [15,16]. Active living is an integral part of current strategies for managing obesity including healthy eating, pharmacotherapy, and bariatric surgery in selected cases [1,17–19]. Yet, limited evidence suggests that certain obesity conditions, such as PWS, may cause reductions in lean body mass relative to overall fat mass [20,21]. This may undermine obesity management efforts by limiting participation in physical activity and related lifestyle modification.

PWS is the most common syndromic obesity condition, which stems from cytogenetic mutation at chromosome 15q11.2-q13 [22–24]. It is characterized by relative increased subcutaneous adiposity, lower visceral adiposity, reduced lean body mass, decreased muscle tone (hypotonia), lower basal metabolic rate and daily energy expenditure, and poor motor proficiency that limits physical activity in the face of hyperphagia [5,6,23,25–29]. PWS occurs in 1 in 100,000 to 300,000 children with differences in frequency and severity of impulse control, adaptive behavior, and intellectual ability depending on genotype [22,23,26]. Genotype is determined based on the primary mechanism causing cytogenetic mutation at chromosome 15q11.2-q13; deletion (approximately 75% of cases), uniparental disomy (UPD) (approximately 25% of cases), or imprinting defect (approximately 1–3% of cases) [22–24]. Deletion occurs via deletion of paternal genes from the 4–6 Mb region chromosome 15q11.2-q13 [22–24]. Imprinting defect is caused by the microdeletion of the imprinting center of chromosome 15q11.2-q13 [22–24]. UPD occurs via inheritance of two copies of a genetic locus from only one parent [30] and may present with higher IQ and less behavior problems, but higher rates of psychosis and co-occurring autism spectrum disorder compared to the deletion genotype [31–33].

NAFLD, on the other hand, is a common condition of non-syndromic obesity in which excess fat builds up in the liver and is characterized by total and central obesity with hyperinsulinemia, insulin resistance, altered liver function, and cardiometabolic dysregulation [34–37]. While underlining obesity may not have a specific genetic cause, several genes, including Phospholipase Domain-containing 3 (PNPLA3), are associated with NAFLD pathogenesis and affect predisposition to, progression, and severity of NAFLD by facilitating hepatic adipose accumulation which impacts lipid and glucose metabolism, resulting in liver damage [38–40]. Furthermore, microRNAs (miRNA) involved in lipid metabolism regulation, including miR-122, miR-192 and miR-375 [41], may predispose individuals to developing or progressing NAFLD due to gene expression alteration caused by environmental factors [41,42]. Prevalence of NAFLD in children is estimated at 13% (9.8% adjusted) and has increased significantly in the last decade given the worsening obesity epidemic [43,44]. NAFLD occurs in 1 in 3 male children and 1 in 4 female children with overweight and obesity [45,46].

PWS and NAFLD represent models of obesity but vary in genetic influence, body composition and cardiometabolic health, which may impact muscle strength, muscle functionality, and associated physical activity levels [47–49], further complicating identification and management strategies. Compared to the central adiposity characterized in NAFLD, those with PWS are known to have relative increased subcutaneous adiposity but lower visceral adiposity and lean body mass [23,25–27,47–49] and better metabolic profiles with increased insulin sensitivity [27]. Therefore, NAFLD is model of obesity with metabolic dysfunction whereas PWS is a model of obesity with relatively functional metabolism. However, no published studies have directly compared these two disorders to understand their etiologic differences. This pilot study was thus designed to examine associations between measures of body composition and cardiometabolic dysfunction with muscle

2. Results

2.1. Demography, Anthropometry, and Body Composition

Demographic and anthropometric data are summarized in Table 1. Twelve healthy controls and 2 children with PWS had body weights within healthy reference ranges. None of the children with NAFLD had body weights within normal reference ranges. Waist circumferences (WC) were within healthy reference ranges for 15 healthy controls, 6 PWS, and 4 NAFLD children ($p < 0.001$). Children with PWS have significantly less skeletal muscle mass, absolute and Z-scores, respectively, compared to children with NAFLD (11.5 ± 4.7 and -1.7 ± 0.9 vs. 20.9 ± 7.2 and 0.9 ± 0.9) ($p > 0.01$).

Table 1. Demographic, Anthropometric and Related Measurements.

	HC (n = 16) [1]	PWS (n = 9) [1]	NAFLD (n = 14) [1]	HC vs. PWS p Value [2]	HC vs. NAFLD p Value [2]	PWS vs. NAFLD p Value [2]
Gender (M:F)	9:7	2:7	8:6	NS	NS	NS
Age (years)	12.7 (10.8, 14.5)	13.0 (9.8, 15.1)	13.6 (11.6, 15.4)	NS	NS	NS
Weight (kg)	41.7 (37.3, 55.7)	42.5 (33.2, 63.2)	88.4 (67.8, 101.7)	NS	<0.0001	0.002
Height (cm)	154 (144, 167)	143 (129, 154)	162 (151, 168)	NS	NS	0.007
BMI (kg/m^2)	17.9 (16.8, 20.1)	21.3 (18.5, 28.1)	32.8 (27.8, 37.3)	0.02	<0.0001	0.007
Weight Z-score [3]	0.51 (−0.19, 0.87)	0.6 (−0.22, 1.5)	3 (2.2, 2.9)	<0.0001	<0.0001	NS
Height Z-score [3]	0.48 (−0.11, 1.43)	−1.3 (−1.9, −0.37)	0.05 (−0.13, 1.5)	0.0007	NS	0.002
BMI Z-score [3]	−0.1 (−0.79, 0.56)	1.2 (−0.67, 2.22)	2.9 (2.5, 2.9)	0.004	<0.0001	0.0003
Waist (cm)	65.7 (62, 71.4)	75.5 (66.4, 87.6)	95.7 (88.9, 114.7)	0.04	<0.0001	0.003
Waist Z-score [3]	−0.3 (−0.52, 0.27)	0.8 (0.31, 1.3)	1.8 (1.5, 2.1)	0.005	<0.0001	0.0002
WHtR [4]	0.42 (0.41, 0.45)	0.5 (0.5, 0.6)	0.6 (0.5, 07)	<0.0001	<0.0001	0.04
WHtR [4] Z-score [3]	−0.67 (−1.0, −0.09)	1.0 (0.5, 1.6)	1.8 (1.4, 2.0)	<0.0001	<0.0001	0.01
Systolic BP Z-score	0.78 (0.019, 1.0)	1.2 (0.4, 2.5)	1.6 (1.2, 1.9)	NS	NS	0.006
Diastolic BP Z-score	0.15 (−0.2, 0.57)	0.9 (0.6, 1.6)	1.0 (0.7, 1.3)	NS	0.01	NS
Handgrip Strength (kg)	18.3 (16.7, 29.2)	9 (3.9, 12.8)	23.7 (17.7, 32.2)	0.002	0.001	NS
6MWT (m)	603 (569, 634)	436 (379, 459)	489 (460, 522)	NS	NS	NS
Muscle Quality [5]	n/a	3.4 (3.1, 3.6)	4.4 (3.0, 5.8)	n/a	n/a	0.05

[1] Values are expressed as median (IQR). [2] p values <0.017 are considered statistically significant with correction (Bonferroni) for multiple pairwise corrections. [3] Determined using World Health Organization anthropometric calculator (Canada, 2014 revision). [4] Waist-to-height ratio (WHtR) calculated as waist circumference (cm)/height (cm). [5] Muscle quality calculated as muscle strength (dominant arm)/total arm lean muscle. Abbreviations: BMI, body mass index; HC, healthy controls; Ht-to-Wt, height-to-weight ratio; NAFLD, non-alcoholic fatty liver disease; PWS, Prader-Willi syndrome; n/a: not available; NS, not significant.

Somatotype data is summarized in Table 2 and Figure 1. All 16 healthy controls, 5 PWS, and 1 NAFLD had somatotypes within normal healthy reference ranges. Healthy controls had a mixed distribution of endo-ecto-meso-morphic body habitus, and all had somatotypes within healthy reference ranges. Healthy controls had significantly lower endomorphic habitus compared to PWS and NAFLD ($p < 0.001$). Both NAFLD and PWS had meso-endomorph body habitus; but NAFLD more so than PWS ($p < 0.001$). There was a significant difference between mesomorph habitus in healthy controls and NAFLD ($p < 0.001$) and between endomorph habitus in children and PWS and NAFLD ($p < 0.001$). Five PWS children and 1 NAFLD had somatotypes within normal healthy reference ranges. Children with PWS had relative overall adiposity, and significantly lower indices of lean body mass, particularly in the lower extremities (Table 3).

Table 2. Somatotypes of Children with Prader-Willi Syndrome (PWS) and Non-Alcoholic Fatty Liver Disease (NAFLD) and Healthy Controls (HC).

	HC (n = 16)[1]	PWS (n = 9)[1]	NAFLD (n = 12)[1]	HC vs. PWS p Value[2]	HC vs. NAFLD p Value[2]	PWS vs. NAFLD p Value[2]
Endomorph	3.2 (2.8–4.1)	5.7 (5.0–6.2)	7.1 (6.4–7.4)	0.0085	<0.001	<0.001
Ectomorph	3.9 (2.8–4.7)	0.9 (0.3–1.9)	0.1 (0.04–0.6)	<0.001	<0.001	0.21
Mesomorph	3.5 (2.9–4.2)	4.7 (3.5–6.7)	7.6 (5.4–8.8)	0.002	<0.001	0.06

[1] Values are expressed median (IQR). [2] p-value of <0.017 was considered significant; p values are corrected for post hoc pairwise comparisons using Bonferroni correction. Abbreviations: PWS, Prader-Willi syndrome; NAFLD, non-alcoholic fatty liver disease; HC, healthy controls.

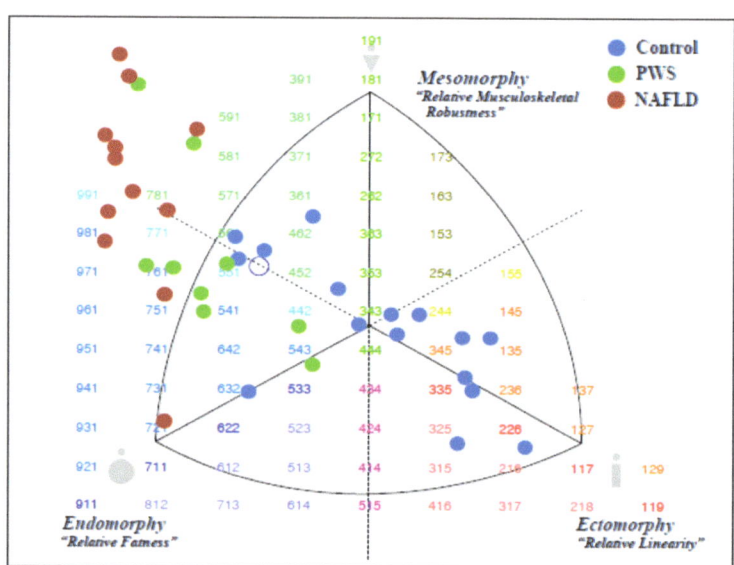

Figure 1. Somatoplot of Children with PWS, NAFLD, and the Healthy Controls. Ten different anthropometric measurements (height, weight, two circumferences [flexed arm and calf]), two bone breadths (humerus and femur), and four skinfolds (triceps, subscapular, supraspinal and medial calf) were entered into the Somatotype 1.2.5 software. The magnitude of the endomorphy, mesomorphy, and ectomorphy were plotted for healthy controls ($n = 16$), PWS ($n = 9$) and NAFLD ($n = 12$). Abbreviations: PWS, Prader-Willi syndrome; NAFLD, non-alcoholic fatty liver disease.

Table 3. Body Composition in Children with PWS and NAFLD as measured by DXA.

Variable	PWS (n = 8) [1]	NAFLD (n = 7) [1]	p Value
Adipose Indices			
Fat mass total (kg)	22.9 ± 11.0	35.4 ± 14.4	NS
Fat mass/Height^2 (kg/m^2)	11.1 ± 4.2	13.7 ± 3.6	NS
Fat mass/Height^2 Z-score	1.2 ± 0.6	1.7 ± 0.3	NS
Android/Gynoid ratio	0.9 ± 0.1	1.1 ± 0.1	0.006
Trunk/Limb fat mass ratio	0.8 ± 0.2	0.9 ± 0.2	NS
Trunk/Limb fat mass ratio z-score	0.5 ± 1.1	1.5 ± 0.6	NS
Fat Mass Index	10.8 ± 4.1	13.5 ± 3.4	NS
Lean Indices			
Lean mass total (kg)	27.3 ± 8.8	43.6 ± 13.0	0.01
Lean Mass/Height^2 (kg/m^2)	13.2 ± 2.4	17.2 ± 2.6	0.009
Lean Mass/Height z-score	−0.2 ± 0.9	1.2 ± 1.1	0.03
Lean Body Mass Index	12.9 ± 2.4	16.9 ± 2.5	0.008
Skeletal Muscle Mass (kg)	11.5 ± 4.7	20.9 ± 7.2	0.009
Skeletal Muscle Mass Z-score	−1.7 ± 0.9	0.9 ± 0.9	0.0001
Appendicular Lean/Height^2 (kg/m^2)	5.3 ± 1.2	7.6 ± 1.2	0.003
Appendicular Lean/Height^2 Z-score	−0.7 ± 0.9	1.3 ± 0.5	0.0003
Lean Mass to Fat Mass Ratio			
Left Arm	1.0 ± 0.2	1.1 ± 0.2	NS
Right Arm	0.9 ± 0.2	1.0 ± 0.2	NS
Trunk	1.5 ± 0.5	1.4 ± 0.3	NS
Left Leg	1.0 ± 0.1	1.2 ± 0.1	0.01
Right Leg	0.9 ± 0.1	1.2 ± 0.1	0.001
Total	1.3 ± 0.2	1.3 ± 0.2	NS

[1] Values are means ± SD (range). T-tests were used to compare differences in means with significance considered at p value < 0.05. Abbreviations: DXA, dual-x ray absorptiometry; NAFLD, non-alcoholic fatty liver disease; PWS, Prader-Willi syndrome; NS, not significant.

There were no significant associations between anthropometrics (weight, weight-z, height, height-z, BMI, BMI-z, WC, WC-z, skinfold measures/circumferences), somatotype characterization, or gender (p > 0.05). No other associations were observed between total/segmental (absolute or percent) measures of body composition.

2.2. Markers of Cardiometabolic Dysregulation and Liver Dysfunction

Serum alanine aminotransferase (ALT) concentrations above 20 U/L were observed in two children with PWS and all children with NAFLD (p = 0.02) (Table 4). Hyperinsulinemia (>20 mU/L) was observed in 2 PWS vs. 11 NAFLD children, while homeostasis model assessment for insulin resistance (HOMA-IR > 3) was observed in 3 PWS vs. 12 NAFLD children. One healthy control (age ~ 14.5 years) had both elevated serum insulin and HOMA-IR, likely secondary to pubertal development. Elevated serum fasting triglycerides (TG) levels were observed in 5 NAFLD children, 2 PWS children, and 1 healthy control (p < 0.05).

Table 4. Biochemical Measures of Liver and Cardiometabolic Dysfunction.

	HC (n = 16) [1]	PWS (n = 9) [1]	NAFLD (n = 14) [1]	HC vs. PWS p Value [2]	HC vs. NAFLD p Value [2]	PWS vs. NAFLD p Value [2]	Reference Values [3]
ALT (U/L)	15 (14, 16.5)	20 (13, 28)	45 (37, 84)	NS	<0.0001	0.0003	<20
AST (U/L)	23 (21, 26)	26 (21, 33)	32 (27, 51)	NS	0.001	NS	2–9 yrs: <50 ≥10 yrs: <40
GGT (U/L)	5 (5, 5)	5 (4, 9)	7 (4.9, 28)	NS	0.005	NS	Male: <70 Female: <55
ALP (U/L)	230 (181, 274)	169 (123, 223)	152 (117, 227)	NS	NS	NS	5–17 yrs 100–500
Glucose (mmol/L)	5.1 (4.7, 5.2)	4.9 (4.7, 5.1)	4.9 (4.6, 5.4)	NS	NS	NS	3.3–6.0
Insulin (mU/L)	5.9 (4.2, 9.4)	13.5 (9.9, 21.4)	29 (21, 50)	NS	<0.0001	0.009	5.0–20.0
HOMA-IR	1.2 (0.9, 2.1)	3.0 (2.1, 4.8)	5.9 (3.9, 12.8)	NS	<0.0001	0.01	3.16
TG (mmol/L)	0.7 (0.6, 1.0)	1.1 (0.6, 1.5)	1.4 (1.0, 2.3)	NS	0.02	NS	<1.5
TC (mmol/L)	3.9 (3.5, 4.2)	4.2 (3.7, 5.3)	4.4 (3.7, 4.7)	NS	NS	NS	<4.4
HDL-C (mmol/L)	1.4 (1.3, 1.6)	1.2 (1.1, 1.7)	1.1 (0.9, 2.3)	NS	0.001	0.02	>1.0
LDL-C (mmol/L)	2.0 (1.8, 2.4)	2.4 (1.8, 3.4)	2.5 (2.1, 2.7)	NS	NS	NS	<2.8
Albumin (g/L)	47 (45, 48)	46 (43, 47)	43 (42, 46)	NS	0.02	NS	35–50
Urate (umol/L)	244 (211, 294)	310 (243, 365)	346 (321, 411)	NS	0.0003	NS	≤9 yrs: 100–300 10–17 yrs: Male: 135–510 Female: 180–450 ≥18 yrs: Male: 180–500 Female: 150–400
CRP (mg/L)	0.4 (0.1, 0.7)	2.0 (0.6, 6.9)	2.2 (1.6, 3.9)	NS	<0.0001	NS	≤10

[1] Values are expressed median (IQR). [2] p-values < 0.016 was considered statistically significant to account for multiple pairwise comparisons. [3] Pediatric reference ranges obtained from Alberta Health Services: http://www.albertahealthservices.ca/assets/wf/lab/wf-lab-chemistry-reference-intervals.pdf (accessed 1 August 2022). There were missing values for urate in the control group (n = 1) and GGT in the NAFLD group (n = 1). Abbreviations: ALT, alanine aminotransferase; ALP, alkaline phosphatase; AST, aspartate transaminase; BP: blood pressure; CRP, C-reactive protein; GGT, gamma-glutamyl transferase; HC, healthy controls; HOMA-IR, homeostatic model assessment of insulin resistance; HDL-C, high density lipoprotein cholesterol; LDL-C, low density lipoprotein cholesterol; NAFLD, non-alcoholic fatty liver disease; PWS, Prader-Willi syndrome; TC, total cholesterol; TG, triglyceride.

Compared to children with serum ALT < 20 U/L, those with serum ALT >20 U/L had significantly higher HOMA-IR (6.7 ± 1.7 vs. 1.9 ± 1.1; $p < 0.001$), TG (1.5 ± 1.0 vs. 0.9 ± 0.5 mmol/L; $p = 0.02$) and lower high density lipoprotein cholesterol (HDL-C) (1.1 ± 0.3 vs. 1.4 ± 0.3 mmol/L; $p = 0.005$).

2.3. Measures of Handgrip Strength, Six Minute-Walk-Test, Blood Pressure, Muscle Quality and Habitual Physical Activity

Resting systolic blood pressure (BP) was significantly higher in the NAFLD group (126 ± 8 mmHg) relative to the PWS (116 ± 16 mmHg) and HC (115 ± 9 mmHg) groups ($p = 0.01$). Handgrip strength and 6-minute walk test (6MWT) results are presented in Figure 2. Children with PWS had significantly lower handgrip strength and 6MWT distances than children with NAFLD or healthy controls ($p < 0.05$). Muscle quality in children with PWS, 3.4 (3.1, 3.6), was significantly lower than those with NAFLD, 4.4 (3.0, 5.8) ($p = 0.05$) (Table 1).

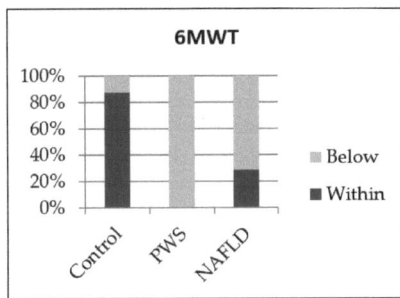
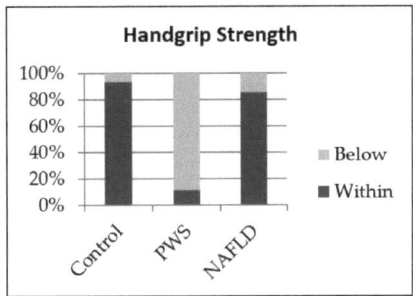

Figure 2. 6MWT and Handgrip Strength Normative Values for Age and Gender. 6MWT distances were compared to reference values. Average handgrip strength scores of three trials for each hand were compared to Jamar® Hydraulic Hand Dynamometer normative values. Scores < 2 standard deviations of the average value for age and gender were considered abnormal. Healthy controls ($n = 16$), PWS ($n = 9$) and NAFLD ($n = 12$). Abbreviations: 6MWT, six minute-walk-tests; PWS, Prader-Willi syndrome; NAFLD, non-alcoholic fatty liver disease.

Physical activity is shown in Figure 3. Mean time spent in sedentary activities was 8.5 ± 0.68 (HC), 8.4 ± 1.9 (PWS), 7.9 ± 1.1 (NAFLD) hours/day ($p > 0.05$). Eight healthy controls and 3 children with NAFLD met current physical activity guidelines (60 min/day) for participation in active physical activity ($p < 0.05$). None of the children with PWS met current guidelines for time spent in active physical activity [50]. In addition, children with PWS had higher values for percentage of weekdays spent inactive ($p = 0.02$) and percentage of weekend days spent inactive ($p = 0.007$) compared to controls. Control children had a higher percentage of Saturday spent active compared to children with PWS ($p = 0.04$).

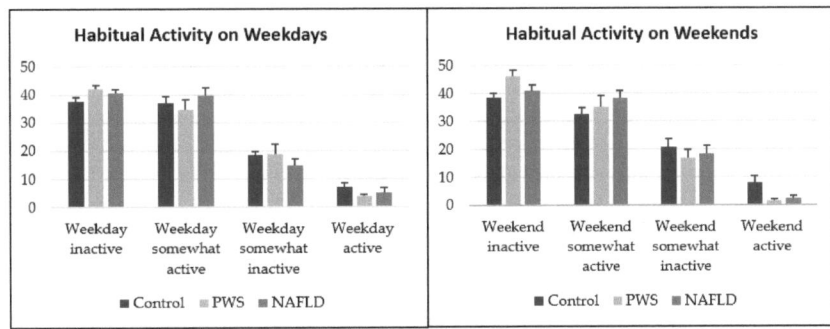

Figure 3. Percentage of Habitual Physical Activity on Weekdays and Weekends. Results are presented as percentage of hours for each day spent at four different activity levels: inactive (lying down), somewhat inactive (sitting), somewhat active (walking) and active (running). Healthy controls ($n = 16$), PWS ($n = 9$) and NAFLD ($n = 12$). Abbreviations: PWS, Prader-Willi syndrome; NAFLD, non-alcoholic fatty liver disease.

2.4. Associations between Anthropometric, Body Composition, and CardioMetabolic Markers

No significant associations were observed between somatotype phenotypes and serum markers of cardiometabolic dysregulation ($p > 0.05$). Body composition was not associated with time spent being active ($p > 0.05$). Endomorphic predominant phenotypes were associated with abnormal diastolic BP and systolic BP Z-scores ($p < 0.05$). Higher trunk-to-limb ratio was associated with serum TG > 1.5 mmol/L and HOMA-IR > 3 ($p = 0.05$).

Increased android/gynoid ratios was associated with serum ALT > 20 U/L ($p = 0.03$). Significant inverse associations were observed between lean indices (appendicular-height, lean-height and lean body mass index) and time spent during the week on sedentary activities ($p < 0.05$).

Children with low 6MWT distance had higher insulin (26.2 ± 22.3 vs. 10.5 ± 8.9; $p = 0.002$), HOMA IR (6.1 ± 6.5 vs. 2.4 ± 2.1; $p = 0.004$) and diastolic BP (73.7 ± 8.7 mmHg vs. 67.9 ± 7.8 m; $p = 0.04$). However, children with both handgrip strength and 6MWT results outside of the reference ranges for age and gender had lower indices of lean body mass, lean height (absolute/Z-scores), skeletal muscle mass (absolute/Z-scores) and higher fat mass index (FMI) ($p < 0.05$). They also had increased serum concentrations of insulin (>20 mU/L), HOMA-IR >3 and ALT > 20 U/L ($p < 0.05$).

2.5. Associations between Genotype and Outcome Measures

DNA polymorphism analysis determined that 5 participants had UPD; fluorescence in situ hybridization (FISH) analysis determined that 3 participants had deletion genotype; and 1 genotype remained unknown. No additional testing, such as imprinting center microdeletion analysis [22], was requested to identify the unknown genotype due to the small sample size for this group. Diastolic BP Z-scores were significantly different between deletion and UPD genotypes, (1.78 (0.76–2.7) vs. 0.82 (0.38–1.5); $p = 0.04$). However, findings show that PWS children with deletion vs. UPD were older, 15.8 ± 2.7 vs. 10.7 ± 2.3, respectively, with expected differences in absolute anthropometric measurements due to age. There were no significant differences in sex, weight Z-score, height Z-score, WC Z-score, waist-to-hip ratio, systolic BP Z-score, and all laboratory measures between genotypes.

3. Discussion

We examined associations between body composition, muscle strength and physical activity in children with syndromic obesity with relatively functional metabolism (PWS), children with non-syndromic obesity with metabolic dysfunction (NAFLD), and healthy children (controls). Children with PWS had significantly lower measures of lean body mass and skeletal muscle mass compared to those with NAFLD. Reductions in lean body mass and skeletal muscle mass in children with PWS were associated with significant impairments in upper and lower muscle strength measures (i.e., handgrip, 6MWT tests) and reduced muscle quality, which translated to more time spent in sedentary activity when compared to NAFLD and healthy children. Notwithstanding, children with PWS had a better metabolic profile, including increased insulin sensitivity compared to the children with NAFLD [27], even though they had higher adiposity. Our study corroborates previous findings of characteristic visceral adiposity, low muscle mass and healthy metabolism observed in PWS [5,6,23,25–29] and the centralized adiposity, robust musculature, and metabolic dysfunction typical of NAFLD compared to healthy children [34–37].

Children with PWS primarily exhibited endomorphic phenotypes that indicate relative overall body fatness even when body weights were within normal reference ranges. Findings of predominantly endomorphic phenotypes, which is associated with large fat deposits and rounded (pear) body shape among children with PWS in this study, is consistent with the characteristic atypical body composition and fatness patterns featuring reduced lean tissue and increased adiposity in PWS [51]. The characteristic reduction in lean body mass, strength, flexibility, overall balance, and poor motor efficiency in the lower limbs has also been associated with reduced exercise capacity and participation and related high levels of sedentary behaviors [28,29]. Growth hormone therapy has been used to induce significant improvements in muscle size and lean body mass after two years in adults with PWS [52], with similar results reported in children [53]. However, our findings suggest that even after ongoing growth hormone therapy for >6 months, participants with PWS presented with significant impairments in muscle strength/functionality. Previous findings have shown that while growth hormone therapy enhances muscle thickness, both muscle growth and training effects (including weight bearing activities such as walking) were the more significant factors influencing overall muscle growth and motor development in infants and toddlers with PWS [54]. Furthermore, excessive adiposity may cause lipid infiltration in the muscle leading to decreased muscle quality and function [55–57]. Children with PWS may require targeted obesity management interventions including physical activity focused on muscle training to modify the characteristic body composition associated with the PWS to improve their quality of life.

Children with NAFLD, comparatively, displayed predominantly mesomorphic phenotypes which may explain the higher muscle strength observed among this group, enhancing their ability to meet physical activity guidelines when compared to children with PWS. Predominantly mesomorphic phenotypes are characterized by relative musculoskeletal robustness, little subcutaneous fat, broad shoulders and chest, small abdomen, and muscular and strong limbs. However, most of the children with NAFLD in our study had body weights outside normal references ranges with increased trunk/limb ratios and associated central adiposity, a phenotype typical of NAFLD [58]. The increased android/gynoid ratios found in children with NAFLD may also be an indicator for insulin resistance [59], which was supported by our findings. Hyperinsulinemia and insulin resistance were observed in a higher proportion of children with NAFLD, as well as significantly higher serum ALT concentrations and resting systolic BP compared to children with PWS and healthy controls. These findings are consistent with established cardiometabolic dysregulation and liver dysfunction in children with NAFLD [60]. Obesity, a marker of adiposity, remains a key predictor of NAFLD in children. As such, changing the anthropometric dimensions such as weight via targeted interventions including diet and physical activity may improve liver dysfunction and systolic BP, which is a predictor of cardiometabolic health.

BMI is utilized in clinical settings as the primary screening tool for obesity risk but has significant limitations as it cannot measure body composition or account for racial and sex differences [61,62]. Dual-x ray absorptiometry (DXA), a direct measures of body composition, is a more accurate screening tool for obesity but is not practical for clinical use due to cost, accessibility, and restrictions of use on healthy children, limiting its ability as an early identification tool for obesity. Our findings support somatotyping as a potential screening tool for obesity in children or adolescents. While somatotyping has been widely used to characterize body morphology and composition in order to determine performance and success in sporting competitions [63–66], its application in non-athletes remains poorly studied. Anthropometric dimensions impact the ability to perform physical activity, which in turn influences body dimensions and composition. This, and the impact of diet on body size and composition, form the basis for the growing interest among physicians, nutritionists, and sports specialists to employ somatotyping as a viable strategy for evaluating changes to an individuals' body composition and shape for improved recovery from health disorders, quality of life and enhancing sports performance [67–70]. Our findings for the predominant endomorphic habitus of PWS and mesomorphic habitus of NAFLD support somatotyping as potential screening tool for assessing the level and location of adiposity, musculoskeletal development, and corresponding physical activity levels and sedentariness. Given that the anthropometric dimensions used for categorizing somatotypes respond to changes in diet and physical activity [36,67,68,71], future investigations are needed to validate somatotyping as a quick, global measure of changes in body composition in response to lifestyle, (e.g., diet and physical activity) and pharmacological (e.g., growth hormone or anti-obesity therapy) interventions. These unique differences in body composition combined with the differences in muscle strength and physical performance have potential implications for rehabilitation and therapy in children with these conditions.

This is one of the first studies to compare PWS and NAFLD as contrasting models of obesity, including the objective measurement of body dimensions and biochemical tests that assess various cardiometabolic parameters. These variables helped to address biases associated with self-reports. We were able to recruit a relatively sizable cohort of children with PWS despite the rarity of this syndromic obesity condition. PWS is a rare genetic condition, which makes recruitment of a larger number of participants difficult. Therefore, the participants were not precisely matched for the case–control design. Additionally, phenotypic expression of PWS may vary depending on genotype but we may have failed to detect such differences due to a limited sample size. As such, our relatively small sample size limited sub-analysis of data to examine patterns. However, a post hoc power analysis revealed sufficient power to determine associations between body composition and measures of muscle strength/function ($\alpha = 0.05$ and $\beta = 0.8$). A larger sample size would allow for better case–control matches and permit assessment of factors such as gut microbiome, which has shown alterations previously in children PWS and NAFLD [72,73]. Additionally, genomic and transcriptomic analyses may be conducted in future investigations to gain insights into the underlying mechanisms influencing obesity in NAFLD and PWS [74–76]. Clinical identification of validated genetic NAFLD risk variants [38–40] and associated miRNA [41,77,78] as well as identification and validation of currently unknown NAFLD-associated genetics may assist in developing a robust genetic profile to enhance our understanding of NAFLD pathogenesis, aid in identifying new therapeutic targets, and improve precision medicine. Previous findings suggest that there may be a distinct miRNA profile for PWS compared to general obesity [74–76]. Analysis of miRNA in PWS may elucidate genetic similarities and differences between PWS genotypes which would enhance our understanding of the mechanisms underlying PWS. Further investigations should be conducted on larger cohorts to unravel clinically relevant differences that may exist between and within groups to enhance the genetic, metabolic, and phenotypic profiles of these models of obesity to aid in early detection and development of targeted obesity management interventions.

4. Materials and Methods

4.1. Participants

Healthy controls ($n = 18$), with healthy lipid panels and body weights within normal reference ranges [1] were recruited from the community via recruitment posters that were posted on community bulletin boards and social media. The recruitment fliers were approved by the Human Research Ethics Board at the University of Alberta. Two healthy controls were excluded from data analysis due to abnormal fasting lipid panel. No significant differences in anthropometric and demographic features were observed between healthy controls ($n = 16$) included in the analysis and those who were excluded ($p > 0.05$).

Children, 7–17 years old, with clinically diagnosed NAFLD ($n = 14$) were prospectively recruited from the Liver Clinic at the Stollery Children's Hospital, Alberta Health Services between 2015 to 2017. Children attending the Liver Clinics for echogenic hepatic ultrasounds also underwent comprehensive metabolic and serological workup. The diagnosis of NAFLD was made in children based on elevated liver enzymes (ALT; aspartate aminotransferase, AST), the presence of hyperinsulinemia and hyperlipidemia, evidence of steatosis on liver ultrasound, liver biopsy where clinically indicated, and exclusion of other known causes of steatosis such as metabolic inborn errors of metabolism, alpha 1-antitrypsin deficiency, Wilson's disease, hepatitis B or C and autoimmune hepatitis [36,37].

Children, 7–17 years old, with a clinical diagnosis of PWS ($n = 9$) and receiving recombinant growth hormone therapy for >6 months were prospectively recruited from the Endocrine Clinic at the Stollery Children's Hospital, Alberta Health Services between 2015 to 2017. DNA methylation polymerase chain reaction (PCR) analysis was used to confirm the clinical diagnosis of PWS by detecting abnormalities within the imprinting region of chromosome 15q11.2-q13 [22–24]. FISH testing was used to identify the deletion genotype by analyzing the number, size, and location of DNA segments at chromosome 15q11.2-q13 [22]. UPD was also identified via DNA polymorphism analysis of chromosome 15q11.2-q13 of the parents and affected child [22]. If indicated, imprinting defect may be confirmed via specialized testing.

Children (1) with a history of a known primary liver disease associated with steatohepatitis not related to NAFLD (e.g., metabolic inborn errors of metabolism, alpha 1-antitrypsin deficiency, Wilson's disease, hepatitis B or C and autoimmune hepatitis); (2) with a known primary diagnosis of type 2 diabetes mellitus or those on insulin; (3) on medications known to cause hepatic steatosis (e.g., corticosteroids, statins) or (4) with a history of comorbid conditions including other liver disorders or gastrointestinal disorders such as celiac disease were excluded from the study. This study was approved by the Health Research Ethics Board at the University of Alberta and all participants provided written informed consent (parents) and assent (participants) prior to participating in this study (Pro00056649).

4.2. Anthropometric Measurements

Height and weight were measured to the nearest 0.1 cm and 0.1 kg, respectively. Weight, height, and BMI were converted into Z-scores/percentiles using the World Health Organization standards [50]. Waist circumference was measured following the World Health Organization criteria and converted into Z-scores/percentiles [79].

4.3. Body Composition

4.3.1. Dual-Energy X-ray Absorptiometry (DXA)

Whole body composition (i.e., total, percent, and regional lean mass; fat mass; and total mass) were measured using a Hologic Densitometer (4500A or Discovery A with Apex System 2.4.2, Waltham, MA, USA). DXA was performed as part of routine clinical care during annual evaluations for children with PWS ($n = 8$) and NAFLD ($n = 7$). Due to University of Alberta ethical restrictions, DXA was not performed for healthy children. Skeletal Muscle Mass (SMM) Z-scores were calculated according to age-gender reference populations [80]. FMI and lean body mass index were calculated as total fat mass or lean mass divided by height^2 (m^2) and were compared to reference values for age and gender [81] (Table 3).

4.3.2. Skinfold and Bone Breadth Tests

Calf circumferences, skinfolds and bone breadths were measured according to standard procedures [36]. Trunk-to-extremity ratio (TER) was used as a measure of relative subcutaneous adipose tissue distribution and was calculated using the following equation:

$$TER = \frac{\text{SubscapularSkinfold} + \text{SupraspinalSkinfold} + \text{IliacSkinfold} + \text{AbdominalSkinfold}}{\text{BicepSkinfold} + \text{TricepSkinfold} + \text{CalfSkinfold}}$$

For this study, skinfolds were measured using a large skinfold caliper (Beta Technology, Santa Cruz, CA) while humerus and femur diameters were measured using a small bone caliper (Calibres Argentinos). All measurements were made by one investigator, (KM), according to the International Society for the Advancement of Kinanthropometry (ISAK) methodology. A technical error of <5% for skinfold and <2% for circumferences was accepted.

4.3.3. Somatotyping

Somatotyping has been used to aid the qualitative description of the relative risk for cardiometabolic dysregulation in various populations [36,67,68,71]. Briefly, somatotypes (i.e., ectomorph, mesomorph, and endomorph) are physical characterization of body morphology and composition. Ectomorphs tend to have relatively linear or slender frame, with low levels of fat and muscular tissue, broad and drooping shoulders, long thin limbs, and narrow thorax and abdomen. Mesomorphs have relative musculoskeletal robustness, little subcutaneous fat, broad shoulders and chest, small abdomen, and muscular and strong limbs. Endomorphs have relative adiposity, with large fat deposits, rounded body (pear) shape, large abdomen, rounded shoulders and head [68]. For this study, somatotyping was completed using the Somatotype 1.2.5 software (Sweat Technologies, Australia) [36,71]. Using the Heath-Carter approach, the software uses anthropometric measurements to evaluate somatotype and presents the individual's classification in the somatotype graph. These measurements include height, body mass, bi-epicondylar breadths of the humerus and femur, girths of the arm's calf and bicep in both flexion and tension, and skin folds (i.e., triceps, biceps, subscapular, supraspinal, suprailiac, abdominal, and calf). Skinfolds were measured using a Lange skinfold caliper (Beta Technology, Santa Cruz, CA). Humerus and femur diameters were measured using a small bone caliper (Calibres Argentinos). These measures were conducted as part of the research protocol according to the ISAK methodology and were measured by 1 investigator (KM) certified in this methodology [36,67,68,71]. A technical error of <5% for skinfold and <2% for circumferences was accepted.

4.4. Surrogate Markers of Liver and Metabolic Disease

Metabolic markers, including TG, HDL-C, low density lipoprotein cholesterol (LDL-C), total cholesterol (TC), insulin, glucose, ALT, aspartate amino transferase (AST), gamma-glutamyl transferase (ϒGT), alkaline phosphatase (ALP), albumin, urate, and C-reactive protein (CRP), were analyzed at the Core Laboratory of Alberta Health Services using standard methods [20]. ALT values >20 U/L were considered abnormal [82]. The homeostasis model assessment for insulin resistance (HOMA-IR) was used as an index of insulin resistance [83] using the following equation:

$$HOMAIR = \frac{fastingglucose\left(\frac{mmol}{L}\right) * fastinginsulin\left(\frac{mU}{L}\right)}{22.5}$$

4.5. Muscle Strength, Six Minute-Walk-Test, Blood Pressure, Muscle Quality and Habitual Physical Activity

Handgrip strength was assessed using a Jamar® Hydraulic Hand Dynamometer (Patterson Medical, Mississauga, ON, Canada). Six-minute walk tests were performed using standard procedures and scores below two standard deviations (SD) for age and gender were considered abnormal [84,85]. BP and heart rate were measured immediately before (after 10 min rest) and after the 6MWT using an Adview® 9000 modular diagnostic station (American Diagnostic Corporation, NY, USA). BP was converted to Z-scores/percentiles [86]. Muscle quality of the upper arms was expressed as the muscle strength (dominant arm)/total arm lean muscle [87]. Physical activity was assessed using the validated Habitual Activity Estimation Scale questionnaire and children were asked to report physical activity on two days and a weekend within two weeks of the study visit [88].

4.6. PWS Genotyping

Genotyping was confirmed for eight out of nine participants with PWS via FISH testing for the deletion genotype and DNA polymorphism analysis for UDP [22–24,30,89]. Briefly, genotype identification is based on the primary mechanism causing cytogenetic mutation at chromosome 15q11.2-q13; mainly deletion, UDP, or imprinting defect [22–24,30]. FISH testing may be used to identify the deletion genotype by analyzing the number, size, and location of DNA segments at chromosome 15q11.2-q13 [22]. UPD may be identified via DNA polymorphism analysis of chromosome 15q11.2-q13 for the parents and affected child [22]. Imprinting defect may be confirmed via specialized testing if required. Since only 1 genotype was not identified via FISH or DNA polymorphism analysis, imprinting defect was suspected but further testing was not requested due to the small sample size for that genotype group.

4.7. Statistical Analysis

Data analysis was completed using the SAS 9.0 statistical software (SAS, Version 9.4; SAS Institute Inc., Cary, NC, USA). Data was expressed as median (interquartile range) for most intra- and inter-group assessments. Mean (standard deviation) was expressed for parametric data assessing the DXA results and the cohort. Data was assessed for normality using the Shapiro–Wilks test. Non-parametric variables were log transformed. Between group (HC vs. PWS vs. NAFLD) were performed using analysis of variance (ANOVA). Primary outcome variables including Z-scores for body composition measures, BP, handgrip strength, and 6MWT were adjusted for age and gender. *T*-tests were performed to compare segmental total body composition measured by DXA in PWS and NAFLD only. Univariate analyses were performed to assess associations between each variable, except DXA, for each group (PWS, NAFLD, and HC) and for the entire cohort. Multivariate analyses were performed to assess associations between body compositions measures, anthropometric measures, muscle strength/functionality, and cardiometabolic markers for the entire cohort. Statistical significance was considered at p value <0.05.

5. Conclusions

In summary, children with PWS in this pilot study exhibited relatively healthy metabolic profiles with body compositions that typify relative body fatness and reduced skeletal muscle which manifests as hypotonia, characterized by decreased muscle strength, muscle quality and increased sedentary activity. Comparatively, children with NAFLD exhibited body compositions that were reflective of relative muscular robustness and central adiposity, body weights outside healthy reference ranges, and associated liver and cardiometabolic dysfunction, which manifests as hyperinsulinemia, insulin resistance, and an increased risk for developing comorbidities such as type 2 diabetes mellitus. Clinical assessment of the genetic, metabolic, and phenotypic profiles for children with PWS and NAFLD is critical in determining the underlying mechanisms contributing to obesity in order to develop targeted screening tools and obesity management interventions for these conditions. Somatotype characterization may be an effective non-invasive tool within the clinical setting for identifying children with excessive adiposity that are at risk for muscle strength deficits; it is easy to perform and can provide important information regarding body composition changes over development and throughout treatment. Future studies of larger cohorts including additional genetic and metabolomic analysis and gut microbial assessment, may aid in developing well-rounded, robust profiles of these models of obesity. This will help to improve detection and management of pediatric obesity and associated comorbidities. Early identification of children with overweight and obesity that may have potential cardiometabolic dysfunction and/or deficits in muscle strength and functionality is necessary to ensure effective rehabilitation strategies are developed to optimize physical activity in children based on their model of obesity.

Author Contributions: Conceptualization, D.R.M. and A.M.H.; Formal analysis, D.R.M., K.M., J.Y. and A.M.H.; Funding acquisition, D.R.M. and A.M.H.; Investigation, K.M. and A.M.H.; Methodology, D.R.M., H.M.A., J.Y., K.S. and A.M.H.; Project administration, H.M.A. and A.M.H.; Resources, D.R.M., H.M.A. and A.M.H.; Software, D.R.M. and K.M.; Supervision, D.R.M. and K.S.; Validation, K.M., J.Y. and K.S.; Visualization, K.M.; Writing—original draft, D.R.M., H.M.A., K.M. and A.M.H.; Writing—review and editing, D.R.M., H.M.A., R.L.D., E.C.D., K.M., J.Y., K.S. and A.M.H. All authors have read and agreed to the published version of the manuscript.

Funding: This research was funded by Vitamin Fund (grant 01, 2016), Department of Department of Agricultural Food and Nutritional Sciences, University of Alberta; The Wirtanen Graduate Scholarship, Alberta Diabetes Institute (2014); Women and Children's Health Research Institute Graduate Scholarship (2016), University of Alberta; and the Food and Health Innovation Initiative, University of Alberta (2016).

Institutional Review Board Statement: The study was conducted in accordance with the Declaration of Helsinki and approved by the Institutional Review Board of the University of Alberta (Pro00056649, 4 August 2015).

Informed Consent Statement: Informed consent was obtained from all subjects involved in the study.

Data Availability Statement: Not applicable.

Acknowledgments: The authors wish to acknowledge Leslie Seto, Leanne Shirton, and Barbara Butler for their assistance with data collection. Financial support from the Wirtanen Graduate Scholarship, Alberta Diabetes Institute (KM) and Women and Children's Health Research Institute Graduate Scholarship, University of Alberta, and the Food & Health Innovation Initiative (AH/DM), University of Alberta. The authors gratefully acknowledge the contribution of the children and families who participated in this research.

Conflicts of Interest: The authors declare no conflict of interest. The funders had no role in the design of the study; in the collection, analyses, or interpretation of data; in the writing of the manuscript; or in the decision to publish the results.

Abbreviations

6MWT	Six minute-walk-test
ALP	Alkaline phosphatase
ALT	Alanine aminotransferase
AST	Aspartate aminotransferase
BMI	Body mass index
BP	Blood pressure
CRP	C-reactive protein
DXA	Dual-energy x-ray absorptiometry
FISH	Fluorescence in situ hybridization
FMI	Fat mass index
ISAK	International Society for the Advancement of Kinanthropometry
ΥGT	Gamma-glutamyl transferase
HDL-C	High density lipoprotein cholesterol
HOMA-IR	Homeostasis model assessment for insulin resistance
LDL-C	Low density lipoprotein cholesterol
miRNA	microRNA
NAFLD	Non-alcoholic fatty liver disease
NS	Not significant
PCR	Polymerase chain reaction
PNPLA3	Patatin-like Phospholipase Domain-containing 3
PWS	Prader-Willi syndrome
SSM	Skeletal muscle mass
SD	Standard deviation
TC	Total cholesterol
TER	Trunk-to-extremity ratio
TG	Fasting triglycerides
UPD	Uniparental disomy
WC	Waist circumference
WHtR	Waist to height ratio

References

1. World Health Organization. Overweight and Obesity. Available online: https://www.who.int/news-room/fact-sheets/detail/obesity-and-overweight (accessed on 25 August 2022).
2. Freemark, M.S. *Pediatric Obesity: Etiology, Pathogenesis and Treatment*; Humana Press: Totowa, NJ, USA, 2018.
3. Murphy, S. Understanding childhood and adolescent obesity. *Clin. Integr. Care* **2022**, *13*, 100114. [CrossRef]
4. Dhaliwal, K.K.; Avedzi, H.M.; Richard, C.; Zwaigenbaum, L.; Haqq, A.M. Brief Report: Plasma Leptin and Mealtime Feeding Behaviors Among Children with Autism Spectrum Disorder: A Pilot Study. *J. Autism Dev. Disord.* **2022**, 1–8. [CrossRef]
5. Goldstone, A.P.; Beales, P.L. Genetic Obesity Syndromes. *Front. Horm. Res.* **2008**, *36*, 37–60.
6. Huvenne, H.; Dubern, B.; Clément, K.; Poitou, C. Rare Genetic Forms of Obesity: Clinical Approach and Current Treatments in 2016. *Obes. Facts* **2016**, *9*, 158–173. [CrossRef]
7. Malik, V.S.; Willett, W.C.; Hu, F.B. Global obesity: Trends, risk factors and policy implications. *Nat. Rev. Endocrinol.* **2013**, *9*, 13–27. [CrossRef] [PubMed]
8. Charakida, M.; E Deanfield, J. BMI trajectories from childhood: The slippery slope to adult obesity and cardiovascular disease. *Eur. Heart J.* **2018**, *39*, 2271–2273. [CrossRef] [PubMed]
9. Park, M.H.; Falconer, C.; Viner, R.M.; Kinra, S. The impact of childhood obesity on morbidity and mortality in adulthood: A systematic review. *Obes. Rev.* **2012**, *13*, 985–1000. [CrossRef] [PubMed]

10. Turer, C.B.; Brady, T.M.; de Ferranti, S.D. Obesity, Hypertension, and Dyslipidemia in Childhood Are Key Modifiable Antecedents of Adult Cardiovascular Disease: A Call to Action. *Circulation* **2018**, *137*, 1256–1259. [CrossRef]
11. Weihrauch-Blüher, S.; Wiegand, S. Risk Factors and Implications of Childhood Obesity. *Curr. Obes. Rep.* **2018**, *7*, 254–259. [CrossRef]
12. Reilly, J.J.; Kelly, J. Long-term impact of overweight and obesity in childhood and adolescence on morbidity and premature mortality in adulthood: Systematic review. *Int. J. Obes.* **2011**, *35*, 891–898. [CrossRef]
13. Romanelli, R.; Cecchi, N.; Carbone, M.G.; Dinardo, M.; Gaudino, G.; Del Giudice, E.M.; Umano, G.R. Pediatric obesity: Prevention is better than care. *Ital. J. Pediatr.* **2020**, *46*, 103. [CrossRef] [PubMed]
14. Singh, A.S.; Mulder, C.; Twisk, J.W.R.; Van Mechelen, W.; Chinapaw, M.J.M. Tracking of childhood overweight into adulthood: A systematic review of the literature. *Obes. Rev.* **2008**, *9*, 474–488. [CrossRef] [PubMed]
15. Au, N. The Health Care Cost Implications of Overweight and Obesity during Childhood. *Health Serv. Res.* **2012**, *47*, 655–676. [CrossRef]
16. Trasande, L.; Chatterjee, S. The Impact of Obesity on Health Service Utilization and Costs in Childhood. *Obes. (Silver Spring)* **2009**, *17*, 1749–1754. [CrossRef]
17. World Health Organization. National Institute for Health and Clinical Excellence: Guidance London. 2006. Available online: https://www.ncbi.nlm.nih.gov/pubmed/22497033 (accessed on 25 August 2022).
18. Flynn, M.A.T.; McNeil, D.A.; Maloff, B.; Mutasingwa, D.; Wu, M.; Ford, C.; Tough, S.C. Reducing obesity and related chronic disease risk in children and youth: A synthesis of evidence with 'best practice' recommendations. *Obes. Rev.* **2006**, *7* (Suppl. 1), 7–66. [CrossRef] [PubMed]
19. Khandelwal, S. Obesity in midlife: Lifestyle and dietary strategies. *Climacteric* **2020**, *23*, 140–147. [CrossRef] [PubMed]
20. Orsso, C.E.; Mackenzie, M.; Alberga, A.S.; Sharma, A.M.; Richer, L.; Rubin, D.A.; Prado, C.M.; Haqq, A.M. The use of magnetic resonance imaging to characterize abnormal body composition phenotypes in youth with Prader–Willi syndrome. *Metabolism* **2017**, *69*, 67–75. [CrossRef]
21. Tovo, C.; A Fernandes, S.; Buss, C.; A De Mattos, A. Sarcopenia and non-alcoholic fatty liver disease: Is there a relationship? A systematic review. *World J. Hepatol.* **2017**, *9*, 326–332. [CrossRef]
22. Cassidy, S.B.; Forsythe, M.; Heeger, S.; Nicholls, R.D.; Schork, N.; Benn, P.; Schwartz, S. Comparison of phenotype between patients with Prader-Willi syndrome due to deletion 15q and uniparental disomy 15. *Am. J. Med. Genet.* **1997**, *68*, 433–440. [CrossRef]
23. Cassidy, S.B.; Schwartz, S.; Miller, J.L.; Driscoll, D.J. Prader-Willi syndrome. *Genet. Med.* **2012**, *14*, 10–26.
24. Costa, R.A.; Ferreira, I.R.; Cintra, H.A.; Gomes, L.H.F.; Guida, L.D.C. Genotype-Phenotype Relationships and Endocrine Findings in Prader-Willi Syndrome. *Front. Endocrinol.* **2019**, *10*, 864. [CrossRef] [PubMed]
25. AlSaif, M.; A Elliot, S.; Mackenzie, M.; Prado, C.M.; Field, C.J.; Haqq, A.M. Energy Metabolism Profile in Individuals with Prader-Willi Syndrome and Implications for Clinical Management: A Systematic Review. *Adv. Nutr. Int. Rev. J.* **2017**, *8*, 905–915. [CrossRef] [PubMed]
26. Brambilla, P.; Crinò, A.; Bedogni, G.; Bosio, L.; Cappa, M.; Corrias, A.; Delvecchio, M.; Di Candia, S.; Gargantini, L.; Grechi, E. Metabolic syndrome in children with Prader–Willi syndrome: The effect of obesity. *Nutr. Metab. Cardiovasc. Dis.* **2011**, *21*, 269–276. [CrossRef] [PubMed]
27. Fintini, D.; Inzaghi, E.; Colajacomo, M.; Bocchini, S.; Grugni, G.; Brufani, C.; Cappa, M.; Nobili, V.; Cianfarani, S.; Crinò, A. Non-Alcoholic Fatty Liver Disease (NAFLD) in children and adolescents with Prader-Willi Syndrome (PWS). *Pediatr. Obes.* **2016**, *11*, 235–238. [CrossRef]
28. Gross, I.; Hirsch, H.J.; Constantini, N.; Nice, S.; Pollak, Y.; Genstil, L.; Eldar-Geva, T.; Tsur, V.G. Physical activity and maximal oxygen uptake in adults with Prader–Willi syndrome. *Eat. Weight Disord.* **2018**, *23*, 615–620. [CrossRef]
29. Lam, M.Y.; Rubin, D.A.; Duran, A.T.; Chavoya, F.A.; White, E.; Rose, D.J. A Characterization of Movement Skills in Obese Children With and Without Prader-Willi Syndrome. *Res. Q. Exerc. Sport* **2016**, *87*, 245–253. [CrossRef]
30. Nicholls, R.D. Genomic imprinting and uniparental disomy in Angelman and Prader-Willi syndromes: A review. *Am. J. Med. Genet.* **1993**, *46*, 16–25. [CrossRef]
31. Duker, A.L.; Ballif, B.C.; Bawle, E.V.; Person, R.E.; Mahadevan, S.; Alliman, S.; Thompson, R.; Traylor, R.; Bejjani, B.A.; Shaffer, L.G.; et al. Paternally inherited microdeletion at 15q11.2 confirms a significant role for the SNORD116 C/D box snoRNA cluster in Prader-Willi syndrome. *Eur. J. Hum. Genet.* **2010**, *18*, 1196–1201. [CrossRef]
32. Jauregi, J.; Arias, C.; Vegas, O.; Alén, F.; Martinez, S.; Copet, P.; Thuilleaux, D. A neuropsychological assessment of frontal cognitive functions in Prader? Willi syndrome. *J. Intellect. Disabil. Res.* **2007**, *51*, 350–365. [CrossRef]
33. Sahoo, T.; Del Gaudio, D.; German, J.R.; Shinawi, M.; Peters, S.U.; Person, R.E.; Garnica, A.; Cheung, S.W.; Beaudet, A.L. Prader-Willi phenotype caused by paternal deficiency for the HBII-85 C/D box small nucleolar RNA cluster. *Nat. Genet.* **2008**, *40*, 719–721. [CrossRef]
34. Gariani, K.; Philippe, J.; Jornayvaz, F. Non-alcoholic fatty liver disease and insulin resistance: From bench to bedside. *Diabetes Metab.* **2013**, *39*, 16–26. [CrossRef] [PubMed]
35. Mager, D.R.; Patterson, C.; So, S.; Rogenstein, C.D.; Wykes, L.J.; A Roberts, E. Dietary and physical activity patterns in children with fatty liver. *Eur. J. Clin. Nutr.* **2010**, *64*, 628–635. [CrossRef]

36. Mager, D.R.; Yap, J.; Rodriguez-Dimitrescu, C.; Mazurak, V.; Ball, G.; Gilmour, S. Anthropometric Measures of Visceral and Subcutaneous Fat Are Important in the Determination of Metabolic Dysregulation in Boys and Girls at Risk for Nonalcoholic Fatty Liver Disease. *Nutr. Clin. Pract.* **2013**, *28*, 101–111. [CrossRef] [PubMed]
37. Vos, M.B.; Abrams, S.H.; Barlow, S.E.; Caprio, S.; Daniels, S.R.; Kohli, R.; Mouzaki, M.; Sathya, P.; Schwimmer, J.B.; Sundaram, S.S.; et al. NASPGHAN Clinical Practice Guideline for the Diagnosis and Treatment of Nonalcoholic Fatty Liver Disease in Children: Recommendations from the Expert Committee on NAFLD (ECON) and the North American Society of Pediatric Gastroenterology, Hepatology and Nutrition (NASPGHAN). *J Pediatr. Gastroenterol. Nutr.* **2017**, *64*, 319–334. [PubMed]
38. Anstee, Q.M.; Day, C.P. The genetics of NAFLD. *Nat. Rev. Gastroenterol. Hepatol.* **2013**, *10*, 645–655. [CrossRef] [PubMed]
39. Del Campo, J.A.; Gallego-Duran, R.; Gallego, P.; Grande, L. Genetic and Epigenetic Regulation in Nonalcoholic Fatty Liver Disease (NAFLD). *Int. J. Mol. Sci.* **2018**, *19*, 911. [CrossRef] [PubMed]
40. Trépo, E.; Valenti, L. Update on NAFLD genetics: From new variants to the clinic. *J. Hepatol.* **2020**, *72*, 1196–1209. [CrossRef]
41. Dongiovanni, P.; Meroni, M.; Longo, M.; Fargion, S.; Fracanzani, A.L. miRNA Signature in NAFLD: A Turning Point for a Non-Invasive Diagnosis. *Int. J. Mol. Sci.* **2018**, *19*, 3966. [CrossRef]
42. Umano, G.R.; Martino, M.; Santoro, N. The Association between Pediatric NAFLD and Common Genetic Variants. *Children* **2017**, *4*, 49. [CrossRef]
43. Sahota, A.K.; Shapiro, W.L.; Newton, K.P.; Kim, S.T.; Chung, J.; Schwimmer, J.B. Incidence of Nonalcoholic Fatty Liver Disease in Children: 2009–2018. *Pediatrics* **2020**, *146*, e20200771. [CrossRef]
44. Schwimmer, J.B.; Deutsch, R.; Kahen, T.; Lavine, J.E.; Stanley, C.; Behling, C. Prevalence of Fatty Liver in Children and Adolescents. *Pediatrics* **2006**, *118*, 1388–1393. [CrossRef] [PubMed]
45. Jimenez-Rivera, C.; Hadjiyannakis, S.; Davila, J.; Hurteau, J.; Aglipay, M.; Barrowman, N.; Adamo, K.B. Prevalence and risk factors for non-alcoholic fatty liver in children and youth with obesity. *BMC Pediatr.* **2017**, *17*, 113. [CrossRef] [PubMed]
46. Sartorio, A.; Del Col, A.; Agosti, F.; Mazzilli, G.; Bellentani, S.; Tiribelli, C.; Bedogni, G. Predictors of non-alcoholic fatty liver disease in obese children. *Eur. J. Clin. Nutr.* **2007**, *61*, 877–883. [CrossRef]
47. Castner, D.M.; Rubin, D.A.; Judelson, D.A.; Haqq, A.M. Effects of Adiposity and Prader-Willi Syndrome on Postexercise Heart Rate Recovery. *J. Obes.* **2013**, *2013*, 384167. [CrossRef] [PubMed]
48. Castner, D.M.; Tucker, J.M.; Wilson, K.S.; Rubin, D.A. Patterns of habitual physical activity in youth with and without Prader-Willi Syndrome. *Res. Dev. Disabil.* **2014**, *35*, 3081–3088. [CrossRef] [PubMed]
49. Woods, S.G.; Knehans, A.; Arnold, S.; Dionne, C.; Hoffman, L.; Turner, P.; Baldwin, J. The associations between diet and physical activity with body composition and walking a timed distance in adults with Prader–Willi syndrome. *Food Nutr. Res.* **2018**, *62*. [CrossRef]
50. Tremblay, M.S.; Carson, V.; Chaput, J.-P.; Gorber, S.C.; Dinh, T.; Duggan, M.; Faulkner, G.; Gray, C.E.; Gruber, R.; Janson, K.; et al. Canadian 24-Hour Movement Guidelines for Children and Youth: An Integration of Physical Activity, Sedentary Behaviour, and Sleep. *Appl. Physiol. Nutr. Metab.* **2016**, *41* (Suppl. 3), S311–S327. [CrossRef]
51. Theodoro, M.F.; Talebizadeh, Z.; Butler, M.G. Body Composition and Fatness Patterns in Prader-Willi Syndrome: Comparison with Simple Obesity. *Obesity* **2006**, *14*, 1685–1690. [CrossRef]
52. Lafortuna, C.; Minocci, A.; Capodaglio, P.; Gondoni, L.; Sartorio, A.; Vismara, L.; Rizzo, G.; Grugni, G. Skeletal Muscle Characteristics and Motor Performance After 2-Year Growth Hormone Treatment in Adults With Prader-Willi Syndrome. *J. Clin. Endocrinol. Metab.* **2014**, *99*, 1816–1824. [CrossRef]
53. Edge, R.; la Fleur, P.; Adcock, L. Human Growth Hormone Treatment for Children with Prader-Willi Syndrome: A Review of Clinical Effectiveness, Cost-Effectiveness, and Guidelines. In *CADTH Rapid Response Reports*; NCBI Bookshelf: Ottawa, ON, Canada, 2018.
54. Rubin, D.A.; Castner, D.; Pham, H.; Ng, J.; Adams, E.; Judelson, D.A. Hormonal and Metabolic Responses to a Resistance Exercise Protocol in Lean Children, Obese Children, and Lean Adults. *Pediatr. Exerc. Sci.* **2014**, *26*, 444–454. [CrossRef]
55. Forsberg, A.M.; Nilsson, E.; Werneman, J.; Bergström, J.; Hultman, E. Muscle composition in relation to age and sex. *Clin. Sci.* **1991**, *81*, 249–256. [CrossRef] [PubMed]
56. Fragala, M.S.; Kenny, A.M.; Kuchel, G.A. Muscle Quality in Aging: A Multi-Dimensional Approach to Muscle Functioning with Applications for Treatment. *Sports Med.* **2015**, *45*, 641–658. [CrossRef] [PubMed]
57. Goodpaster, B.H.; Carlson, C.L.; Visser, M.; Kelley, D.E.; Scherzinger, A.; Harris, T.B.; Stamm, E.; Newman, A.B. Attenuation of skeletal muscle and strength in the elderly: The Health ABC Study. *J. Appl. Physiol. (1985)* **2001**, *90*, 2157–2165. [CrossRef] [PubMed]
58. Samsell, L.; Regier, M.; Walton, C.; Cottrell, L. Importance of Android/Gynoid Fat Ratio in Predicting Metabolic and Cardiovascular Disease Risk in Normal Weight as well as Overweight and Obese Children. *J. Obes.* **2014**, *2014*, 846578. [CrossRef] [PubMed]
59. Aucouturier, J.; Meyer, M.; Thivel, D.; Taillardat, M.; Duché, P. Effect of Android to Gynoid Fat Ratio on Insulin Resistance in Obese Youth. *Arch. Pediatr. Adolesc. Med.* **2009**, *163*, 826–831. [CrossRef]
60. Sweeny, K.F.; Lee, C.K. Nonalcoholic Fatty Liver Disease in Children. *Gastroenterol. Hepatol. (N. Y.)* **2021**, *17*, 579–587. [PubMed]
61. Adab, P.; Pallan, M.; Whincup, P.H. Is BMI the best measure of obesity? *BMJ* **2018**, *360*, k1274. [CrossRef]
62. Kipping, R.R.; Jago, R.; Lawlor, D.A. Obesity in children. Part 1: Epidemiology, measurement, risk factors, and screening. *BMJ* **2008**, *337*, a1824. [CrossRef]

63. Buśko, K.; Lewandowska, J.; Lipińska, M.; Michalski, R.; Pastuszak, A. Somatotype-variables related to muscle torque and power output in female volleyball players. *Acta Bioeng. Biomech.* **2013**, *15*, 119–126.
64. Carter, J.E. The somatotypes of athletes—A review. *Hum. Biol.* **1970**, *42*, 535–569.
65. Stepnicka, J. *Somatotype in Relation to Physical Performance, Sports and Body Posture*; E and FN Spon: London, UK, 1986.
66. Lewandowska, J.; Buśko, K.; Pastuszak, A.; Boguszewska, K. Somatotype Variables Related to Muscle Torque and Power in Judoists. *J. Hum. Kinet.* **2011**, *30*, 21–28. [CrossRef] [PubMed]
67. Ryan-Stewart, H.; Faulkner, J.; Jobson, S. The influence of somatotype on anaerobic performance. *PLoS ONE* **2018**, *13*, e0197761. [CrossRef] [PubMed]
68. Silva CAD, d.S.M.D.; Oliveira, E.; Almeida, H.A.; Ascenso, R.M.T. BodyShifter–Software to Determine and Optimize an Individual's Somatotype. *Procedia Technol.* **2014**, *16*, 1456–1461. [CrossRef]
69. Carter, J.E.; Phillips, W.H. Structural changes in exercising middle-aged males during a 2-year period. *J. Appl. Physiol.* **1969**, *27*, 787–794. [CrossRef] [PubMed]
70. Norton, K.O.T.; Olive, S.; Craig, N. *Anthropometry and Sports Performance*; CBS Publishers & Distributors: Delhi, India, 1996.
71. Heath, B.H.; Carter, J.E.L. A modified somatotype method. *Am. J. Phys. Anthropol.* **1967**, *27*, 57–74. [CrossRef] [PubMed]
72. Peng, Y.; Tan, Q.; Afhami, S.; Deehan, E.; Liang, S.; Gantz, M.; Triador, L.; Madsen, K.; Walter, J.; Tun, H.; et al. The Gut Microbiota Profile in Children with Prader–Willi Syndrome. *Genes* **2020**, *11*, 904. [CrossRef] [PubMed]
73. Schwimmer, J.B.; Johnson, J.S.; Angeles, J.E.; Behling, C.; Belt, P.H.; Borecki, I.; Bross, C.; Durelle, J.; Goyal, N.P.; Hamilton, G.; et al. Microbiome Signatures Associated With Steatohepatitis and Moderate to Severe Fibrosis in Children With Nonalcoholic Fatty Liver Disease. *Gastroenterology* **2019**, *157*, 1109–1122. [CrossRef]
74. Bochukova, E.G.; Lawler, K.; Croizier, S.; Keogh, J.M.; Patel, N.; Strohbehn, G.; Lo, K.K.; Humphrey, J.; Hokken-Koelega, A.; Damen, L.; et al. A Transcriptomic Signature of the Hypothalamic Response to Fasting and BDNF Deficiency in Prader-Willi Syndrome. *Cell Rep.* **2018**, *22*, 3401–3408. [CrossRef]
75. Ferrante, S.C.; Nadler, E.P.; Pillai, D.K.; Hubal, M.; Wang, Z.; Wang, J.M.; Gordish-Dressman, H.; Koeck, E.; Sevilla, S.; Wiles, A.A.; et al. Adipocyte-derived exosomal miRNAs: A novel mechanism for obesity-related disease. *Pediatr. Res.* **2015**, *77*, 447–454. [CrossRef]
76. Pascut, D.; Tamini, S.; Bresolin, S.; Giraudi, P.; Basso, G.; Minocci, A.; Tiribelli, C.; Grugni, G.; Sartorio, A. Differences in circulating microRNA signature in Prader–Willi syndrome and non-syndromic obesity. *Endocr. Connect.* **2018**, *7*, 1262–1274. [CrossRef]
77. Cheung, O.; Puri, P.; Eicken, C.; Contos, M.J.; Mirshahi, F.; Maher, J.W.; Kellum, J.M.; Min, H.; Luketic, V.A.; Sanyal, A.J. Nonalcoholic steatohepatitis is associated with altered hepatic MicroRNA expression. *Hepatology* **2008**, *48*, 1810–1820. [CrossRef] [PubMed]
78. Ng, R.; Wu, H.; Xiao, H.; Chen, X.; Willenbring, H.; Steer, C.J.; Song, G. Inhibition of microRNA-24 expression in liver prevents hepatic lipid accumulation and hyperlipidemia. *Hepatology* **2014**, *60*, 554–564. [CrossRef] [PubMed]
79. Patry-Parisien, J.; Shields, M.; Bryan, S. Comparison of waist circumference using the World Health Organization and National Institutes of Health protocols. *Health Rep.* **2012**, *23*, 53–60. [PubMed]
80. Webber, C.E.; Barr, R.D. Age- and gender-dependent values of skeletal muscle mass in healthy children and adolescents. *J. Cachex. Sarcopenia Muscle* **2011**, *3*, 25–29. [CrossRef] [PubMed]
81. Butler, M.G.; Bittel, D.C.; Kibiryeva, N.; Talebizadeh, Z.; Thompson, T. Behavioral Differences Among Subjects With Prader-Willi Syndrome and Type I or Type II Deletion and Maternal Disomy. *Pediatrics* **2004**, *113*, 565–573. [CrossRef]
82. Schwimmer, J.B.; Dunn, W.; Norman, G.; Pardee, P.E.; Middleton, M.S.; Kerkar, N.; Sirlin, C. SAFETY Study: Alanine Aminotransferase Cutoff Values Are Set Too High for Reliable Detection of Pediatric Chronic Liver Disease. *Gastroenterology* **2010**, *138*, 1357–1364.e2. [CrossRef]
83. Matthews, D.R.; Hosker, J.P.; Rudenski, A.S.; Naylor, B.A.; Treacher, D.F.; Turner, R.C. Homeostasis model assessment: Insulin resistance and beta-cell function from fasting plasma glucose and insulin concentrations in man. *Diabetologia* **1985**, *28*, 412–419. [CrossRef]
84. Geiger, R.; Strasak, A.; Treml, B.; Gasser, K.; Kleinsasser, A.; Fischer, V.; Geiger, H.; Loeckinger, A.; Stein, J.I. Six-Minute Walk Test in Children and Adolescents. *J. Pediatr.* **2007**, *150*, 395–399.e2. [CrossRef]
85. McQuiddy, V.A.; Scheerer, C.R.; Lavalley, R.; McGrath, T.; Lin, L. Normative Values for Grip and Pinch Strength for 6- to 19-Year-Olds. *Arch. Phys. Med. Rehabil.* **2015**, *96*, 1627–1633. [CrossRef]
86. National High Blood Pressure Education Program Working Group on High Blood Pressure in C, Adolescents. The fourth report on the diagnosis, evaluation, and treatment of high blood pressure in children and adolescents. *Pediatrics* **2004**, *114* (Suppl. 2), 555–576. [CrossRef]
87. Chiles Shaffer, N.; Fabbri, E.; Ferrucci, L.; Shardell, M.; Simonsick, E.M.; Studenski, S. Muscle Quality, Strength, and Lower Extremity Physical Performance in the Baltimore Longitudinal Study of Aging. *J. Frailty Aging* **2017**, *6*, 183–187. [CrossRef] [PubMed]
88. Hay, J.A.; University, B.; Cairney, J. Development of the Habitual Activity Estimation Scale for Clinical Research: A Systematic Approach. *Pediatr. Exerc. Sci.* **2006**, *18*, 193–202. [CrossRef]
89. Smith, A.; Hung, D. The dilemma of diagnostic testing for Prader-Willi syndrome. *Transl. Pediatr.* **2017**, *6*, 46–56. [CrossRef] [PubMed]

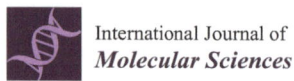 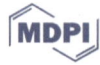

Article

Preserved Sleep for the Same Level of Respiratory Disturbance in Children with Prader-Willi Syndrome

Qiming Tan [1,2], Xiao Tian (Tim) He [1], Sabrina Kang [1], Andrea M. Haqq [1,2,3] and Joanna E. MacLean [1,2,3,*]

[1] Department of Pediatrics, Faculty of Medicine & Dentistry, University of Alberta, Edmonton, AB T6G 1C9, Canada
[2] Women & Children's Health Research Institute, Faculty of Medicine & Dentistry, University of Alberta, Edmonton, AB T6G 1C9, Canada
[3] Stollery Children's Hospital, Edmonton, AB T6G 2B7, Canada
* Correspondence: maclean5@ualberta.ca

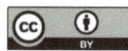

Citation: Tan, Q.; He, X.T.; Kang, S.; Haqq, A.M.; MacLean, J.E. Preserved Sleep for the Same Level of Respiratory Disturbance in Children with Prader-Willi Syndrome. *Int. J. Mol. Sci.* **2022**, *23*, 10580. https://doi.org/10.3390/ijms231810580

Academic Editors: David E. Godler and Olivia J. Veatch

Received: 8 August 2022
Accepted: 8 September 2022
Published: 13 September 2022

Publisher's Note: MDPI stays neutral with regard to jurisdictional claims in published maps and institutional affiliations.

Copyright: © 2022 by the authors. Licensee MDPI, Basel, Switzerland. This article is an open access article distributed under the terms and conditions of the Creative Commons Attribution (CC BY) license (https://creativecommons.org/licenses/by/4.0/).

Abstract: Debate remains as to how to balance the use of recombinant human growth hormone (rhGH) as an important treatment in Prader-Willi syndrome (PWS) with its potential role in obstructive sleep apnea. This single-center, retrospective study assessed differences in overnight polysomnography results between children with and without PWS and changes in respiratory parameters before and after the initiation of rhGH treatment in those with PWS. Compared with age-, sex-, and body-mass-index-matched controls (n = 87), children with PWS (n = 29) had longer total sleep time (434 ± 72 vs. 365 ± 116 min; $p < 0.01$), higher sleep efficiency (86 ± 7 vs. 78 ± 15%; $p < 0.05$), and lower arousal events (8.1 ± 4.5 vs. 13.0 ± 8.9 events/h; $p < 0.05$). Mean oxygen saturation was lower in PWS children (94.3 ± 6.0 vs. 96.0 ± 2.0%; $p < 0.05$), with no other differences in respiratory parameters between groups. Eleven children with PWS (38%) met the criteria for further analyses of the impact of rhGH; polysomnography parameters did not change with treatment. Compared with other children undergoing polysomnography, children with PWS had more favorable markers of sleep continuity and lower oxygen saturation for the same level of respiratory disturbance. rhGH administration was not associated with changes in respiratory parameters in PWS.

Keywords: sleep-related breathing disorders; obstructive sleep apnea; polysomnography; growth hormone; before-after comparison

1. Introduction

Prader-Willi syndrome (PWS) is a multisystem neurodevelopmental disorder, with an incidence of 1/10,000 to 1/25,000 live births, caused by an absence of a functionally active paternal contribution in the chromosome 15q11.2-q13 region [1]. Clinical manifestations of PWS include infantile lethargy and hypotonia, contributing to poor feeding and failure to thrive, followed by excess weight gain and hyperphagia in early childhood, as well as hypogonadism, global developmental delay, intellectual impairment, and minor facial abnormalities. Management of PWS is multidisciplinary, with the goal of controlling weight, monitoring and treating comorbid conditions, and replacing hormone deficiencies, including recombinant human growth hormone (rhGH) [1]. Sleep disorders, including sleep-related breathing disorders, are common comorbid conditions in PWS [2].

Sleep-related breathing disorders in PWS present as early as infancy, with central sleep apnea (CSA) most commonly manifesting in infancy and obstructive sleep apnea (OSA) in childhood [3]. The prevalence of sleep-related breathing disorders in PWS is difficult to estimate as definitions of CSA and OSA vary across studies. While the prevalence of OSA in children with PWS is uncertain, it has been observed to be higher than in the general pediatric population, with OSA prevalence being as high as 80% in children with PWS of certain ages [4,5]. Sleep-related breathing disorders in PWS also show clinical characteristics that are different from those found in age- and body mass index (BMI) z-score-matched children without PWS [6]. Adenotonsillar hypertrophy, hypotonia, respiratory muscle weakness, pharyngeal narrowing, and hypothalamic dysfunction are important predisposing factors that may coexist in individuals with PWS [2]. Untreated OSA in PWS is associated with poorer neurocognitive outcomes and psychosocial deficits in children with PWS, who already face cognitive and behavioral challenges. Respiratory causes account for more than 50% of the deaths in children and adults with PWS, with some reported cases of sudden death occurring at night [7,8]. Therefore, early recognition and aggressive treatment of sleep-related breathing disorders are important to preserve cardiovascular health, improve daytime functioning, limit the risk of severe respiratory events during sleep, and improve quality of life in this population.

GH therapy is the only approved pharmacotherapy for PWS to date, with proven efficacy to normalize linear growth, significantly improve body composition and body mass index, and modify the natural history of PWS with a good safety profile [9]. Increasing evidence supports that rhGH therapy leads to better cognition and motor development in young infants and toddlers with PWS, while continued rhGH therapy into later childhood and adulthood may be beneficial for maintaining the improved body composition in adult patients [9,10]. Some early studies have also demonstrated favorable effects of rhGH therapy on sleep quality and respiratory function [11–13]. Unfortunately, several sudden death incidents during the initial phase of rhGH treatment, caused by suspected airway obstruction, were reported in the first few years after approval. rhGH therapy was thought to exacerbate underlying respiratory conditions in patients with PWS, which led to these incidents [14–17]. In a few cases, patients on long-term rhGH therapy had to discontinue the treatment due to the occurrence of severe OSA [18,19]. However, further studies revealed that PWS syndrome itself predisposes the individual to a risk of sudden death (with or without concurrent rhGH administration) [20,21]. This still raises a question about how to balance the use of rhGH as an important treatment in PWS with its potential role in OSA. The aims of this study were (i) to identify unique features in the clinical presentations of sleep-related breathing disorders and polysomnography (PSG) results of children with PWS and (ii) to determine what changes occur in these features after starting rhGH therapy.

2. Results

We identified 29 children with PWS who underwent PSG and matched them to 87 comparison children. Molecular genetics for the children with PWS showed deletion ($n = 15$, 52%), uniparental disomy ($n = 7$, 24%), imprinting defect ($n = 3$, 10%), and translocation ($n = 1$, 3%), with a specific defect not available for 3 children (10%). Children with PWS were matched with control children with respect to age, sex, and BMI z-score; children with PWS had lower height z-score (Table 1). Indications for PSG differed only related in relation to rhGH, with no difference in the frequency of other common indications. The only sleep-related symptoms that differed between children with PWS and matched controls were restless sleep and attention concerns, which were less common in children with PWS (Table 2). Within PWS, sleep symptoms did not differ by molecular genetics (data not shown).

Analysis of PSG variables from the initial study showed that children with PWS had longer total sleep time, higher sleep efficiency, and less arousals from sleep compared with the matched comparison group (Table 3). The proportion of sleep time spent in REM sleep did not differ by group. The only respiratory variable that differed between the groups was mean pulse oxygen saturation (SpO_2), which was lower in PWS children. Hypoventilation, as measured by the percent time with end tidal carbon dioxide ($ETCO_2$) > 50 mmgh (%TST with $ETCO_2$ > 50 mmHg), did not differ between groups. There was no difference in the occurrence of OSA (PWS 59% vs. comparison 60%, OR 1.04, [95% CI: 0.55, 1.96]) or distribution of OSA severity between groups (PWS: no OSA 41.4%, mild OSA 31.0%, moderate OSA 17.2%, and severe OSA 10.3%; matched comparison group: no OSA 40.2%, mild OSA 33.3%, moderate OSA 10.3%, and severe OSA 16.1%; chi square 1.4, p = ns). On univariate analysis, the only demographic variable demonstrating a significant association with any OSA or moderate/severe OSA was boys having higher rates of any OSA (girls 48% vs. boys 73%, OR 1.56 [95% CI: 1.13, 2.15]) and moderate/severe OSA (girls 16% vs. boys 40%, OR 1.97 [95% CI: 1.15, 3.36]). Within the PWS group, molecular genetics were not associated with risk of any OSA (deletion: 59%, uniparental disomy 23%, translocation 0%, imprinting defect 0%, and not reported 18%; chi square 5.21, p = ns) or moderate/severe OSA (deletion: 62%, uniparental disomy 13%, translocation 0%, imprinting defect 0%, and not reported 25%; chi square 5.21, p = ns). Given the low number of children and uneven distribution of groups, this analysis could not rule out OSA risk difference by molecular genetic subtypes.

Table 1. Demographic characteristics of children with PWS and the matched comparison group.

Parameter	Prader-Willi Syndrome (n = 29)	Matched Comparison Group (n = 87)
Age at PSG (years, mean ± SD)	4.4 ± 5.2	4.4 ± 5.1
Sex (F:M, % female)	17:12 (59%)	47:40 (54%)
Weight z-score ± SD	−0.99 ± 1.90	−0.12 ± 2.28
Height z-score ± SD **	−2.09 ± 1.99	−0.80 ± 2.08
BMI z-score	0.28 ± 2.28	0.38 ± 1.88
Indications for PSG (n, %) [†]:		
Recombinant human growth hormone [‡]	6 (21%)	0
Obstructive sleep apnea	22 (76%)	54 (65%)
Central sleep apnea	1 (3%)	2 (2%)
Excessive daytime sleepiness	1 (3%)	3 (3%)
Other	0	2 (2%)
Not reported	3 (10%)	5 (6%)

[†] More than one indication for some children. ** $p < 0.01$, [‡] $p < 0.0001$. BMI, body mass index; PSG, polysomnography; recombinant human growth hormone, rhGH; F:M, female to male ratio.

Table 2. Sleep-related symptoms in children with Prader-Willi syndrome and matched comparison group.

Symptom	Prader-Willi Syndrome (n = 20)	Matched Comparison Group (n = 60)
Snoring	48%	47%
Witnessed apnea	14%	12%
Restless sleep **	14%	41%
Nighttime awakening	21%	28%
Morning headache	0%	11%
Mouth breathing	45%	52%
Daytime sleepiness	28%	27%
Poor school performance	21%	17%
Attention concerns *	0%	13%

* $p < 0.05$, ** $p < 0.01$.

Of the 29 children with PWS, 24 (82%) had PSG prior to starting rhGH. Of these 24 children, 5 (21%) did not have follow-up studies, and 7 (29%) were started on noninvasive ventilation (i.e., continuous or bilevel positive airway pressure) before rhGH so subsequent studies were treatment studies. This left 12 children with PSGs before and after starting rhGH with 1 excluded as the follow-up study had a TST < 2 h, leaving 11 children with diagnostic PSG results before and after initiation of rhGH therapy. Overall, there was no change in any PSG parameters 6.8 (95% CI 2.0, 11.7) months after starting rhGH with a mean difference of 1.0 (95% CI 1.3, 0.80) years between PSG measurements (Table 4). Both increases and decreases in respiratory events were seen after the administration of rhGH (Figure 1). Of the six children that did not meet the criteria for OSA prior to initiation of rhGH, three met the criteria after starting treatment, with two having mild OSA (obstructive-mixed apnea-hypopnea index [OMAHI] 1.50 to 2.20 and 0.80 to 3.70 events/h) and one having moderate OSA (OMAHI 0 to 8.8 events/h), and three continued to not meet the OSA criteria with OMAHI < 1 event/h before and after treatment. Of the five children who met the criteria for OSA prior to initiation of rhGH, two did not meet the criteria after starting treatment (OMAHI 5.10 to 0.7 and 4.5 to 1.7 events/h) and three continued to meet the criteria for OSA (OMAHI 10.0 to 5.0, 3.1 to 8.8, and 4.40 to 10.7 events/h). None met the criteria for hypoventilation.

Table 3. Polysomnography results for children with Prader-Willi syndrome and matched comparison group.

	Prader-Willi Syndrome	Matched Comparison Group
Total sleep time (min) **	434 ± 72	370 ± 118
Sleep efficiency (%) *	86 ± 7	78 ± 15
N3 sleep (%)	29 ± 15	31 ± 13
REM sleep (%)	27 ± 10	26 ± 13
Arousal index (events/h) *	8.1 ± 4.5	13.0 ± 8.9
AHI (median (IQR), events/h)	7.3 (11.8)	6.0 (13.8)
OMAHI (median (IQR), events/h)	3.2 (6.7)	2.5 (7.0)
Central index (median (IQR), events/h)	2.9 (10.1)	1.8 (5.4)
ODI (median (IQR), events/h)	3.6 (12.6)	4.7 (22.7)
Mean SpO$_2$ (%) *	94.3 ± 6.0	96.0 ± 2.0
Minimum SpO$_2$ (%)	82.9 ± 6.1	84.0 ± 11.1
%TST with SpO$_2$ < 90% (%)	3.1 ± 7.3	4.2 ± 15.1
Mean ETCO$_2$ (mmHg)	41.6 ± 58	41.5 ± 5.4
Maximum ETCO$_2$ (mmHg)	51.9 ± 8.0	51.3 ± 8.8
%TST with ETCO$_2$ > 50 mmHg (%)	3.1 ± 8.7	3.5 ± 14.5

* $p < 0.05$, ** $p < 0.01$ AHI, apnea-hypopnea index; CI, confidence interval; ETCO$_2$, end tidal carbon dioxide; max, maximum; Max, maximum; Min, minimum; N3, slow wave sleep; ODI, oxygen desaturation index; OMAHI, obstructive-mixed apnea-hypopnea index; REM, rapid eye movement; SpO$_2$, pulse oxygen saturation; TST, total sleep time. Data are presented as mean ± SD.

Table 4. Comparison of polysomnography results before and after initiation of recombinant human growth hormone.

Parameter	Before Starting rhGH	After Starting rhGH	Mean Difference (95% CI) or Wilcoxon Test Statistic
Age (years) ***	3.2 ± 3.3	4.3 ± 5.6	−1.0 (−1.3, −0.80)
Total sleep time (min)	467 ± 50	477 ± 38	−10.0 (−49.6, 29.3)
Sleep efficiency (%)	89 ± 5	88 ± 7	1.2 (−3.4, 5.8)
N3 sleep (%)	26 ± 15	29 ± 14	−2.9 (−17.3, 11.6)
REM sleep (%)	30 ± 13	22 ± 7	8.1 (−0.44, 16.2)
Arousal index (events/h)	11.4 ± 8.8	6.2 ± 2.5	5.2 (−1.2, 11.6)
AHI (median (IQR), events/h)	5.7 (5.3)	2.0 (0.0)	−0.58
OMAHI (median (IQR), events/h)	1.8 (3.5)	2.2 (8.0)	−1.07
Central index (median (IQR), events/h)	3.6 (8.5)	1.8 (3.5)	−1.89
ODI (median (IQR), events/h)	2.9 (13.4)	7.8 (12.3)	−1.58
Mean SpO$_2$ (%)	93.5 ± 9.7	95.1 ± 1.9	−1.6 (−8.4, 5.1)
Min SpO$_2$ (%)	85.0 ± 4.9	74.9 ± 23.1	10.1 (−4.6, 24.8)
%TST with SpO$_2$ < 90% (%)	0.39 ± 0.35	3.3 ± 8.4	−2.9 (−8.5, 2.7)
Mean ETCO$_2$ (mmHg)	39.7 ± 7.3	42.7 ± 2.7	−3.0 (−7.3, 1.4)
Max ETCO$_2$ (mmHg)	48.8 ± 4.4	49.6 ± 7.1	−0.78 (−7.3, 5.7)
%TST with ETCO$_2$ > 50 mmHg (%)	0.12 ± 0.18	2.0 ± 4.8	−1.8 (−5.1, 1.4)

*** $p < 0.001$ AHI, apnea-hypopnea index; CI, confidence interval; ETCO$_2$, end tidal carbon dioxide; max, maximum; Max, maximum; Min, minimum; N3, slow wave sleep; ODI, oxygen desaturation index; OMAHI, obstructive-mixed apnea-hypopnea index; REM, rapid eye movement; SpO$_2$, pulse oxygen saturation; TST, total sleep time. Data are presented as mean ± SD or as median (interquartile range).

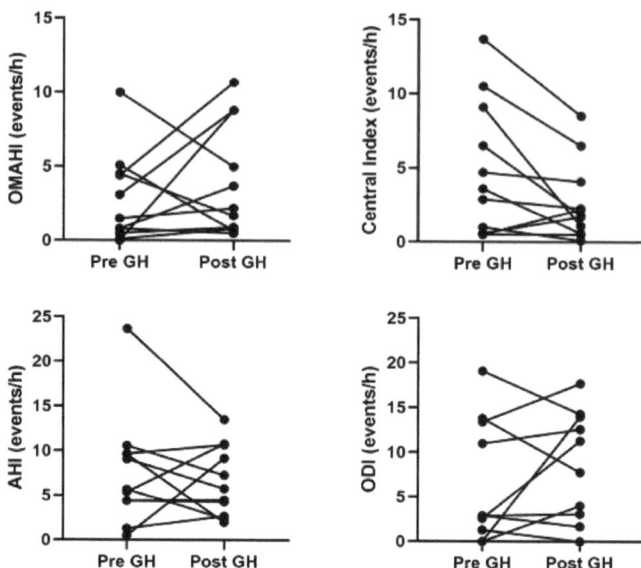

Figure 1. Analysis of summary polysomnography variables before and after starting recombinant human growth hormone showed no differences. AHI, apnea-hypopnea index; ODI, oxygen desaturation index; OMAHI, obstructive-mixed apnea hypopnea index.

3. Discussion

The results from this retrospective review showed that children with PWS have more favorable sleep symptoms, with less restless sleep and attention concern reported by parents, and more favorable PSG sleep parameters, including longer total sleep time, higher sleep efficiency, and less arousals from sleep, compared with contemporary age-, sex-, and BMI-matched children who also underwent PSG. These differences are in the context of a similar index of respiratory events and carbon dioxide parameters with lower mean SpO_2. PWS was not associated with an altered risk of OSA, suggesting that the risk of OSA and the severity of OSA are similar for PWS and other children undergoing PSG. Overall, being male sex was shown to be a risk factor for OSA with neither PWS nor BMI z-score altering this risk. Finally, PSG parameters overall did not differ before and after initiation of treatment with rhGH. Of note, just under one-third of children with PWS were started on noninvasive ventilation prior to starting rhGH, and one child developed severe OSA after starting rhGH.

Defining the risk of and risk factors for OSA in children with PWS is challenging because of differences in the definition of OSA, Refs. [22–25], with some studies reporting respiratory events from PSG without defining OSA, Refs. [26,27] as well differences in age and growth parameters. With no clear PSG standards for the identification of OSA in infants, OSA may be over-reported in infants if the pediatric criteria are applied to this younger age group [12,28,29]. Two studies reported rates of 27% and 44% based on obstructive AHI > 1.5 and >1 event/h, respectively, prior to rhGH therapy [24]. The findings of studies looking at risk factors for OSA in children with PWS are inconsistent, with some identifying association with older age, higher BMI, and adenotonsillar hypertrophy, while others failed to replicate these same findings [24,30]. In the present study, OSA incidence and severity did not differ from that of a matched comparison group. While PWS may confer a higher risk of OSA compared with otherwise healthy children, risk factors for OSA for PWS likely overlap with unselected children undergoing PSG. Further work is needed to understand OSA pathophysiology and its ensuing risk factors in children with PWS.

OSA is a multifactorial and heterogeneous disorder where airway compromise can be mitigated or worsened by an individual's arousal response, upper airway response, and response to change in oxygen and carbon dioxide. Sleep in PWS has been characterized by a higher propensity for sleep, as measured by shorter sleep and REM latency, as well as longer sleep time on PSG, shorter mean sleep latency test scores, and excessive daytime sleepiness or hypersomnolence on validated questionnaires [31–33]. Studies measuring the arousal response have shown a higher arousal threshold to hypercapnia as well as abnormal arousal and cardiorespiratory response to hypoxia compared with controls, with a hypothalamic abnormality as a prime target to link hypersomnolence and abnormality in ventilatory control [34–36]. In the present study, we demonstrated that children with PWS had more favorable sleep symptoms and PSG sleep characteristics, including less restless sleep, longer TST, higher sleep efficiency, and lower arousal index compared with matched comparison children. This was despite similar respiratory event parameters and a lower mean SpO_2. This suggests that children with PWS, for the same level of respiratory events, are less likely to experience arousal from sleep or may awaken from sleep later during respiratory events compared with other children with suspected OSA. Impairments in arousal or awakening responses, including responses to respiratory events or changes in oxygen and carbon dioxide, increase the risk of OSA even with a relatively uncompromised airway and may contribute to the risk of sudden death in the context of illness or other physiological disruption.

While there is controversy about a link between rhGH therapy and sudden death, there is widespread agreement on the benefits of starting rhGH treatment prior to obesity onset (typically by age 2 years), and emerging evidence supports very early initiation between 4 and 6 months of age in patients with PWS [37]. Reports of initial sudden death associated with rhGH therapy raised concerns over rhGH safety; postmortem findings suggested that the treatment might have led to OSA, respiratory infection, and sudden death in those patients [38]. In the largest study of adverse events in children with PWS receiving rhGH (N = 675), five children, aged 2.1 to 15.8 years, died, and two teens developed apnea [38]. In response, PSG has become a standard examination before initiating and during rhGH treatment. There are studies where symptoms of OSA developed or worsened during rhGH use in some children, though few ceased treatment or had dose reductions [24,39]. Several longitudinal studies, including the present one, demonstrated no association between rhGH treatment and increased risk of OSA in children with PWS [12,22,23,26]. Of note, there is no standard definition of what constitutes a clinically important change in OSA measurement; this may differ across the spectrum of mild-to-severe OSA as well as for different groups with OSA including PWS. Given that the risk of OSA during sleep in individual patients is multifactorial and changes in symptoms do not always reflect OSA, PSG before and after initiation of rhGH and if sleep symptoms worsen is prudent. For many years, as the only approved therapy for PWS, rhGH treatment has proven its long-term safety and efficacy in improving patients' final height, body composition, and quality of life [37]. While OSA might be a risk factor for sudden death in children with PWS, it is not the only factor, as children without OSA experience sudden death as well [22,38,40]. Despite uncertainties, deciding against or delaying rhGH treatment because of the concern for rare serious adverse events must be balanced with the risk of developing complications in a child with PWS untreated with rhGH.

The unique cause of PWS may account for a component of the observed phenotypic variability in sleep problems in children with PWS. A large cohort study found that children with PWS had less parent-reported sleep problems, daytime sleepiness, and symptoms of sleep-disordered breathing than those with Rett and Angelman syndromes [41]. Similarly, in our study, children with PWS tended to have a less-worse sleep profile compared with their age-, sex-, and BMI-matched control subjects. Although we did not find any differences in sleep symptoms between molecular genetics, the potential direct and indirect contribution of PWS candidate genes to OSA and other sleep problems is worth further investigation. For instance, *MAGEL2*, an imprinted gene within the Prader-Willi critical region, has been shown to be important for the coordination of circadian rhythm in hypothalamic neurons [42–44], whereas circadian clock disruption might be a key contributing factor to OSA complications [45]. In addition, dysfunction of the autonomic nervous system is also present in patients with PWS [46]. There is evidence indicating a bidirectional relationship between sleep and autonomic activity [47]. Chronic sleep disruption impairs autonomic coordination, whereas the dysregulation of autonomic functions interferes with the initiation and maintenance of sleep. Future studies may consider exploring this bidirectionality in children with PWS, as it may play a crucial role in the pathophysiology of various sleep disorders, including OSA [47].

The limitations of the study must be acknowledged. As with any retrospective chart review, it is subject to selection bias and limited by the quality of the medical records. To maximize the numbers for a relatively rare condition, a broad time frame was used across which clinical practice, both with respect to PWS and OSA, had likely changed. To account for this in the comparison of PWS with a matched comparison group, children were matched for both demographic characteristics as well as the date of their PSG. In our study cohort, only one child with PWS and two children in the comparison group had a diagnosis of CSA, with no difference in the central index between the PWS and matched comparison group. With a relatively broad age range in our sample, further work is needed to understand the pathogenesis of previously described central sleep apnea associated with PWS. Additionally, the number of patients who had repeated PSG was small; thus, the statistical power to detect differences in PSG results before and after rhGH initiation was limited. A prospective trial comparing PSG results before and during rhGH treatment in a larger cohort of children with PWS across a broad age range is needed to confirm the results of the present study.

4. Materials and Methods

This study was a retrospective single-center chart review of children with PWS who underwent overnight PSG in a tertiary care pediatric sleep laboratory (Stollery Children's Hospital, Edmonton, AB, Canada). Sleep laboratory records were screened to identify children who had undergone diagnostic PSG from January 2005 to September 2021; this time frame was chosen as PSG records were available from 2005. Health administrative data were also searched using International Classification of Disease codes for PWS, and this list was cross-referenced against sleep laboratory records. The final list was reviewed to confirm that all identified children had a genetically confirmed diagnosis of PWS. Each child with PWS was matched for age, sex, and BMI as well as date of diagnostic PSG, with three children undergoing PSG who did not have PWS. This matched comparison group did not exclude children with known risk factors for OSA or medical comorbidity. Data were extracted from sleep laboratory records and medical records. The study protocol and waiver of informed consent were approved by the University of Alberta human research ethics boards (Pro00064982).

Data collection included demographics, anthropometric measures, medical history, and PSG results. Height was measured using a stadiometer, and weight was measured on a digital scale. Height, weight, and BMI were converted to z-scores using available normative data [48]. Ethnicity was described by the parent/guardian. Presenting symptoms and medical history were extracted from medical charts and sleep laboratory questionnaires.

Diagnostic PSG was performed in accordance with clinical protocols at the time of the PSG, which included adherence to the standards of the American Academy of Sleep Medicine guidelines [49,50]. This included the determination of sleep state using electroencephalography, electrooculography, and submental electromyography. Channels to evaluate respiratory status included SpO_2, nasal/oral air flow by thermistor, nasal pressure, and chest and abdominal wall movement using respiratory inductance plethysmography. CO_2 was monitored using $ETCO_2$ monitoring. Cardiac monitoring included electrocardiography.

Analysis of PSG data was completed by experienced scorers using the criteria of the American Academy of Sleep Medicine available at the time of the study [49,50]. Measures of sleep continuity included total sleep time (TST), sleep efficiency (percent time of time in bed spent in sleep), arousal index (number of arousals per hour of TST), and proportion of TST spent in stage 3 and rapid-eye-movement sleep (N3 and REM sleep, respectively). AHI was calculated based on the number of apneas and hypopneas during sleep divided by the total sleep time (TST). Oxygen desaturation index (ODI) was calculated based on the number of oxygen desaturation events $\geq$ 3% during sleep divided by the TST. An OMAHI index $\geq$ 1 events/h was used to define the presence of OSA [51]. The severity of OSA was further characterized as mild (OMAHI 1–4.9 events/h), moderate (OMAHI 5.0–9.9 events/h), or severe (OMAHI $\geq$ 10 events/h). As there are no clear parameters for the identification of OSA in infants, this pediatric OSA classification was used for infants as well to facilitate group comparisons, recognizing that this may over-represent OSA in children under 1 year of age [29]. Hypoventilation was identified by a CO_2 > 50 mmHg for >25% of the TST. Studies were excluded from the analysis if the TST was <2 h.

The study data were managed using REDCap electronic data capture tools hosted by the Women & Children's Health Research Institute, University of Alberta, Edmonton, AB, Canada. Statistical analysis was performed using the IBM© SPSS © Statistics (IBM Corp. Released 2019. IBM SPSS Statistics for Windows, Version 26.0. Armonk, NY, USA: IBM Corp). Student's t-tests and Wilcoxon sign-ranked test were used to analyze paired and unpaired comparisons for parametric and nonparametric data, respectively. Categorical variables were analyzed using chi-square analysis, likelihood ratio (LR), or odds ratio (OR), as appropriate. A p-value < 0.05 indicated statistically significant effects. Binary regression analysis was used to assess potential demographic predictors of any and moderate/severe OSA, with covariates selection for multivariable analysis based on univariate analysis with p < 0.10.

5. Conclusions

This retrospective study found that, for the same level of respiratory events, sleep was preserved in children with PWS compared with other children, suggesting that arousal mechanisms may be altered in PWS and may contribute to the risk of OSA and sudden death. rhGH therapy was not associated with increased risk of OSA in children with PWS; this finding supports the recommendation that the treatment should be continued for as long as benefits outweigh risks. Future studies to better understand the pathophysiology of OSA and the consequences of OSA in PWS are needed. This includes establishing consistent definitions of OSA for children with PWS and evidence-based guidelines to support the management of OSA in this population.

Author Contributions: Conceptualization, J.E.M. and A.M.H.; methodology, J.E.M. and A.M.H.; formal analysis, Q.T., X.T.H., S.K., A.M.H. and J.E.M.; resources, J.E.M. and A.M.H.; data curation, J.E.M. and A.M.H.; writing—original draft preparation, J.E.M. and Q.T.; writing—review and editing, Q.T., X.T.H., S.K., A.M.H and J.E.M.; visualization, X.T.H., S.K. and J.E.M.; supervision, J.E.M. All authors have read and agreed to the published version of the manuscript.

Funding: This research received no external funding.

Institutional Review Board Statement: The study was conducted in accordance with the Declaration of Helsinki and approved by the Institutional Review Board of the University of Alberta (Pro00064982).

Informed Consent Statement: Patient consent was waived as the study was retrospective with no contact with the participants. The request to waive the documentation of informed consent was reviewed and approved by the University of Alberta Research Ethics Boards.

Data Availability Statement: Data sharing is not applicable to this article.

Acknowledgments: This research has been facilitated by the Women and Children's Health Research Institute through the Stollery Children's Hospital Foundation.

Conflicts of Interest: The authors declare no conflict of interest.

References

1. Butler, M.G.; Miller, J.L.; Forster, J.L. Prader-Willi Syndrome—Clinical Genetics, Diagnosis and Treatment Approaches: An Update. *Curr. Pediatr Rev.* **2019**, *15*, 207–244. [CrossRef] [PubMed]
2. Khayat, A.; Narang, I.; Bin-Hasan, S.; Amin, R.; Al-Saleh, S. Longitudinal evaluation of sleep disordered breathing in infants with Prader-Willi syndrome. *Arch. Dis. Child.* **2017**, *102*, 634–638. [CrossRef] [PubMed]
3. Cataldi, M.; Arnaldi, D.; Tucci, V.; De Carli, F.; Patti, G.; Napoli, F.; Pace, M.; Maghnie, M.; Nobili, L. Sleep disorders in Prader-Willi syndrome, evidence from animal models and humans. *Sleep Med. Rev.* **2021**, *57*, 101432. [CrossRef] [PubMed]
4. Sedky, K.; Bennett, D.S.; Pumariega, A. Prader Willi syndrome and obstructive sleep apnea: Co-occurrence in the pediatric population. *J. Clin. Sleep Med.* **2014**, *10*, 403–409. [CrossRef]
5. Trosman, I. Childhood obstructive sleep apnea syndrome: A review of the 2012 American Academy of Pediatrics guidelines. *Pediatr Ann.* **2013**, *42*, 195–199. [CrossRef]
6. Lecka-Ambroziak, A.; Wysocka-Mincewicz, M.; Świercz, A.; Jędrzejczak, M.; Szalecki, M. Comparison of Frequency and Severity of Sleep-Related Breathing Disorders in Children with Simple Obesity and Paediatric Patients with Prader-Willi Syndrome. *J. Pers. Med.* **2021**, *11*, 141. [CrossRef]
7. Tauber, M.; Diene, G.; Molinas, C.; Hébert, M. Review of 64 cases of death in children with Prader-Willi syndrome (PWS). *Am. J. Med. Genet A* **2008**, *146A*, 881–887. [CrossRef]
8. Alfaro, D.L.P.; Lemoine, P.; Ehlinger, V.; Molinas, C.; Diene, G.; Valette, M.; Pinto, G.; Coupaye, M.; Poitou-Bernert, C.; Thuilleaux, D.; et al. Causes of death in Prader-Willi syndrome: Lessons from 11 years' experience of a national reference center. *Orphanet J. Rare. Dis.* **2019**, *14*, 238. [CrossRef]
9. Passone, C.G.B.; Franco, R.R.; Ito, S.S.; Trindade, E.; Polak, M.; Damiani, D.; Bernardo, W.M. Growth hormone treatment in Prader-Willi syndrome patients: Systematic review and meta-analysis. *BMJ Paediatr Open* **2020**, *4*, e000630. [CrossRef]
10. Bakker, N.E.; Lindberg, A.; Heissler, J.; Wollmann, H.A.; Camacho-Hübner, C.; Hokken-Koelega, A.C.; Committee, K.S. Growth Hormone Treatment in Children With Prader-Willi Syndrome: Three Years of Longitudinal Data in Prepubertal Children and Adult Height Data From the KIGS Database. *J. Clin. Endocrinol. Metab.* **2017**, *102*, 1702–1711. [CrossRef]
11. Lindgren, A.C.; Hellström, L.G.; Ritzén, E.M.; Milerad, J. Growth hormone treatment increases CO(2) response, ventilation and central inspiratory drive in children with Prader-Willi syndrome. *Eur. J. Pediatr* **1999**, *158*, 936–940. [CrossRef] [PubMed]
12. Haqq, A.M.; Stadler, D.D.; Jackson, R.H.; Rosenfeld, R.G.; Purnell, J.Q.; LaFranchi, S.H. Effects of growth hormone on pulmonary function, sleep quality, behavior, cognition, growth velocity, body composition, and resting energy expenditure in Prader-Willi syndrome. *J. Clin. Endocrinol. Metab.* **2003**, *88*, 2206–2212. [CrossRef] [PubMed]
13. Miller, J.; Silverstein, J.; Shuster, J.; Driscoll, D.J.; Wagner, M. Short-term effects of growth hormone on sleep abnormalities in Prader-Willi syndrome. *J. Clin. Endocrinol. Metab.* **2006**, *91*, 413–417. [CrossRef] [PubMed]
14. Nordmann, Y.; Eiholzer, U.; l'Allemand, D.; Mirjanic, S.; Markwalder, C. Sudden death of an infant with Prader-Willi syndrome–not a unique case? *Biol. Neonate* **2002**, *82*, 139–141. [CrossRef]
15. Van Vliet, G.; Deal, C.L.; Crock, P.A.; Robitaille, Y.; Oligny, L.L. Sudden death in growth hormone-treated children with Prader-Willi syndrome. *J. Pediatr* **2004**, *144*, 129–131. [CrossRef]
16. Grugni, G.; Livieri, C.; Corrias, A.; Sartorio, A.; Crinò, A.; Genetic Obesity Study Group of the Italian Society of Pediatric Endocrinology and Diabetology. Death during GH therapy in children with Prader-Willi syndrome: Description of two new cases. *J. Endocrinol. Invest.* **2005**, *28*, 554–557. [CrossRef]
17. Riedl, S.; Blümel, P.; Zwiauer, K.; Frisch, H. Death in two female Prader-Willi syndrome patients during the early phase of growth hormone treatment. *Acta. Paediatr* **2005**, *94*, 974–977. [CrossRef]
18. Al-Saleh, S.; Al-Naimi, A.; Hamilton, J.; Zweerink, A.; Iaboni, A.; Narang, I. Longitudinal evaluation of sleep-disordered breathing in children with Prader-Willi Syndrome during 2 years of growth hormone therapy. *J. Pediatr* **2013**, *162*, 263–268.e261. [CrossRef]
19. Nixon, G.M.; Rodda, C.P.; Davey, M.J. Longitudinal association between growth hormone therapy and obstructive sleep apnea in a child with Prader-Willi syndrome. *J. Clin. Endocrinol. Metab.* **2011**, *96*, 29–33. [CrossRef]
20. Nagai, T.; Obata, K.; Tonoki, H.; Temma, S.; Murakami, N.; Katada, Y.; Yoshino, A.; Sakazume, S.; Takahashi, E.; Sakuta, R.; et al. Cause of sudden, unexpected death of Prader-Willi syndrome patients with or without growth hormone treatment. *Am. J. Med. Genet A* **2005**, *136*, 45–48. [CrossRef]
21. Eiholzer, U. Deaths in children with Prader-Willi syndrome. A contribution to the debate about the safety of growth hormone treatment in children with PWS. *Horm Res.* **2005**, *63*, 33–39. [CrossRef] [PubMed]
22. Festen, D.A.; de Weerd, A.W.; van den Bossche, R.A.; Joosten, K.; Hoeve, H.; Hokken-Koelega, A.C. Sleep-related breathing disorders in prepubertal children with Prader-Willi syndrome and effects of growth hormone treatment. *J. Clin. Endocrinol. Metab.* **2006**, *91*, 4911–4915. [CrossRef] [PubMed]
23. Salvatoni, A.; Veronelli, E.; Nosetti, L.; Berini, J.; de Simone, S.; Iughetti, L.; Bosio, L.; Chiumello, G.; Grugni, G.; Delu, G.; et al. Short-term effects of growth hormone treatment on the upper airways of non severely obese children with Prader-Willi syndrome. *J. Endocrinol. Investig.* **2009**, *32*, 601–605. [CrossRef]
24. Vandeleur, M.; Davey, M.J.; Nixon, G.M. Are sleep studies helpful in children with Prader-Willi syndrome prior to commencement of growth hormone therapy? *J. Paediatr. Child Health* **2013**, *49*, 238–241. [CrossRef] [PubMed]

25. Polytarchou, A.; Katsouli, G.; Tsaoussoglou, M.; Charmandari, E.; Kanaka-Gantenbein, C.; Chrousos, G.; Kaditis, A.G. Obstructive events in children with Prader-Willi syndrome occur predominantly during rapid eye movement sleep. *Sleep Med.* **2019**, *54*, 43–47. [CrossRef] [PubMed]
26. Katz-Salamon, M.; Lindgren, A.C.; Cohen, G. The effect of growth hormone on sleep-related cardio-respiratory control in Prader-Willi syndrome. *Acta. Paediatr.* **2012**, *101*, 643–648. [CrossRef]
27. Miller, J.L.; Shuster, J.; Theriaque, D.; Driscoll, D.J.; Wagner, M. Sleep disordered breathing in infants with Prader-Willi syndrome during the first 6 weeks of growth hormone therapy: A pilot study. *J. Clin. Sleep Med.* **2009**, *5*, 448–453. [CrossRef]
28. Daftary, A.S.; Jalou, H.E.; Shively, L.; Slaven, J.E.; Davis, S.D. Polysomnography Reference Values in Healthy Newborns. *J. Clin. Sleep Med.* **2019**, *15*, 437–443. [CrossRef]
29. Dehaan, K.L.; Seton, C.; Fitzgerald, D.A.; Waters, K.A.; MacLean, J.E. Polysomnography for the diagnosis of sleep disordered breathing in children under 2 years of age. *Pediatric Pulmonol.* **2015**, *50*, 1346–1353. [CrossRef]
30. Canora, A.; Franzese, A.; Mozzillo, E.; Fattorusso, V.; Bocchino, M.; Sanduzzi, A. Severe obstructive sleep disorders in Prader-Willi syndrome patients in southern Italy. *Eur. J. Pediatrics* **2018**, *177*, 1367–1370. [CrossRef]
31. Joo, E.Y.; Hong, S.B.; Sohn, Y.B.; Kwak, M.J.; Kim, S.J.; Choi, Y.O.; Kim, S.W.; Paik, K.H.; Jin, D.K. Plasma adiponectin level and sleep structures in children with Prader-Willi syndrome. *J. Sleep Res.* **2010**, *19*, 248–254. [CrossRef] [PubMed]
32. Priano, L.; Grugni, G.; Miscio, G.; Guastamacchia, G.; Toffolet, L.; Sartorio, A.; Mauro, A. Sleep cycling alternating pattern (CAP) expression is associated with hypersomnia and GH secretory pattern in Prader-Willi syndrome. *Sleep Med.* **2006**, *7*, 627–633. [CrossRef] [PubMed]
33. Ghergan, A.; Coupaye, M.; Leu-Semenescu, S.; Attali, V.; Oppert, J.M.; Arnulf, I.; Poitou, C.; Redolfi, S. Prevalence and Phenotype of Sleep Disorders in 60 Adults With Prader-Willi Syndrome. *Sleep* **2017**, *40*, 1. [CrossRef] [PubMed]
34. Livingston, F.R.; Arens, R.; Bailey, S.L.; Keens, T.G.; Ward, S.L. Hypercapnic arousal responses in Prader-Willi syndrome. *Chest* **1995**, *108*, 1627–1631. [CrossRef]
35. Arens, R.; Gozal, D.; Burrell, B.C.; Bailey, S.L.; Bautista, D.B.; Keens, T.G.; Ward, S.L. Arousal and cardiorespiratory responses to hypoxia in Prader-Willi syndrome. *Am. J. Respir. Crit. Care Med.* **1996**, *153*, 283–287. [CrossRef]
36. Manni, R.; Politini, L.; Nobili, L.; Ferrillo, F.; Livieri, C.; Veneselli, E.; Biancheri, R.; Martinetti, M.; Tartara, A. Hypersomnia in the Prader Willi syndrome: Clinical-electrophysiological features and underlying factors. *Clin. Neurophysiol.* **2001**, *112*, 800–805. [CrossRef]
37. Deal, C.L.; Tony, M.; Höybye, C.; Allen, D.B.; Tauber, M.; Christiansen, J.S.; 2011 Growth Hormone in Prader-Willi Syndrome Clinical Care Guidelines Workshop Participants. GrowthHormone Research Society workshop summary: Consensus guidelines for recombinant human growth hormone therapy in Prader-Willi syndrome. *J. Clin. Endocrinol. Metab.* **2013**, *98*, E1072–E1087. [CrossRef]
38. Craig, M.E.; Cowell, C.T.; Larsson, P.; Zipf, W.B.; Reiter, E.O.; Wikland, K.A.; Ranke, M.B.; Price, D.A.; Board, K.I. Growth hormone treatment and adverse events in Prader-Willi syndrome: Data from KIGS (the Pfizer International Growth Database). *Clin. Endocrinol.* **2006**, *65*, 178–185. [CrossRef]
39. Berini, J.; Russotto, V.S.; Castelnuovo, P.; Di Candia, S.; Gargantini, L.; Grugni, G.; Iughetti, L.; Nespoli, L.; Nosetti, L.; Padoan, G.; et al. Growth hormone therapy and respiratory disorders: Long-term follow-up in PWS children. *J. Clin. Endocrinol. Metab.* **2013**, *98*, E1516–E1523. [CrossRef]
40. Pomara, C.; D'Errico, S.; Riezzo, I.; de Cillis, G.P.; Fineschi, V. Sudden cardiac death in a child affected by Prader-Willi syndrome. *Int. J. Legal Med.* **2005**, *119*, 153–157. [CrossRef]
41. Veatch, O.J.; Malow, B.A.; Lee, H.S.; Knight, A.; Barrish, J.O.; Neul, J.L.; Lane, J.B.; Skinner, S.A.; Kaufmann, W.E.; Miller, J.L.; et al. Evaluating Sleep Disturbances in Children With Rare Genetic Neurodevelopmental Syndromes. *Pediatr Neurol* **2021**, *123*, 30–37. [CrossRef] [PubMed]
42. Kozlov, S.V.; Bogenpohl, J.W.; Howell, M.P.; Wevrick, R.; Panda, S.; Hogenesch, J.B.; Muglia, L.J.; Van Gelder, R.N.; Herzog, E.D.; Stewart, C.L. The imprinted gene Magel2 regulates normal circadian output. *Nat. Genet.* **2007**, *39*, 1266–1272. [CrossRef] [PubMed]
43. Bischof, J.M.; Stewart, C.L.; Wevrick, R. Inactivation of the mouse Magel2 gene results in growth abnormalities similar to Prader-Willi syndrome. *Hum. Mol. Genet.* **2007**, *16*, 2713–2719. [CrossRef] [PubMed]
44. Mercer, R.E.; Kwolek, E.M.; Bischof, J.M.; van Eede, M.; Henkelman, R.M.; Wevrick, R. Regionally reduced brain volume, altered serotonin neurochemistry, and abnormal behavior in mice null for the circadian rhythm output gene Magel2. *Am. J. Med. Genet. B Neuropsychiatr Genet.* **2009**, *150B*, 1085–1099. [CrossRef]
45. Gabryelska, A.; Turkiewicz, S.; Karuga, F.F.; Sochal, M.; Strzelecki, D.; Białasiewicz, P. Disruption of Circadian Rhythm Genes in Obstructive Sleep Apnea Patients-Possible Mechanisms Involved and Clinical Implication. *Int. J. Mol. Sci.* **2022**, *23*, 709. [CrossRef]
46. Haqq, A.M.; DeLorey, D.S.; Sharma, A.M.; Freemark, M.; Kreier, F.; Mackenzie, M.L.; Richer, L.P. Autonomic nervous system dysfunction in obesity and Prader-Willi syndrome: Current evidence and implications for future obesity therapies. *Clin. Obes.* **2011**, *1*, 175–183. [CrossRef]
47. Kim, J.; Jung, H.R.; Kim, J.B.; Kim, D.J. Autonomic Dysfunction in Sleep Disorders: From Neurobiological Basis to Potential Therapeutic Approaches. *J. Clin. Neurol* **2022**, *18*, 140–151. [CrossRef]
48. Centers for Disease Control and Prevention. CDC Growh Charts. Available online: http://www.cdc.gov/growthcharts/cdc_charts.htm (accessed on 5 July 2017).

49. Iber, C.; Ancoli-Israel, S.; Cheeson, A.L.; Quan, S.F. *The AASM Manual for the Scoring of Sleep and Associated Events: Rules, Terminology and Technical Specifications*; American Academy of Sleep Medicine: Westchester, IL, USA, 2007.
50. The AASM Manual for the Scoring of Sleep and Associated Events. Available online: https://aasm.org/clinical-resources/scoring-manual/ (accessed on 3 January 2022).
51. Sateia, M.J. International Classification of Sleep Disorders-Third Edition. *Chest* **2014**, *146*, 1387–1394. Available online: https://journal.chestnet.org/article/S0012-3692(15)52407-0/fulltext (accessed on 7 August 2022). [CrossRef]

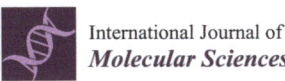

Article

Evaluation of Autonomic Nervous System Dysfunction in Childhood Obesity and Prader–Willi Syndrome

Lawrence P. Richer [1], Qiming Tan [1], Merlin G. Butler [2], Hayford M. Avedzi [1], Darren S. DeLorey [3], Ye Peng [4], Hein M. Tun [4], Arya M. Sharma [5], Steven Ainsley [1], Camila E. Orsso [6], Lucila Triador [1], Michael Freemark [7] and Andrea M. Haqq [1,7,*]

1. Department of Pediatrics, University of Alberta, Edmonton, AB T6G 2R3, Canada
2. Departments of Psychiatry & Behavioral Sciences and Pediatrics, Kansas University Medical Center, Kansas City, KS 66160, USA
3. Faculty of Kinesiology, Sport, and Recreation, University of Alberta, Edmonton, AB T6G 2R3, Canada
4. JC School of Public Health, Faculty of Medicine, The Chinese University of Hong Kong, Hong Kong 999077, China
5. Department of Medicine, University of Alberta, Edmonton, AB T6G 2R3, Canada
6. Department of Agricultural Food & Nutritional Science, University of Alberta, Edmonton, AB T6G 2R3, Canada
7. Division of Pediatric Endocrinology, Duke University Medical Center, Durham, NC 27705, USA
* Correspondence: haqq@ualberta.ca

Abstract: The autonomic nervous system (ANS) may play a role in the distribution of body fat and the development of obesity and its complications. Features of individuals with Prader–Willi syndrome (PWS) impacted by PWS molecular genetic classes suggest alterations in ANS function; however, these have been rarely studied and presented with conflicting results. The aim of this study was to investigate if the ANS function is altered in PWS. In this case-control study, we assessed ANS function in 20 subjects with PWS (6 males/14 females; median age 10.5 years) and 27 body mass index (BMI) z-score-matched controls (19 males/8 females; median age 12.8 years). Standardized non-invasive measures of cardiac baroreflex function, heart rate, blood pressure, heart rate variability, quantitative sudomotor axon reflex tests, and a symptom questionnaire were completed. The increase in heart rate in response to head-up tilt testing was blunted ($p < 0.01$) in PWS compared to controls. Besides a lower heart rate ratio with Valsalva in PWS ($p < 0.01$), no significant differences were observed in other measures of cardiac function or sweat production. Findings suggest possible altered sympathetic function in PWS.

Keywords: autonomic nervous system (ANS); childhood obesity; genetics; Prader–Willi syndrome (PWS)

1. Introduction

Childhood obesity, regardless of the cause, increases risks for early onset cardio-metabolic morbidity, premature mortality, and higher healthcare costs [1–3]. Prader–Willi syndrome (PWS) is the most common syndromic form of obesity and recognized as an extreme model in humans. PWS is a multisystem genetic disorder that occurs in all races and ethnicities with comparable rates in males and females [4,5]. PWS is due to errors in genomic imprinting, most often by a paternal loss of expression of imprinted genes in the 15q11-q13 region [6–8].

Approximately 60% of individuals with PWS show a paternally derived 15q11-q13 deletion (DEL15), 35% have uniparental disomy 15 (UDP15), or both 15s from the mother; while the remaining have imprinting center defects, translocations or inversions involving chromosome 15 [8]. Clinical and behavioral differences have been identified in those with PWS having the 15q11-q13 deletion or with maternal disomy 15. Those with maternal disomy 15 have a higher verbal IQ, delayed diagnosis, and more psychosis or autistic behavior than those with the deletion [9–11]. The individuals with PWS and the deletion are more prone to have compulsions, self-injury, higher pain threshold and hypopigmentation compared with those having maternal disomy 15 [9,12–16].

Dozens of genes and/or transcripts are identified between chromosome 15q11-q13 breakpoints associated with PWS and are prone to non-homologous recombination leading to 15q11-q13 deletions observed in PWS. Genes in the 15q11-q13 region contain both imprinted (NDN, MAGEL2, MKRN3, SNURF-SNRPN, SNORDs, UBE3A, ATP10A) and non-imprinted (NIPA1, NIPA2, CYFIP1, TUBGCP5, GABA receptors, OCA2) genes [6–8]. These genes and their encoded protein functions are implicated in neurodevelopment, motor control, behavioral issues, learning disabilities, autism, hyperphagia, obesity, hypogonadism, infertility, precocious puberty, sleep disturbances, skin pigment production, and hormone and metabolic disturbances (Figure 1) [6–9,16,17].

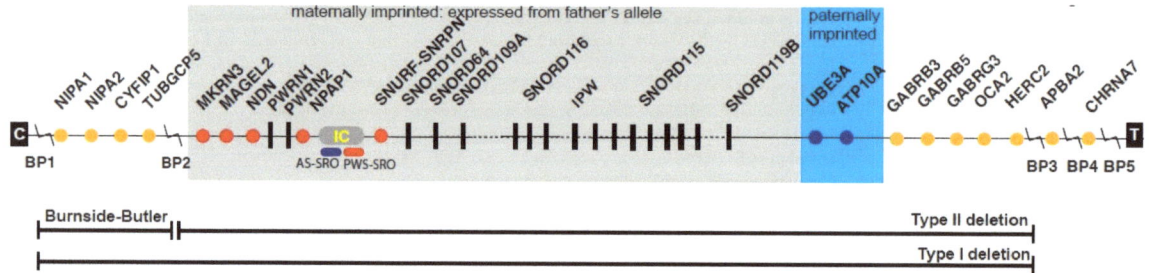

Figure 1. Linear order of genes and transcripts with their location from the proximal long arm of chromosome 15 in Prader–Willi syndrome (PWS). Three recognized deletions are shown including the larger typical 15q11-q13 Type I deletion involving breakpoints BP1 and BP3, and smaller typical 15q11-q13 Type II deletion involving BP2 and BP3, both causing PWS and Angelman syndrome (AS) depending on the parent of origin. The 15q11.2 BP1-BP2 deletion (Burnside–Butler) involves only BP1 and BP2. Nonimprinted genes are shown in orange while maternally imprinted genes (paternally expressed) are shown in red and paternally imprinted genes (maternally expressed) are shaded in blue. Abbreviations: BP, breakpoint; IC, imprinting center; PWS-SRO, PWS smallest region of overlap; AS-SRO, AS smallest region of overlap; C and T, centromere and telomere locations (from Butler, Lee, and Whitman [9] with permission from publisher).

The autonomic nervous system (ANS) involvement in the pathogenesis of obesity and PWS has been summarized previously [18,19]. The ANS, composed of the central autonomic network and peripheral components (i.e., sympathetic, parasympathetic, and enteric nervous systems), maintains homeostasis by regulating essential physiological processes such as heart rate, blood pressure, breathing, digestion, body temperature, hormone production, and sexual arousal with many of these features disturbed in PWS [20]. Individuals with PWS often exhibit oropharyngeal and bowel dysmotility, abnormal temperature regulation (reduction in core temperature in response to cold stress), altered sleep control (excessive daytime somnolence, a primary abnormality of the circadian rhythm of rapid eye movement sleep, and insensitivity to hypoxia and hypercarbia), altered perception of pain (markedly altered cold and heat pain sensations not attributed to peripheral nerve involvement) [21], and decreased salivation [22,23]. Functional magnetic resonance imaging (MRI) studies of adults with PWS have shown significant delay in activation of areas subserving satiety and autonomic function including the hypothalamus, insula, ventromedial prefrontal cortex, and nucleus accumbens [24]. Other investigations have shown alternation in the medial prefrontal cortex (MPFC)/inferior parietal lobe (IPL), MPFC/precuneus, IPL/precuneus, and IPL/hippocampus, and other regions in the resting state.

Prefrontal circuitry is an important factor determining hunger and satiety. When compared with simple obesity and healthy weight controls, those with PWS demonstrated higher activity in the reward/limbic regions (nucleus accumbens, amygdala) and lower activity in the hypothalamus and hippocampus in response to food versus non-food images before food consumption [25–29]. In PWS, hyperactivations in subcortical reward circuitry and hypoactivations in cortical inhibitory regions were found after eating which provided evidence of neural substrates associated with variable abnormal food motivation phenotypes in PWS and those with simple obesity. The results point to distinct neural mechanisms associated with hyperphagia in PWS. These studies lend evidence for the role of the ANS in obesity and specifically in PWS. PWS is recognized as an extreme form of obesity in humans and can serve as a unique model to study the functional connectivity in brain regions implicated in eating, reward, and ANS function with alterations in PWS [30].

Startle response as an involuntary reflex activated by the ANS has been investigated in PWS [31]. This reflex is in response to sudden or disturbed auditory/visual stimuli which may be modulated by the emotional valence of concurrently viewed visual stimuli. The subjective ratings of food images and urge to eat were significantly higher in PWS than controls and did not significantly decline post meal. Acoustic startle response was detected in PWS but was significantly lower than controls under all conditions. Abnormal responses to food images in PWS were attenuated relative to other picture types with potentially abnormal emotional modulation of responses to non-food images which contrasted self-reported picture ratings. A stable positive emotional valence to food images was observed pre-and post-feeding with a sustained urge to consume food in PWS. Possibly, a disruption of the autonomic or sympathetic nervous system functioning reported in PWS may impact on hunger and/or food drive states. These studies support the feasibility of eyeblink startle modulation to assess food motivation in PWS and provide preliminary data to stimulate additional studies. These studies would optimize methodological parameters to judge more objectively hyperphagia in PWS than currently available subjective hyperphagia questionnaire forms in use.

Experimental animal models of PWS suggest specific abnormalities in the development of the sympathetic nervous system [32]. Necdin is one of several proteins that are genetically inactivated in PWS and it is important in the differentiation of sensory neurons. Necdin-null mice have diminished formation, migration, and survival of the sympathetic superior cervical ganglion neurons (the most rostral of the paravertebral sympathetic ganglions innervating the pupil, lacrimal, salivary glands, and cerebral blood vessels) and reduced innervation of target systems [32]. Furthermore, axonal extension is impaired throughout the sympathetic nervous system in necdin-null mice.

Unlike exogenous childhood obesity, which is caused primarily by external modifiable risk factors such as physical inactivity and unhealthy diet, PWS is characterized by certain hormonal and biochemical adaptations that may increase the risk for obesity [19]. For example, adolescents and children with PWS have higher insulin sensitivity than children with comparable body mass index (BMI) z-scores [33] and have higher fasting and post-prandial levels of ghrelin, a circulatory peptide produced in the stomach that stimulates appetite and promotes weight gain [34–36]. Likewise, the ratio between acylated and unacylated ghrelin was elevated in a recent study of 138 children and adults with PWS [37].

Food intake is controlled by the hypothalamus including the melanocortin and neuropeptide Y (NPY) systems in the arcuate nucleus [34,35]. Ghrelin is short-lived but stimulates eating behavior while peptide YY (PYY), released post-prandially in proportion to caloric intake, remains elevated for several hours and decreases eating [36,38]. Ghrelin levels are inversely correlated with body weight, higher during starvation and increased during weight loss in humans [36,38]. Total ghrelin levels are suppressed in non-PWS children and adults with exogenous obesity or with obesity caused by mutations in leptin or the melanocortin-4 receptor [39]. The mechanisms underlying hyperghrelinemia in PWS remain unclear at this time but prohormone convertase PC1 required to cleave inactive prohormones including POMC (pro-opio-melanocortin, key for hypothalamic appetite regulation) into individual active peptides appears abnormal in PWS. It may play a role in hormone production and function in PWS [40]. Yet, two recent open trials of vagus nerve stimulation showed improvements in maladaptive behavior, temperament, social functioning, and food-seeking behavior, but not weight in adults with PWS [41,42]. These findings suggest that increased vagal nerve efferent activity to the gastrointestinal tract in PWS may contribute to the higher concentrations of ghrelin seen in this disorder. Furthermore, gene expression studies of ghrelin detected no differences in the pattern of gene expression in the brain between those with or without PWS [43].

Recent studies have shown that prohormone convertase PC1 disturbances are associated with the PWS clinical phenotype impacting several hormones in PWS. These hormone disturbances lead to hyperphagic obesity, short stature, hypogonadism, growth and other hormone deficiencies, high ghrelin, and relatively low insulin levels thought to be due to impaired prohormone processing [40]. Burnett et al. [40] reported reduced levels and activity of prohormone convertase PC1 in PWS and proposed that humans and mice deficient in PC1 display hyperphagic-related obesity. Many PWS features may be due to impaired prohormone processing and lack of active hormones required for normal multiple organ systems in PWS. For example, POMC is a large prohormone that requires cleavage from an inactive prohormone status to smaller active peptides for normal appetite regulation and eating behavior. Several major abnormal neuroendocrine clinical findings seen in PWS could be due to PC1 deficiency also impacting ANS function [18,33,44,45].

Few human studies have evaluated autonomic regulation in PWS and have typically used only indirect measures of autonomic function [19]. One study reported diminished parasympathetic nervous system function based on findings of higher resting heart rate and reduced increases in diastolic blood pressure upon standing [46]. However, when controlling for BMI, other studies report no differences in the autonomic control of cardiac reflexes on heart rate and blood pressure in PWS subjects [47]. The purpose of the present study was to determine if autonomic symptoms and metrics of cardiac autonomic reflex control and post-ganglionic autonomic innervation of sweat glands differ between children with PWS and age- and BMI z-score-matched controls.

2. Results

2.1. Participant Characteristics

Baseline participant characteristics are summarized in Table 1. Twenty children with PWS (median age and BMI z-score: 10.8 years and 0.7, respectively) participated in this study. We recruited 27 control subjects with age and BMI z-scores as close as possible to participants with PWS (median age and BMI z-score: 12.8 years and 0.2, respectively). Some controls were siblings or friends of the participants with PWS, while others were recruited from the local Pediatric Centre for Weight and Health. Due to random chance, a higher percentage of children with PWS were female (70%) as opposed to the control group (30%). Eleven subjects with PWS were taking recombinant human growth hormone (rhGH) (mean dose 0.02 mg/kg/d) at the time of the study [48]. Referring physicians made the initial decisions whether to treat with rhGH and patients had been receiving GH intervention for at least 1 year at the time of study. There was no significant difference in characteristics between PWS patients and PWS patients on rhGH intervention ($p > 0.05$). All participants with PWS had free thyroxine (T4) and thyroid stimulating hormone (TSH) levels in the normal range (either endogenous or on replacement); three participants with PWS were on thyroid replacement to treat central hypothyroidism.

Table 1. Characteristics of study participants.

	PWS			Controls			p-Values [1]
	n	Median (25th, 75th Percentiles)	Mean (SD)	n	Median (25th, 75th Percentiles)	Mean (SD)	
Age, years	20	10.5 (7.1, 14.3)	10.8 (3.9)	27	12.8 (9.0, 14.0)	12.2 (3.1)	0.17
Male/Female	6/14	-	-	19/8	-	-	0.006 *
Weight, z-score	20	0.3 (−0.4, 1.0)	0.3 (1.3)	27	0.4 (−0.03, 0.9)	0.4 (0.9)	0.77
Height, z-score	20	−0.9 (−1.9, −0.2)	−0.9 (1.1)	27	0.2 (−0.4, 0.8)	0.2 (0.8)	0.0003 *
BMI, z-score	20	0.7 (0.2, 1.5)	0.8 (1.1)	27	0.2 (−0.5, 1.1)	0.3 (1.0)	0.15
WC (cm)	19	71.7 (56.5, 87.2)	76.1 (23.2)	24	67.0 (58.4, 72.4)	67.4 (15.8)	0.39

BMI z-scores were calculated using EpiInfo (CDC, Atlanta, GA). Independent samples *t*-test was used to evaluate differences between groups [1]. Statistically significant ($p < 0.05$) *. Abbreviations: PWS, Prader–Willi syndrome; SD, standard deviation; BMI, body mass index; WC, waist circumference.

2.2. Genetics of PWS Patients

Of the 20 PWS patients, 12 patients had the 15q11-q13 deletion (DEL15) form of the syndrome, 6 patients had uniparental disomy 15 (UPD15), whereas 2 cases were unclear. There was no significant difference between the characteristics for DEL15 patients and UPD15 patients ($p > 0.05$) (Table 2).

Table 2. Genetics of Prader–Willi syndrome participants.

Characteristic	Overall, $n = 18$ [1]	Deletion, $n = 12$ [1]	UPD, $n = 6$ [1]	p-Value [2]
Resting supine HR	74 (64, 82)	66 (60, 80)	81 (72, 85)	0.15
(Missing)	4	3	1	
Max HR	117 (111, 126)	117 (104, 126)	116 (113, 123)	>0.9
(Missing)	4	3	1	
Max change HR	41 (34, 47)	41 (36, 53)	38 (31, 42)	0.2
(Missing)	4	3	1	
Max change in SBP	−38 (−48, −28)	−42 (−55, −33)	−30 (−37, −28)	0.4
(Missing)	5	4	1	
Valsalva–HR ratio	1.61 (1.45, 1.91)	1.80 (1.62, 1.97)	1.50 (1.37, 1.63)	0.3
(Missing)	10	8	2	
Valsalva–HR ratio (per protocol)	1.91 (1.54, 1.92)	1.92 (1.68, 2.01)	1.73 (1.63, 1.82)	0.8
(Missing)	13	9	4	
HR Deep Breathing	22 (18, 28)	23 (19, 28)	20 (17, 21)	0.4
(Missing)	3	2	1	
HR Deep Breathing (per protocol)	22.4 (20.8, 26.1)	22.8 (21.1, 25.1)	21.9 (20.5, 29.8)	>0.9
(Missing)	8	5	3	
Duration of HRDB	45.0 (43.0, 45.0)	45.0 (37.5, 45.0)	45.0 (44.0, 45.5)	0.6
(Missing)	8	5	3	

Data presented as Median (Inter-Quartile Range (IQR)) [1]. Wilcoxon rank sum test and Wilcoxon rank sum exact test were used to evaluate differences between groups. *p*-value for independent groups *t*-test (approximately normal distribution); Mann–Whitney U test (non-normal distribution) [2]. Statistically significant ($p < 0.05$). Abbreviations: UPD, uniparental disomy; HR, heart rate; SBP, systolic blood pressure, HRDB, heart rate deep breathing.

2.3. Autonomic Symptom Questionnaire

An ANS symptom questionnaire was used to describe the self-reported presence and frequency of symptoms on an ordinal scale: 0 = never, 1 = <once per month, 2 = 2–4 times per month, 3 = 5–7 times per month, 4 = most days, and 5 = daily. Of this cohort, 90% ($n = 18$) of the participants with PWS and 70% ($n = 19$) of the controls completed their ANS evaluation. Comparison of results in PWS individuals versus controls is shown in a heatmap (Figure 2). There were significant differences in the presence and frequency of various domains, including cardiovascular (i.e., discoloration of hands or feet), gastrointestinal (i.e., dry mouth, decreased saliva secretion, bloating, feeding difficulty, and

food preoccupation), thermoregulation (i.e., flush, low temperature, and excess sweat), neurological (i.e., lack of coordination in movement, fatigue, excessive daytime sleepiness, pain tolerance, sleeping issues, feeling of weakness, and pain in hands/feet), and psychological (excessive/inappropriate emotional reactions, anxiety, socialization, memory, confusion, learning disability, school performance, and tics) symptoms between the two groups. Dry mouth and decreased saliva secretion, lack of coordination in movement, and excessive/inappropriate emotional reactions were particularly common in PWS.

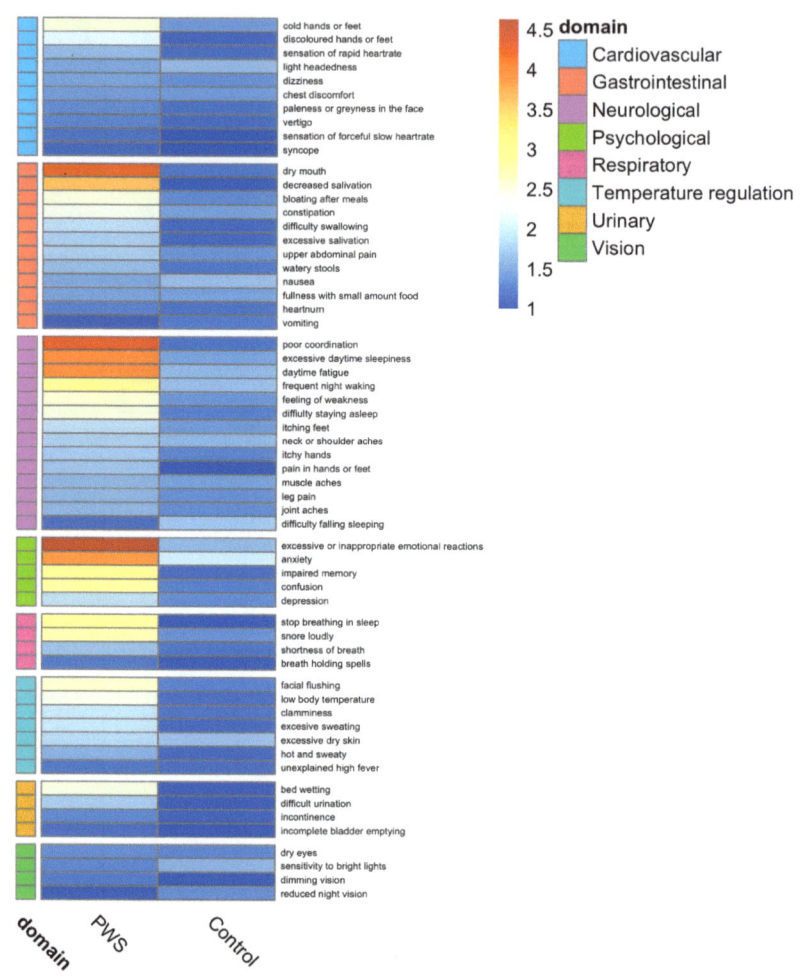

Figure 2. Evaluation of the presence and frequency of cardiovagal, gastrointestinal, thermoregulatory, neuropathic, and psychological symptoms in Prader–Willi Syndrome and control groups. Ordinal frequency scale: 0 = never, 1 = <once per month, 2 = 2–4 times per month, 3 = 5–7 times per month, 4 = most days, and 5 = daily.

2.4. Clinical Autonomic Cardiac Reflex Testing

Results of the clinical autonomic cardiac reflex tests, including 70 degrees head-up tilt (HUT), Valsalva maneuver, and heart rate deep breathing (HRDB), and associated heart rate and non-invasive blood pressure and group comparisons are shown in Table 3. There was a significant difference between PWS and control groups in the maximum change in heart rate from baseline on the HUT test ($p < 0.01$). On Valsalva maneuver, the median heart rate ratio with Valsalva was significantly lower in the PWS group ($p < 0.01$) compared with controls at 1.68 (95% CI 1.45, 1.92). However, the heart rate ratio in the PWS group was above the normal threshold of 1.20 used in our clinical laboratory. In the per protocol analysis, the heart rate ratio with Valsalva was 1.92 (95% CI 1.63, 2.06) in the PWS group, and the difference between groups was no longer significant ($p = 0.059$). The average heart rate difference between inspiration and expiration with HRDB was not significantly different between groups (Table 3).

Table 3. Clinical Autonomic Cardiac Reflex Testing: Head-up tilt, Valsalva, Heart Rate Deep Breathing, and Quantitative Sudomotor Axon Reflex Test and group comparisons.

Characteristic	Group [1]		p-Values [2]
	Control n = 19	PWS n = 18	
	Head-Up Tilt		
Resting supine HR			0.2
Median (IQR)	66 (61, 74)	74 (65, 82)	
(Missing)	1	2	
Max HR			0.12
Median (IQR)	124 (118, 132)	117 (112, 124)	
(Missing)	1	2	
Max change HR			0.002 *
Median (IQR)	55 (49, 60)	41 (35, 50)	
(Missing)	1	2	
Max change in SBP			0.4
Median (IQR)	−44 (−64, −34)	−38 (−47, −27)	
(Missing)	1	3	
	Valsalva and Deep Breathing		
Valsalva—HR ratio			0.007 *
Median (IQR)	2.28 (1.94, 2.44)	1.68 (1.45, 1.92)	
(Missing)	1	9	
Valsalva—HR ratio (per protocol)			0.059
Median (IQR)	2.29 (2.00, 2.46)	1.92 (1.63, 2.06)	
(Missing)	2	12	
HR Deep Breathing			0.7
Median (IQR)	26 (20, 31)	22 (18, 29)	
(Missing)	1	1	
HR Deep Breathing (per protocol)			0.7
Median (IQR)	24 (18, 31)	23 (21, 27)	
(Missing)	3	7	
Duration of HRDB			0.12
Median (IQR)	45.0 (44.8, 46.2)	45.0 (42.5, 45.0)	
(Missing)	3	7	

Data presented as Median (Inter-Quartile Range (IQR) [1]. p-value for independent groups t-test (approximately normal distribution); Mann–Whitney U test (non-normal distribution); Wilcoxon rank sum test and Wilcoxon rank sum exact test were used to evaluate differences between groups [2]. Statistically significant ($p < 0.05$) *. Abbreviations: PWS, Prader–Willi syndrome; HR, Heart rate; SBP, systolic blood pressure; HRDB, heart rate deep breathing.

2.5. Heart Rate Variability

Heart rate variability, which provides a secondary measure of sympathetic and parasympathetic tone on heart rate during the short term (5 min) component of HUT and 5 min of supine rest, was not significantly different between groups. Time domain metrics, included RMSSD, NN50, pNN50 [49], were not significantly different between groups at rest or HUT. Frequency domain measures included low frequency (LF)/high frequency (HF) power and were not significantly different between groups at rest (Controls 1.18 (95% CI 0.48, 2.02) and PWS 1.36 (95% CI 0.64, 1.88); $p = 0.8$) but were significantly different with HUT (Controls 1.34 (95% CI 0.99, 2.28) and PWS 2.57 (95% CI 1.52, 4.62); $p = 0.035$).

2.6. Quantitative Sudomotor Axon Reflex Test

The volume of quantitative sudomotor axon reflex test (QSART) was not well tolerated among participants with missing data at one or more testing among 19 of 20 in the control group and 23 of 24 in the PWS group. The forearm and proximal leg sites had fewer participants missing with 2 in the control group and 12 in the PWS group. Non-parametric analysis of available data showed no statistically significant difference between groups, but the frequency of missing data and low power makes interpretation problematic. Potential group differences in stroke volume were not measured.

2.7. Pupillometry

The pupillometry procedure was also poorly tolerated among participants and many refused the procedure. With available data, the mean increase in pupil size (mydriasis) following the application of 5% cocaine to the conjunctiva was normally distributed and not significantly different ($p = 0.532$) between groups, with a mean of 1.51 mm (SD 0.85, $n = 9$) for the controls and 1.28 mm (SD 0.71, $n = 10$) for participants with PWS. There was, however, a significant difference in the baseline pupil size ($p = 0.038$); the control group members had a larger baseline pupil size (mean 5.21 mm, SD 0.52) than the PWS group members (mean 4.59 mm, SD 0.67).

3. Discussion

This study investigated the clinical autonomic phenotype, cardiac autonomic reflexes, and peripheral small nerve fiber sudomotor (sweat) function of 47 participants, including 20 individuals with PWS and 27 BMI z-score-matched controls. The most striking observation was the notable participant and parent-reported differences in the frequency of signs and symptoms often associated with peripheral autonomic nerve dysfunction like dry mouth, decreased salivation, pain insensitivity as well as more general symptoms often associated with autonomic dysfunction like fatigue and daytime sleepiness. The study aimed to examine measures of autonomic function including cardiac reflexes, heart rate variability, sudomotor function, and pupillometry. The primary observation was a blunted heart rate response to HUT among PWS participants compared with age and weight-matched controls. This finding may suggest a blunted sympathetically mediated heart rate response to HUT or higher vagally mediated parasympathetic tone. There were no significant associated differences observed in the decrease of systolic blood pressure with HUT, suggesting peripheral autonomic control, including sympathetic control on cardiac output and peripheral vascular resistance, was similar between groups [50]. We did not detect any significant differences between groups in other measures of parasympathetically mediated autonomic control, including Valsalva and HRDB. While a significant difference in the maximum heart rate ratio was observed with Valsalva maneuver, the group mean was above a normal threshold and the difference did not persist in the per protocol analysis. The difference in heart rate variability on the LF/HF ratio with HUT was more likely to have been observed by chance when accounting for multiple comparisons. Finally, the data on sudomotor (sweat) response on QSART was insufficient to draw any conclusions.

Our findings may be consistent with experimental findings reported by other groups. In the mouse model of PWS (necdin-null mouse), loss of necdin impairs the survival and axonal elongation of sympathetic neurons and reduces the innervation of target glands with most rostral of sympathetic ganglia being affected [32]. Necdin appears to be crucial for the rostral migration and survival, but not proliferation, of the sympathetic superior cervical ganglion neurons; axonal extension is also impaired throughout the sympathetic nervous system. Impaired sympathetic function may explain, in part, the blunted heart rate response to HUT in the absence of evident parasympathetic dysfunction in PWS. Castner et al. also observed lower peak heart rate to a bicycle exercise test in PWS as compared with control weight and obese groups [51]. Additionally, in this study, all groups displayed similar heart rate recovery from peak exercise, while control (54 ± 16 beats) and obese group (50 ± 12 beats) subjects exhibited a significantly faster heart rate recovery from submaximal exercise than subjects with PWS (37 ± 14 beats) [51]. A delayed heart rate recovery in PWS from submaximal intensity exercise compared to normal weight controls also suggests possible ANS dysfunction. To the conclusion of the authors, these findings may be consistent with impaired sympathetically mediated heart rate responses to various stimuli in children with PWS. It should be noted that there are deletions of genes other than necdin in PWS; a major target is MAGEL2, which conveys information about autonomic status to the peripheral autonomic system [52]. Therefore, we might predict combined central and peripheral autonomic dysfunction in individuals with PWS.

The heart rate response to orthostatic stress like HUT reflects the combination of increased sympathetic and noradrenergic neurotransmission to the heart, and withdrawal of parasympathetic and vagal transmission. A blunted sympathetic and noradrenergic response in PWS compared with normal controls is one possible explanation of our findings given the absence of parasympathetic or vagally mediated dysfunction in other tests. However, all of the observed reflexes share sympathetic and parasympathetic inputs, and we did not perform specific tests of sympathetic function such as muscle sympathetic nerve activity (MSNA). Differences in peripheral vascular resistance and stroke volume may also contribute to group differences but were not measured.

Our findings also revealed no significant differences in LF and HF cardiac autonomic modulation or in the LF/HF ratio. These findings are in agreement with Baharav et al. who found no differences in cardiac autonomic modulation between patients with PWS and controls [53], and Wade et al., who found no difference in cardiac autonomic function during supine, standing, sitting, exercising or recovery measurements (LF, HF or LF:HF ratio) in 26 children with PWS compared to 26 age-, gender-, and BMI-matched controls [47]. Goldstone et al. reported abnormal (decreased) parasympathetic vagal innervation of the stomach as a possible reason for the elevation in ghrelin seen in PWS [54]. However, besides decreased salivation, we did not observe any evidence for parasympathetic dysfunction in PWS in the present study; interestingly, the necdin-null mice exhibit reduced sympathetic innervation of the intestinal tract but no defects in the parasympathetic innervation [32].

We observed notable differences in the pattern of symptoms reported by PWS and control participants on the ANS symptom questionnaire. Yet, decreased salivation and dry mouth were more frequently reported in PWS, as has been commonly observed [23,55,56]. The secretion of saliva is predominantly under parasympathetic control via the facial and glossopharyngeal cranial nerves [57], so decreased salivation may suggest alterations in parasympathetic control or innervation of the salivary glands.

Pain insensitivity is also a well-documented symptom in PWS. We did not observe any evidence of small fiber nerve dysfunction as assessed by the sudomotor (sweat) function test, but significant missing data make our observations problematic. Priano et al. conducted a detailed neurophysiological battery of tests in 14 adults with PWS, 10 controls with obesity but no diabetes, and 10 age-matched lean controls [21]. Normal electroneurographic, sympathetic skin responses, and somatosensory-evoked potentials were found in all three groups. Thermal and pain thresholds, but not vibration, were significantly elevated in PWS compared to obese or lean controls. They suggested that abnormalities of the small nociceptive neurons of the dorsal root ganglia or hypothalamic region may be implicated.

Other general neurological symptoms including lack of coordination, excessive daytime sleepiness, and fatigue were also commonly reported in PWS. Defects in gross motor performance may develop as a consequence of an abnormal body composition and decreased physical activity. However, growth hormone therapy has been shown to improve motor development and body composition in children with PWS [58,59].

Arousals and respiratory events (central and obstructive sleep apnea) disrupt sleep by producing prolonged awakenings and thus shortening total sleep time, which may cause daytime sleepiness in PWS. However, even when the quantity and quality of sleep appears sufficient, many children with PWS complain of excessive sleepiness and fatigue [60,61], which can be highly disruptive to the daily routines of patients and their families, and affects clinical care and learning [62]. Moreover, excessive sleepiness and circadian disruption can reduce energy expenditure and promote food-seeking behavior [63,64], thereby contributing to the overweight and obesity observed in PWS. The ANS plays key roles in appetite, food intake, hormone production, body temperature, and sleep [63]; thus deficits in ANS function in PWS may require interventions in order to forestall chronic disease. Some case reports suggested that modafinil may effectively treat the sleep disturbances and excessive daytime sleepiness in PWS, but more clinical trials are needed [65,66].

Individuals with PWS exhibited significantly higher levels of psychological dysfunction with multiple areas of disturbance compared to controls. Lack of emotional regulation, anxiety, and difficulties of social adaptation suggest disturbances in social and emotional competencies in these patients [67]. Current knowledge is incomplete, hindering appropriate clinical care; hence, more studies characterizing the emotional/behavioral functioning of people with PWS are required [67].

The unique constellation of symptoms observed in children with PWS based on an autonomic symptom questionnaire could be validated by some objective assessments. In our current study, the rise in heart rate during HUT testing was reduced in children with PWS compared to controls, suggesting possible altered ANS function in PWS and corroborates findings in other studies [50,51]. Given the difficulty and lack of standardized autonomic tests and well-established ranges of normal values for children, and non-availability of testing facilities nor experts [68], complete objective ANS testing could be used in future, to validate the autonomic symptom questionnaire as an alternative screener for detecting ANS function accurately in children with PWS.

Emerging evidence points to specific genetic causes explaining autonomic dysregulation in certain conditions [18,69]. In future, detailed molecular genetic testing might be carried out in order to isolate and identify the genes in question and make early personalized preventative and treatment plans [18,69].

A major strength of the current study is the recruitment and comparison of ANS function in a sizeable sample of children with PWS to controls. Given that PWS is a rare genetic condition, it is often difficult to recruit and administer a battery of tests on individuals who exhibit high levels of anxiety and other psychological and social disturbances.

The strengths of this study notwithstanding, we encountered some limitations as follows. The best standardized battery of tests presently available for testing ANS function were used in this study. However, there are known limitations in the testing of ANS function [68], especially in children. As such, children who participated in this study may have found it difficult adhering to the strict protocol for ANS testing provided in the lab. This may have resulted in some variability; for example, participants had difficulty breathing at the prescribed rate during the HRDB test and also had difficulty achieving and maintaining the required expiratory pressure during the Valsalva test, evidenced by the number of missing data points for each of these assessments (Table 2). Given that our focus, however, was the comparison of PWS and controls under the same conditions, the results are still valid across groups. Finally, we also observed missing data from both the PWS and control groups at random, further highlighting the difficulty associated with testing ANS function in children. Improvements to the comprehensiveness and protocol for testing ANS function in children are therefore needed to enhance reproducibility of tests and results in pediatric populations. Another limitation of the present study was the higher preponderance of female participants in the PWS group compared to controls. This precluded a systematic sex-stratified analysis. Despite more pronounced parasympathetic cardiac regulation, women have been reported to have a higher resting heart rate and lower baroreflex sensitivity [70]. Yet despite the predominance of females in the PWS group, their maximum heart rate responses were lower than those in the control group. Unfortunately, we did not investigate the origins of altered pain perception in participants with PWS.

4. Materials and Methods

4.1. Subjects

Children with genetically confirmed PWS ($n = 20$) were recruited for this study from pediatric endocrinology and genetics clinics at the University of Alberta, University of Calgary, and from across Canada and the United States. Age, weight z-score, and BMI z-score-matched controls ($n = 27$) were recruited from the Pediatric Centre for Weight and Health in Edmonton, Alberta. Potential participants were excluded if they had diabetes mellitus, chronic inflammatory bowel disease, severe liver or kidney disease, neurologic disorder, or claustrophobia. The study protocol was approved by the human research ethics committee of the University of Alberta (Pro00009903). All participants and parents provided written informed consent prior to taking part in the study.

4.2. Autonomic Symptom Questionnaire

An autonomic symptom questionnaire was used to assess symptoms of autonomic function in each of the following organ system domains: cardiovascular, respiratory, gastrointestinal and eating behaviours, urinary, temperature regulation, neurological, psychological, and vision [71–74]. Questions (e.g., "How often does your child experience difficulty emptying the bladder?") were answered based on frequency of symptoms with the following ordinal options: never, <once per month, 2–4 times per month, 5–7 times per month, most days, and daily. Participants were encouraged to seek clarification if there was uncertainty about the question.

4.3. Pupillometry

Pupillometry, a test of sympathetic innervation of the pupil, was performed by applying a topical ophthalmologic solution of 5% cocaine to the conjunctiva of one eye of those participants who consented to the procedure [75,76]. After 15 min, the pupils were photographed without a flash and pupil diameter was measured. The online image processing software, ImageJ.JS 1.53m (https://ij.imjoy.io/ accessed on 10 January 2021), was used for analysis of pupil diameter.

4.4. Clinical Autonomic Cardiac Reflex Testing

A battery of standard ANS clinical assessments, including HRDB, Valsalva maneuver, 70 degrees HUT, and QSART were used to assess both cardiac autonomic reflexes and sudomotor function [71]. The electrocardiogram (ECG) was measured continuously with a digital sampling rate of 200 Hz and heart rate was derived from ECG waveform [77]. Finger arterial blood pressure was measured continuously during each procedure using a finger cuff and infrared plethysmograph (Finometer PRO, Finapress Medical Systems BV, Amsterdam, The Netherlands). All autonomic assessments and signals were captured in an integrated digital recording platform (WR TestWorks®, Stillwater, MN, USA). The HRDB procedure required the participant to follow a metronome to breathe at approximately 6 breaths per minute for a total of 8 breaths [71]. At least two attempts were made with a rest interval of 5 min in between. The average heart rate difference between inspiration and expiration for the best HRDB response was included in the analysis, and the time taken for 5 breaths was recorded. The Valsalva maneuver involved maintaining an expiratory pressure of 40 mm Hg for 15 s, blowing into a mouthpiece with high expiratory outflow resistance to increase intrathoracic pressure transiently [71]. The maximum heart rate during Valsalva and lower heart rate within 30 s after Valsalva was recorded as the heart ratio. The greatest heart rate ratio was included in the analysis from two Valsalva attempts conducted with a 5 min rest interval in between.

In addition, heart rate variability at rest and in response to HUT was assessed using time domain and frequency domain analysis [78]. For frequency domain analysis, the power density spectrum was integrated, and power spectra within the 0.04–0.15 Hz range were defined as LF components, whereas those at 0.15–0.4 Hz frequency were defined as HF components. Autoregressive spectral analysis was used to derive the frequency domain measures in high (HF), low (LF), and very low frequencies (VLF). The LF/HF power ratio was also determined as an indirect measure of sympathovagal balance [78].

QSART [79] was used to quantify postganglionic sweat output resulting from axon reflex stimulation using acetylcholine iontophoresis. The QSART device (Q-Sweat, WR Medical Inc., Stillwater, MN, USA) was used to measure sweat output, indicative of the sudomotor response at the foot, distal leg, proximal leg, and ipsilateral forearm.

4.5. Statistical Analysis

The a priori statistical analysis was performed on all available data. Considerable efforts were made to obtain high quality data from each participant, but the autonomic testing maneuvers described above were performed with variable degrees of adherence. As a quality and sensitivity analysis, a per protocol analysis was also performed where data from procedures with inadequate adherence to the protocol were excluded. Normally distributed continuous variables were represented as mean ± standard deviation (SD); group differences in these variables were compared by Student's t-test. Other continuous variables were represented as medians and 25th and 75th percentiles of the interquartile ranges; group differences in these variables were compared by Wilcoxon's rank test. Categorical variables were described as frequencies and percentages, with the between-group difference tested by means of the chi-square test or Fisher's exact test when the number of events was less than 5. A p-value < 0.05 was considered statistically significant. The Statistical Package for the Social Sciences (SPSS) software (version 20.0; IBM Corp., Armonk, NY, USA) was used to analyze all data. R (version 4.2.2) [80], R-Studio (2022.12.0.353) [81], and tidyverse package [82] were used for the analysis of autonomic outcome measures, and the gtsummary package [83] was used for the formatting of reporting tables.

5. Conclusions

In summary, the increase of heart rate in response to HUT was reduced in children with PWS compared to controls, suggesting possible altered sympathetic function in PWS which is supported by the self- and parent-reported frequency of signs and symptoms associated with peripheral autonomic dysfunction compared to controls. There were no significant differences detected between groups for the other measures of parasympathetically mediated autonomic control, including Valsalva and HRDB. Our findings are supported by both studies in PWS mouse models and clinical trials of individuals with PWS. Future studies are needed to complete detailed molecular genetic testing to isolate and identify genes associated with central and peripheral autonomic dysfunction in PWS. Additionally, longitudinal studies of children and adults with PWS should determine if abnormalities in ANS function progress with age. These future studies may lead to the development of targeted treatment for ANS sympathetic dysfunction in PWS in order to improve exercise tolerance, gastrointestinal and respiratory function, and enhance overall quality of life. Future studies may also be used to validate the autonomic symptom questionnaire as a screening tool for detecting ANS dysfunction in individuals with PWS and enhance clinical care through early detection.

Author Contributions: L.P.R.: conceptualization, methodology, data collection, writing—original draft, and writing—review and editing; A.M.H.: conceptualization, methodology, resources, funding acquisition, supervision, writing—original draft, and writing—review and editing; C.E.O.: data curation, formal analysis; M.G.B., H.M.A., Q.T., D.S.D., Y.P., H.M.T., A.M.S., S.A., L.T. and M.F.: writing—review and editing. All authors have read and agreed to the published version of the manuscript.

Funding: This research was funded by the Canadian Institutes of Health Research (RES0011552, RES0011818); the Women and Children's Health Research Institute (RES0009935, RES0003532); University of Alberta start-up funds (RES0001726), and the Prader–Willi Syndrome Association of Alberta (RES0009325).

Institutional Review Board Statement: This study was conducted in accordance with the Declaration of Helsinki and approved by the Ethics Committee of the University of Alberta (protocol code Pro00009903, approval date of 19 March 2010).

Informed Consent Statement: Informed consent was obtained from all subjects involved in the study.

Data Availability Statement: The data are not publicly available due to ethical restrictions.

Acknowledgments: We thank the participants and families who generously participated in this research. We acknowledge the immense contributions of Michelle L. Mackenzie and Reena Duke to the research and this manuscript.

Conflicts of Interest: The authors declare no conflict of interest.

References

1. Bendor, C.D.; Bardugo, A.; Pinhas-Hamiel, O.; Afek, A.; Twig, G. Cardiovascular morbidity, diabetes and cancer risk among children and adolescents with severe obesity. *Cardiovasc. Diabetol.* **2020**, *19*, 79. [CrossRef]
2. Chung, S.T.; Onuzuruike, A.U.; Magge, S.N. Cardiometabolic risk in obese children. *Ann. N. Y. Acad. Sci.* **2018**, *1411*, 166–183. [CrossRef]
3. Reilly, J.J.; Kelly, J. Long-term impact of overweight and obesity in childhood and adolescence on morbidity and premature mortality in adulthood: Systematic review. *Int. J. Obes.* **2011**, *35*, 891–898. [CrossRef]
4. Angulo, M.A.; Butler, M.G.; Cataletto, M.E. Prader-Willi syndrome: A review of clinical, genetic, and endocrine findings. *J. Endocrinol. Investig.* **2015**, *38*, 1249–1263. [CrossRef]
5. Huvenne, H.; Dubern, B.; Clement, K.; Poitou, C. Rare Genetic Forms of Obesity: Clinical Approach and Current Treatments in 2016. *Obes. Facts* **2016**, *9*, 158–173. [CrossRef] [PubMed]
6. Bittel, D.C.; Butler, M.G. Prader-Willi syndrome: Clinical genetics, cytogenetics and molecular biology. *Expert Rev. Mol. Med.* **2005**, *7*, 1–20. [CrossRef] [PubMed]
7. Butler, M.G. Single Gene and Syndromic Causes of Obesity: Illustrative Examples. *Prog. Mol. Biol. Transl. Sci.* **2016**, *140*, 1–45. [CrossRef] [PubMed]
8. Butler, M.G.; Hartin, S.N.; Hossain, W.A.; Manzardo, A.M.; Kimonis, V.; Dykens, E.; Gold, J.A.; Kim, S.J.; Weisensel, N.; Tamura, R.; et al. Molecular genetic classification in Prader-Willi syndrome: A multisite cohort study. *J. Med. Genet.* **2019**, *56*, 149–153. [CrossRef] [PubMed]
9. Butler, M.; Lee, P.; Whitman, B. *Management of Prader-Willi Syndrome*, 4th ed.; Springer Publishers: New York, NY, USA, 2022.
10. Butler, M.G.; Matthews, N.A.; Patel, N.; Surampalli, A.; Gold, J.A.; Khare, M.; Thompson, T.; Cassidy, S.B.; Kimonis, V.E. Impact of genetic subtypes of Prader-Willi syndrome with growth hormone therapy on intelligence and body mass index. *Am. J. Med. Genet. A* **2019**, *179*, 1826–1835. [CrossRef]
11. Roof, E.; Stone, W.; MacLean, W.; Feurer, I.D.; Thompson, T.; Butler, M.G. Intellectual characteristics of Prader-Willi syndrome: Comparison of genetic subtypes. *J. Intellect. Disabil. Res.* **2000**, *44*, 25–30. [CrossRef]
12. Bittel, D.C.; Kibiryeva, N.; Butler, M.G. Expression of 4 genes between chromosome 15 breakpoints 1 and 2 and behavioral outcomes in Prader-Willi syndrome. *Pediatrics* **2006**, *118*, e1276–e1283. [CrossRef] [PubMed]
13. Butler, M.G.; Bittel, D.C.; Kibiryeva, N.; Talebizadeh, Z.; Thompson, T. Behavioral differences among subjects with Prader-Willi syndrome and type I or type II deletion and maternal disomy. *Pediatrics* **2004**, *113*, 565–573. [CrossRef] [PubMed]
14. Hartley, S.L.; Maclean, W.E., Jr.; Butler, M.G.; Zarcone, J.; Thompson, T. Maladaptive behaviors and risk factors among the genetic subtypes of Prader-Willi syndrome. *Am. J. Med. Genet. A* **2005**, *136*, 140–145. [CrossRef] [PubMed]
15. Zarcone, J.; Napolitano, D.; Peterson, C.; Breidbord, J.; Ferraioli, S.; Caruso-Anderson, M.; Holsen, L.; Butler, M.G.; Thompson, T. The relationship between compulsive behaviour and academic achievement across the three genetic subtypes of Prader-Willi syndrome. *J. Intellect. Disabil. Res.* **2007**, *51*, 478–487. [CrossRef] [PubMed]
16. Butler, M.G. Imprinting disorders in humans: A review. *Curr. Opin. Pediatr.* **2020**, *32*, 719–729. [CrossRef]
17. Nicholls, R.D.; Knepper, J.L. Genome organization, function, and imprinting in Prader-Willi and Angelman syndromes. *Annu. Rev. Genom. Hum. Genet.* **2001**, *2*, 153–175. [CrossRef]
18. Butler, M.G.; Victor, A.K.; Reiter, L.T. Autonomic nervous system dysfunction in Prader-Willi syndrome. *Clin. Auton. Res.* **2022**, in press. [CrossRef]
19. Haqq, A.M.; DeLorey, D.S.; Sharma, A.M.; Freemark, M.; Kreier, F.; Mackenzie, M.L.; Richer, L.P. Autonomic nervous system dysfunction in obesity and Prader-Willi syndrome: Current evidence and implications for future obesity therapies. *Clin. Obes.* **2011**, *1*, 175–183. [CrossRef]
20. Sanchez-Manso, J.C.; Gujarathi, R.; Varacallo, M. Autonomic Dysfunction. In *StatPearls*; StatPearls Publishing: Treasure Island, FL, USA, 2022.
21. Priano, L.; Miscio, G.; Grugni, G.; Milano, E.; Baudo, S.; Sellitti, L.; Picconi, R.; Mauro, A. On the origin of sensory impairment and altered pain perception in Prader-Willi syndrome: A neurophysiological study. *Eur. J. Pain* **2009**, *13*, 829–835. [CrossRef]

22. Driscoll, D.J.; Miller, J.L.; Schwartz, S.; Cassidy, S.B. Prader-Willi Syndrome. In *GeneReviews((R))*; Adam, M.P., Everman, D.B., Mirzaa, G.M., Pagon, R.A., Wallace, S.E., Bean, L.J.H., Gripp, K.W., Amemiya, A., Eds.; University of Washington: Seattle, WA, USA, 1993.
23. Hart, P.S. Salivary abnormalities in Prader-Willi syndrome. *Ann. N. Y. Acad. Sci.* **1998**, *842*, 125–131. [CrossRef]
24. Shapira, N.A.; Lessig, M.C.; He, A.G.; James, G.A.; Driscoll, D.J.; Liu, Y. Satiety dysfunction in Prader-Willi syndrome demonstrated by fMRI. *J. Neurol. Neurosurg. Psychiatry* **2005**, *76*, 260–262. [CrossRef]
25. Bruce, A.S.; Holsen, L.M.; Chambers, R.J.; Martin, L.E.; Brooks, W.M.; Zarcone, J.R.; Butler, M.G.; Savage, C.R. Obese children show hyperactivation to food pictures in brain networks linked to motivation, reward and cognitive control. *Int. J. Obes.* **2010**, *34*, 1494–1500. [CrossRef]
26. Holsen, L.M.; Savage, C.R.; Martin, L.E.; Bruce, A.S.; Lepping, R.J.; Ko, E.; Brooks, W.M.; Butler, M.G.; Zarcone, J.R.; Goldstein, J.M. Importance of reward and prefrontal circuitry in hunger and satiety: Prader-Willi syndrome vs simple obesity. *Int. J. Obes.* **2012**, *36*, 638–647. [CrossRef] [PubMed]
27. Holsen, L.M.; Zarcone, J.R.; Brooks, W.M.; Butler, M.G.; Thompson, T.I.; Ahluwalia, J.S.; Nollen, N.L.; Savage, C.R. Neural mechanisms underlying hyperphagia in Prader-Willi syndrome. *Obesity* **2006**, *14*, 1028–1037. [CrossRef]
28. Holsen, L.M.; Zarcone, J.R.; Chambers, R.; Butler, M.G.; Bittel, D.C.; Brooks, W.M.; Thompson, T.I.; Savage, C.R. Genetic subtype differences in neural circuitry of food motivation in Prader-Willi syndrome. *Int. J. Obes.* **2009**, *33*, 273–283. [CrossRef] [PubMed]
29. Martin, L.E.; Holsen, L.M.; Chambers, R.J.; Bruce, A.S.; Brooks, W.M.; Zarcone, J.R.; Butler, M.G.; Savage, C.R. Neural mechanisms associated with food motivation in obese and healthy weight adults. *Obesity* **2010**, *18*, 254–260. [CrossRef] [PubMed]
30. Zhang, Y.; Zhao, H.; Qiu, S.; Tian, J.; Wen, X.; Miller, J.L.; von Deneen, K.M.; Zhou, Z.; Gold, M.S.; Liu, Y. Altered functional brain networks in Prader-Willi syndrome. *NMR Biomed.* **2013**, *26*, 622–629. [CrossRef] [PubMed]
31. Gabrielli, A.; Poje, A.B.; Manzardo, A.; Butler, M.G. Startle Response Analysis of Food-Image Processing in Prader-Willi Syndrome. *J. Rare Disord.* **2018**, *6*, 18–27.
32. Tennese, A.A.; Gee, C.B.; Wevrick, R. Loss of the Prader-Willi syndrome protein necdin causes defective migration, axonal outgrowth, and survival of embryonic sympathetic neurons. *Dev. Dyn.* **2008**, *237*, 1935–1943. [CrossRef]
33. Haqq, A.M.; Muehlbauer, M.J.; Newgard, C.B.; Grambow, S.; Freemark, M. The metabolic phenotype of Prader-Willi syndrome (PWS) in childhood: Heightened insulin sensitivity relative to body mass index. *J. Clin. Endocrinol. Metab.* **2011**, *96*, E225–E232. [CrossRef]
34. Adrian, T.E.; Bacarese-Hamilton, A.P.; Savage, K.; Wolfe, K.; Besterman, H.S.; Bloom, S.R. Plasma PYY concentrations in gastrointestinal diseases. *Dig. Dis. Sci.* **1984**, *29*, 35–39. [CrossRef]
35. Schwartz, M.W.; Woods, S.C.; Porte, D., Jr.; Seeley, R.J.; Baskin, D.G. Central nervous system control of food intake. *Nature* **2000**, *404*, 661–671. [CrossRef] [PubMed]
36. Tschop, M.; Weyer, C.; Tataranni, P.A.; Devanarayan, V.; Ravussin, E.; Heiman, M.L. Circulating ghrelin levels are decreased in human obesity. *Diabetes* **2001**, *50*, 707–709. [CrossRef] [PubMed]
37. Kuppens, R.J.; Diene, G.; Bakker, N.E.; Molinas, C.; Faye, S.; Nicolino, M.; Bernoux, D.; Delhanty, P.J.; van der Lely, A.J.; Allas, S.; et al. Elevated ratio of acylated to unacylated ghrelin in children and young adults with Prader-Willi syndrome. *Endocrine* **2015**, *50*, 633–642. [CrossRef] [PubMed]
38. Shiiya, T.; Nakazato, M.; Mizuta, M.; Date, Y.; Mondal, M.S.; Tanaka, M.; Nozoe, S.; Hosoda, H.; Kangawa, K.; Matsukura, S. Plasma ghrelin levels in lean and obese humans and the effect of glucose on ghrelin secretion. *J. Clin. Endocrinol. Metab.* **2002**, *87*, 240–244. [CrossRef] [PubMed]
39. Goldstone, A.P.; Patterson, M.; Kalingag, N.; Ghatei, M.A.; Brynes, A.E.; Bloom, S.R.; Grossman, A.B.; Korbonits, M. Fasting and postprandial hyperghrelinemia in Prader-Willi syndrome is partially explained by hypoinsulinemia, and is not due to peptide YY3-36 deficiency or seen in hypothalamic obesity due to craniopharyngioma. *J. Clin. Endocrinol. Metab.* **2005**, *90*, 2681–2690. [CrossRef]
40. Burnett, L.C.; LeDuc, C.A.; Sulsona, C.R.; Paull, D.; Rausch, R.; Eddiry, S.; Carli, J.F.; Morabito, M.V.; Skowronski, A.A.; Hubner, G.; et al. Deficiency in prohormone convertase PC1 impairs prohormone processing in Prader-Willi syndrome. *J. Clin. Investig.* **2017**, *127*, 293–305. [CrossRef]
41. Manning, K.E.; Beresford-Webb, J.A.; Aman, L.C.S.; Ring, H.A.; Watson, P.C.; Porges, S.W.; Oliver, C.; Jennings, S.R.; Holland, A.J. Transcutaneous vagus nerve stimulation (t-VNS): A novel effective treatment for temper outbursts in adults with Prader-Willi Syndrome indicated by results from a non-blind study. *PLoS ONE* **2019**, *14*, e0223750. [CrossRef]
42. Manning, K.E.; McAllister, C.J.; Ring, H.A.; Finer, N.; Kelly, C.L.; Sylvester, K.P.; Fletcher, P.C.; Morrell, N.W.; Garnett, M.R.; Manford, M.R.; et al. Novel insights into maladaptive behaviours in Prader-Willi syndrome: Serendipitous findings from an open trial of vagus nerve stimulation. *J. Intellect. Disabil. Res.* **2016**, *60*, 149–155. [CrossRef]
43. Talebizadeh, Z.; Kibiryeva, N.; Bittel, D.C.; Butler, M.G. Ghrelin, peptide YY and their receptors: Gene expression in brain from subjects with and without Prader-Willi syndrome. *Int. J. Mol. Med.* **2005**, *15*, 707–711. [CrossRef]
44. Cui, H.; Lopez, M.; Rahmouni, K. The cellular and molecular bases of leptin and ghrelin resistance in obesity. *Nat. Rev. Endocrinol.* **2017**, *13*, 338–351. [CrossRef]
45. Davis, J. Hunger, ghrelin and the gut. *Brain. Res.* **2018**, *1693*, 154–158. [CrossRef]
46. DiMario, F.J., Jr.; Dunham, B.; Burleson, J.A.; Moskovitz, J.; Cassidy, S.B. An evaluation of autonomic nervous system function in patients with Prader-Willi syndrome. *Pediatrics* **1994**, *93*, 76–81. [CrossRef] [PubMed]

47. Wade, C.K.; De Meersman, R.E.; Angulo, M.; Lieberman, J.S.; Downey, J.A. Prader-Willi syndrome fails to alter cardiac autonomic modulation. *Clin. Auton. Res.* **2000**, *10*, 203–206. [CrossRef] [PubMed]
48. Irizarry, K.A.; Bain, J.; Butler, M.G.; Ilkayeva, O.; Muehlbauer, M.; Haqq, A.M.; Freemark, M. Metabolic profiling in Prader-Willi syndrome and nonsyndromic obesity: Sex differences and the role of growth hormone. *Clin. Endocrinol.* **2015**, *83*, 797–805. [CrossRef] [PubMed]
49. Camm, A.J.; Malik, M.; Bigger, J.T.; Breithardt, G.; Cerutti, S.; Cohen, R.J.; Coumel, P.; Fallen, E.L.; Kennedy, H.L.; Kleiger, R.E. Heart rate variability: Standards of measurement, physiological interpretation and clinical use. *Task Force Eur. Soc. Cardiol. N. Am. Soc. Pacing Electrophysiol.* **1996**, *93*, 1043–1065.
50. Metzler, M.; Duerr, S.; Granata, R.; Krismer, F.; Robertson, D.; Wenning, G.K. Neurogenic orthostatic hypotension: Pathophysiology, evaluation, and management. *J. Neurol.* **2013**, *260*, 2212–2219. [CrossRef]
51. Castner, D.M.; Rubin, D.A.; Judelson, D.A.; Haqq, A.M. Effects of adiposity and Prader-Willi Syndrome on postexercise heart rate recovery. *J. Obes.* **2013**, *2013*, 384167. [CrossRef]
52. Lee, S.; Kozlov, S.; Hernandez, L.; Chamberlain, S.J.; Brannan, C.I.; Stewart, C.L.; Wevrick, R. Expression and imprinting of MAGEL2 suggest a role in Prader-willi syndrome and the homologous murine imprinting phenotype. *Hum. Mol. Genet.* **2000**, *9*, 1813–1819. [CrossRef]
53. Baharav, A.; Kotagal, S.; Akselrod, S. A noninvasive evaluation of the autonomic nervous system function in children with Prader-Willi syndrome. *Clin. Auton. Res.* **1996**, *6*, 292.
54. Goldstone, A.P. Prader-Willi syndrome: Advances in genetics, pathophysiology and treatment. *Trends Endocrinol. Metab.* **2004**, *15*, 12–20. [CrossRef]
55. Munne-Miralves, C.; Brunet-Llobet, L.; Cahuana-Cardenas, A.; Torne-Duran, S.; Miranda-Rius, J.; Rivera-Baro, A. Oral disorders in children with Prader-Willi syndrome: A case control study. *Orphanet. J. Rare Dis.* **2020**, *15*, 43. [CrossRef]
56. Saeves, R.; Nordgarden, H.; Storhaug, K.; Sandvik, L.; Espelid, I. Salivary flow rate and oral findings in Prader-Willi syndrome: A case-control study. *Int. J. Paediatr. Dent.* **2012**, *22*, 27–36. [CrossRef]
57. Proctor, G.B.; Carpenter, G.H. Regulation of salivary gland function by autonomic nerves. *Auton. Neurosci.* **2007**, *133*, 3–18. [CrossRef]
58. Luo, Y.; Zheng, Z.; Yang, Y.; Bai, X.; Yang, H.; Zhu, H.; Pan, H.; Chen, S. Effects of growth hormone on cognitive, motor, and behavioral development in Prader-Willi syndrome children: A meta-analysis of randomized controlled trials. *Endocrine* **2021**, *71*, 321–330. [CrossRef] [PubMed]
59. Passone, C.G.B.; Franco, R.R.; Ito, S.S.; Trindade, E.; Polak, M.; Damiani, D.; Bernardo, W.M. Growth hormone treatment in Prader-Willi syndrome patients: Systematic review and meta-analysis. *BMJ Paediatr. Open* **2020**, *4*, e000630. [CrossRef] [PubMed]
60. Nixon, G.M.; Brouillette, R.T. Sleep and breathing in Prader-Willi syndrome. *Pediatr. Pulmonol.* **2002**, *34*, 209–217. [CrossRef]
61. Harris, J.C.; Allen, R.P. Is excessive daytime sleepiness characteristic of Prader-Willi syndrome? The effects of weight change. *Arch. Pediatr. Adolesc. Med.* **1996**, *150*, 1288–1293. [CrossRef] [PubMed]
62. Cotton, S.; Richdale, A. Brief report: Parental descriptions of sleep problems in children with autism, Down syndrome, and Prader-Willi syndrome. *Res. Dev. Disabil.* **2006**, *27*, 151–161. [CrossRef]
63. Broussard, J.L.; Van Cauter, E. Disturbances of sleep and circadian rhythms: Novel risk factors for obesity. *Curr. Opin. Endocrinol. Diabetes Obes.* **2016**, *23*, 353–359. [CrossRef]
64. McHill, A.W.; Wright, K.P., Jr. Role of sleep and circadian disruption on energy expenditure and in metabolic predisposition to human obesity and metabolic disease. *Obes. Rev.* **2017**, *18*, 15–24. [CrossRef]
65. De Cock, V.C.; Diene, G.; Molinas, C.; Masson, V.D.; Kieffer, I.; Mimoun, E.; Tiberge, M.; Tauber, M. Efficacy of modafinil on excessive daytime sleepiness in Prader-Willi syndrome. *Am. J. Med. Genet. A* **2011**, *155*, 1552–1557. [CrossRef]
66. Weselake, S.V.; Foulds, J.L.; Couch, R.; Witmans, M.B.; Rubin, D.; Haqq, A.M. Prader-Willi syndrome, excessive daytime sleepiness, and narcoleptic symptoms: A case report. *J. Med. Case. Rep.* **2014**, *8*, 127. [CrossRef]
67. Famelart, N.; Diene, G.; Cabal-Berthoumieu, S.; Glattard, M.; Molinas, C.; Guidetti, M.; Tauber, M. Equivocal expression of emotions in children with Prader-Willi syndrome: What are the consequences for emotional abilities and social adjustment? *Orphanet. J. Rare Dis.* **2020**, *15*, 55. [CrossRef] [PubMed]
68. Longin, E.; Dimitriadis, C.; Shazi, S.; Gerstner, T.; Lenz, T.; Konig, S. Autonomic nervous system function in infants and adolescents: Impact of autonomic tests on heart rate variability. *Pediatr. Cardiol.* **2009**, *30*, 311–324. [CrossRef] [PubMed]
69. Maltese, P.E.; Manara, E.; Beccari, T.; Dundar, M.; Capodicasa, N.; Bertelli, M. Genetic testing for autonomic dysfunction or dysautonomias. *Acta Biomed.* **2020**, *91*, e2020002. [CrossRef]
70. Smetana, P.; Malik, M. Sex differences in cardiac autonomic regulation and in repolarisation electrocardiography. *Pflugers. Arch.* **2013**, *465*, 699–717. [CrossRef]
71. Low, P.A.; Tomalia, V.A.; Park, K.J. Autonomic function tests: Some clinical applications. *J. Clin. Neurol.* **2013**, *9*, 1–8. [CrossRef]
72. Low, P.A. Composite autonomic scoring scale for laboratory quantification of generalized autonomic failure. *Mayo Clin. Proc.* **1993**, *68*, 748–752. [CrossRef] [PubMed]
73. Suarez, G.A.; Opfer-Gehrking, T.; Offord, K.; Atkinson, E.; O'brien, P.; Low, P. The Autonomic Symptom Profile: A new instrument to assess autonomic symptoms. *Neurology* **1999**, *52*, 523. [CrossRef] [PubMed]
74. Sletten, D.M.; Suarez, G.A.; Low, P.A.; Mandrekar, J.; Singer, W. COMPASS 31: A refined and abbreviated Composite Autonomic Symptom Score. *Mayo Clin. Proc.* **2012**, *87*, 1196–1201. [CrossRef]

75. Fotiou, F.; Fountoulakis, K.N.; Goulas, A.; Alexopoulos, L.; Palikaras, A. Automated standardized pupillometry with optical method for purposes of clinical practice and research. *Clin. Physiol.* **2000**, *20*, 336–347. [CrossRef] [PubMed]
76. Muppidi, S.; Adams-Huet, B.; Tajzoy, E.; Scribner, M.; Blazek, P.; Spaeth, E.B.; Frohman, E.; Davis, S.; Vernino, S. Dynamic pupillometry as an autonomic testing tool. *Clin. Auton. Res.* **2013**, *23*, 297–303. [CrossRef] [PubMed]
77. Patel, S.; Harmer, J.A.; Loughnan, G.; Skilton, M.R.; Steinbeck, K.; Celermajer, D.S. Characteristics of cardiac and vascular structure and function in Prader-Willi syndrome. *Clin. Endocrinol.* **2007**, *66*, 771–777. [CrossRef] [PubMed]
78. Pagani, M.; Lombardi, F.; Guzzetti, S.; Rimoldi, O.; Furlan, R.; Pizzinelli, P.; Sandrone, G.; Malfatto, G.; Dell'Orto, S.; Piccaluga, E.; et al. Power spectral analysis of heart rate and arterial pressure variabilities as a marker of sympatho-vagal interaction in man and conscious dog. *Circ. Res.* **1986**, *59*, 178–193. [CrossRef]
79. Low, P.A.; Caskey, P.E.; Tuck, R.R.; Fealey, R.D.; Dyck, P.J. Quantitative sudomotor axon reflex test in normal and neuropathic subjects. *Ann. Neurol.* **1983**, *14*, 573–580. [CrossRef] [PubMed]
80. R Core Team (Ed.) *R: Language and Environment for Statistical Computing*; R Foundation for Statistical Computing: Vienna, Austria, 2022.
81. RStudio. Integrated Development Environment for R. Available online: http://www.posit.co/ (accessed on 10 January 2021).
82. Wickham, H.; Averick, M.; Bryan, J.; Chang, W.; McGowan, L.; François, R.; Grolemund, G.; Hayes, A.; Henry, L.; Hester, J.; et al. Welcome to the Tidyverse. *J. Open Source Softw.* **2019**, *4*, 1686. [CrossRef]
83. Sjoberg, D.; Whiting, K.; Curry, M.; Lavery, J.; Larmarange, J. Reproducible Summary Tables with the gtsummary Package. *R J.* **2021**, *13*, 570–580. [CrossRef]

Disclaimer/Publisher's Note: The statements, opinions and data contained in all publications are solely those of the individual author(s) and contributor(s) and not of MDPI and/or the editor(s). MDPI and/or the editor(s) disclaim responsibility for any injury to people or property resulting from any ideas, methods, instructions or products referred to in the content.

Article

Chromosomal Microarray Study in Prader-Willi Syndrome

Merlin G. Butler [1,*], Waheeda A. Hossain [1], Neil Cowen [2] and Anish Bhatnagar [2]

[1] Department of Psychiatry and Behavioral Sciences, University of Kansas Medical Center, 3901 Rainbow Blvd., MS 4015, Kansas City, KS 66160, USA
[2] Soleno Therapeutics, Inc., Redwood City, CA 94065, USA
* Correspondence: mbutler4@kumc.edu

Abstract: A high-resolution chromosome microarray analysis was performed on 154 consecutive individuals enrolled in the DESTINY PWS clinical trial for Prader-Willi syndrome (PWS). Of these 154 PWS individuals, 87 (56.5%) showed the typical 15q11-q13 deletion subtypes, 62 (40.3%) showed non-deletion maternal disomy 15 and five individuals (3.2%) had separate unexpected microarray findings. For example, one PWS male had Klinefelter syndrome with segmental isodisomy identified in both chromosomes 15 and X. Thirty-five (40.2%) of 87 individuals showed typical larger 15q11-q13 Type I deletion and 52 individuals (59.8%) showed typical smaller Type II deletion. Twenty-four (38.7%) of 62 PWS individuals showed microarray patterns indicating either maternal heterodisomy 15 subclass or a rare non-deletion (epimutation) imprinting center defect. Segmental isodisomy 15 was seen in 34 PWS subjects (54.8%) with 15q26.3, 15q14 and 15q26.1 bands most commonly involved and total isodisomy 15 seen in four individuals (6.5%). In summary, we report on PWS participants consecutively enrolled internationally in a single clinical trial with high-resolution chromosome microarray analysis to determine and describe an unbiased estimate of the frequencies and types of genetic defects and address potential at-risk genetic disorders in those with maternal disomy 15 subclasses in the largest PWS cohort studied to date.

Keywords: Prader-Willi syndrome (PWS); high-resolution chromosomal microarray; PWS molecular genetic classes; typical 15q11-q13 deletion subtypes; maternal disomy 15 subclasses; atypical PWS genetic findings; DESTINY PWS

1. Introduction

Improved genetic testing has been developed over the past four decades and proven helpful to genetically confirm the diagnosis of Prader-Willi syndrome (PWS). The first advances in the early 1980s included high-resolution chromosome karyotypes that led to identification of the first microdeletion seen in PWS involving the 15q11-q13 region and reported by Ledbetter et al. [1]. In the late 1980s the discovery of DNA markers of genes identified in the 15q11-q13 region led to development of commercially available fluorescent in situ hybridization (FISH) in the early 1990s based on fluorescently labeled DNA probes hybridized usually by a single test probe to identify the deletion if the DNA sequence or structure is missing and a single normal control probe in the chromosome outside of the deletion region and may be with a different color visualized microscopically in the non-deleted region [2]. This method resulted in further discoveries of small deletions at the chromosome level for dozens of microdeletion syndromes besides PWS.

Comparative genomic hybridization (CGH) was developed and expanded as an array-CGH method to be used clinically in the 2000s. It provided an interface between thousands of DNA probes and cytogenetics by isolating DNA from the patient under study and normative controls, then fluorescently labeling the DNA aliquots differently (e.g., green or red). When equal labelled DNA quantities from a patient and a normal control with a different fluorescent color were mixed, the resulting computer-generated signals involving multiple probes covering all of the human chromosomes could detect deletions or duplications on each chromosome (e.g., red represented a deletion; green represented a duplication and yellow represented normal) [3].

Further research with the use of copy number and single nucleotide polymorphism DNA probes led to development of high-resolution chromosomal microarrays over the past 10 years were helpful in identifying small deletions or duplications and uniparental disomy as seen in Prader-Willi syndrome and/or other syndromes such as Angelman, Williams and Smith-Magenis along with dozens of other congenital malformation disorders in which the cause was previously unknown [4]. Prior to advances in genetic testing, the detection of subtle genetic anomalies with high precision would not be possible, particularly in identifying clinical genetic syndromes and confirmation of patients presenting with features of a microdeletion syndrome. In addition, regions of homozygosity (ROH) or absence of heterozygosity (AOH) of 3 Mb in size were helpful in determining identical by decent or consanguinity and later loss of heterozygosity (LOH) of 8 Mb in size was proven useful for identification of uniparental disomy such as maternal disomy 15 in PWS [5,6].

Prader-Willi syndrome is recognized as the first example in humans of errors in genomic imprinting and generally due to lack of expression of a cluster of paternally inherited genes on chromosome 15q11-q13 generally from a paternal deletion or by uniparental maternal disomy 15 [6] (e.g., Butler 2016). PWS is recognized by severe hypotonia in infancy with a poor suck, feeding difficulties and failure to thrive, hypogonadism/hypogenitalism, cryptorchidism, short stature and small hands and feet due to growth and other hormone deficiencies and developmental delay. During early childhood, mild intellectual disability is noted along with food seeking and hyperphagia leading to obesity, if not externally controlled. Obesity and behavioral problems present in childhood includes anxiety, temper tantrums, skin picking and compulsions and can contribute to other comorbidities and clinical findings [7]. PWS accounts for one in 15,000 to 20,000 live births with over 400,000 individuals worldwide [8].

There are five recognized chromosome 15q breakpoints (BP1, BP2, BP3, BP4 and BP5) with two typical paternal 15q11-q13 deletions causing PWS and classified as a larger Type I or smaller Type II deletion including the Prader-Willi syndrome critical region (PWSCR). The Type I deletion involves a proximal 15q11 breakpoint BP1 and a distally located 15q13 breakpoint BP3 while the smaller Type II deletion involves a second proximal 15q11 breakpoint BP2 but with the same distal breakpoint BP3 [9,10] (see Figure 1). An average size of the larger Type I deletion is approximately 6 Mb, while the smaller Type II deletion is approximately 5.5 Mb. The larger deletion encompasses four non-imprinted genes (TUBGCP5, CYFIP1, NIPA1 and NIPA2) that reside between BP1 and BP2. Those individuals with PWS and the larger Type I deletion often have more learning and behavioral problems specifically compulsions, maladaptive behaviors and self-injury along with lower cognitive skills when compared to those with PWS having the smaller Type II deletion [11,12]. Specific clinical differences have also been reported in those with the second major cause of PWS, that is, maternal disomy 15 (see Figure 2). Those with PWS and maternal disomy 15 have a higher verbal intelligence quotient (IQ) than those with the paternal 15q11-q13 deletions and less self-injury but with more psychosis and autism [6,13,14].

The PWS cohort was recruited by DESTINY PWS (ClinicalTrials.gov number NCT03440 814), an international, randomized, double-blind, placebo-controlled, parallel-group, Phase 3 study comparing diazoxide choline extended-release tablet (DCCR) to placebo in individuals with PWS [15]. The study enrolled males and females with PWS, aged 4 years and older with hyperphagia, weighing between 20 and 135 kg, in a stable care setting, at 29 sites in the US and UK. High-resolution chromosomal microarrays to analyze DNA samples from individuals enrolled in the study were used to confirm their genetic class.

This report and review will summarize the results of the DESTINY PWS clinical trial and characterize the genetic findings in a large PWS cohort. The importance to increase awareness and confirmation of genetic defects causing PWS will be stressed and discussed including genetic mechanisms and relationships with reported chromosome 15 recessive genes depending on specific PWS molecular subtypes and subclasses with potential novel genetic changes as a component of the PWS diagnosis. This study may stimulate additional research to further understand the genetic causation of PWS, clinical treatment and surveillance along with genetic counseling purposes.

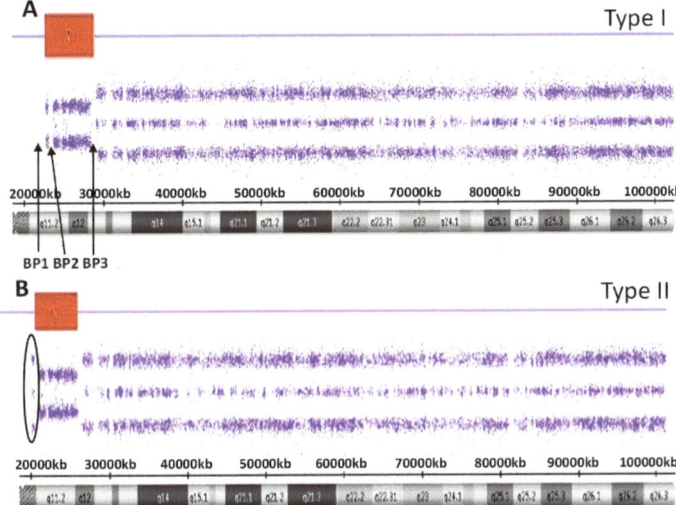

Figure 1. High-resolution chromosome microarray results for the larger typical 15 q11-q13 Type I deletion involving breakpoints BP1 and BP2 (**A**) while the smaller typical 15q11-q13 Type II deletion involving breakpoints BP2 and and BP3 (**B**). The red-colored bars represent the deletion region for both the Type I and Type II deletions.

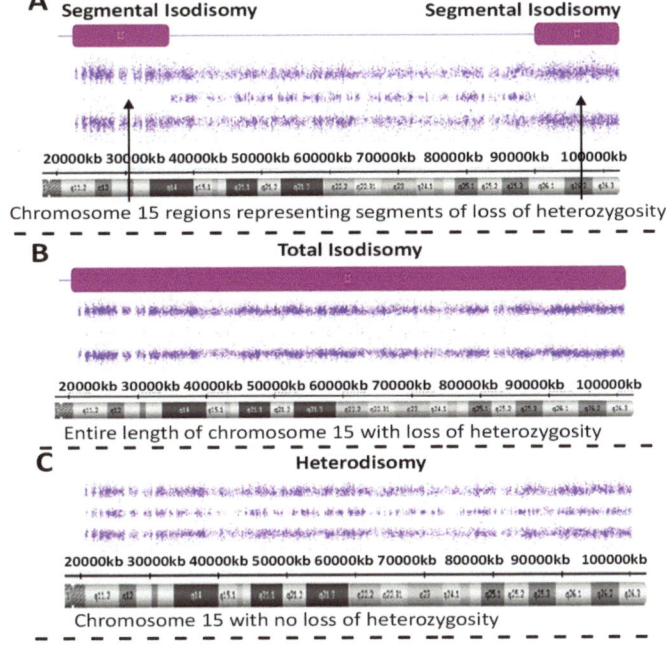

Figure 2. *Cont.*

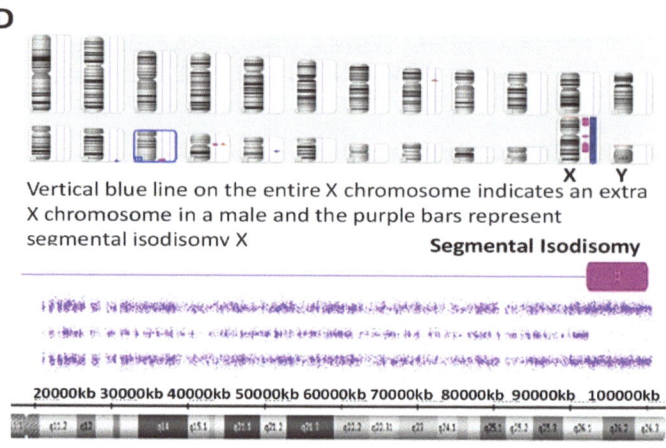

Maternal disomy 15 with segmental isodisomy and an extra X chromosome with segmental isodisomy X in a male with both PWS and Klinefelter syndrome

Figure 2. High-resolution chromosome microarray results showing examples of maternal disomy 15 in four PWS participants (**A–D**). Segmental isodisomy 15 is represented by segments of loss of heterozygosity as a purple-colored bar and found in (**A,D**) while total isodisomy 15 is seen in (**B**). Maternal heterodisomy 15 is shown in (**C**) with no loss of heterozygosity. (**D**) represents a PWS participant with segmental isodisomy 15 and segmental isodisomy X but with an extra X chromosome indicating the presence of Klinefelter syndrome, as well.

2. Results

Of the 154 individuals with PWS, 87 (56.5%) showed a 15q11-q13 deletion with 35 (22.7%) having the larger typical 15q11-q13 Type I deletion subtype. Fifty-two individuals (33.8%) had the smaller typical 15q-q13 Type II deletion subtype (see Figure 1). One (ID #20-055176) of these PWS subjects had the typical Type I deletion, but also a small duplication at 15q13.3 (433 kb in size) that contained two genes (OTUD7A and CHRNA7) residing between breakpoints BP4 and BP5. Deletions of this region are associated with neurodevelopmental problems and seizures (www.omim.org). Of those with the Type II deletion, one (ID #20-058046) had a small duplication at 15q13.1-q13.2 (187 kb in size) and contained two poorly characterized genes (TJP1 and GOLGA8) residing between breakpoints BP4 and BP5.

Sixty-two individuals (40.3%) with PWS had maternal disomy 15 with segmental isodisomy 15 in 34 subjects (22 females, 12 males) or 54.8 percent due to normal cross-over events in female meiosis I with gene segregation (see Figure 2). The average size of the total LOH isodisomic region was 27.06 Mb and each LOH varied in size from 5.57 to 52.22 Mb. The average size of individual isodisomic regions was 18.40 Mb. Twenty-two of these subjects showed one LOH segment, ten showed two separate LOH segments and two showed three LOH segments. LOHs were seen throughout chromosome 15 involving the proximal, middle or distal long arm. Chromosome 15 bands at the terminal (15q26.3; 21 PWS subjects), middle (15q14; 16 PWS subjects) and proximal (15q26.1; 15 PWS subjects) regions were most often involved (see Figure 3). Two subjects had only a proximal LOH segment, four subjects had only a middle LOH segment, eight subjects had only a distal LOH segment, two subjects had both proximal and middle LOH segments, 11 subjects had middle and distal LOH segments, two subjects had both proximal and distal LOH segments, five subjects had proximal and distal LOH segments with one having a long 49 Mb LOH segment, three subjects had two LOH segments each and one subject had three separate LOH segments.

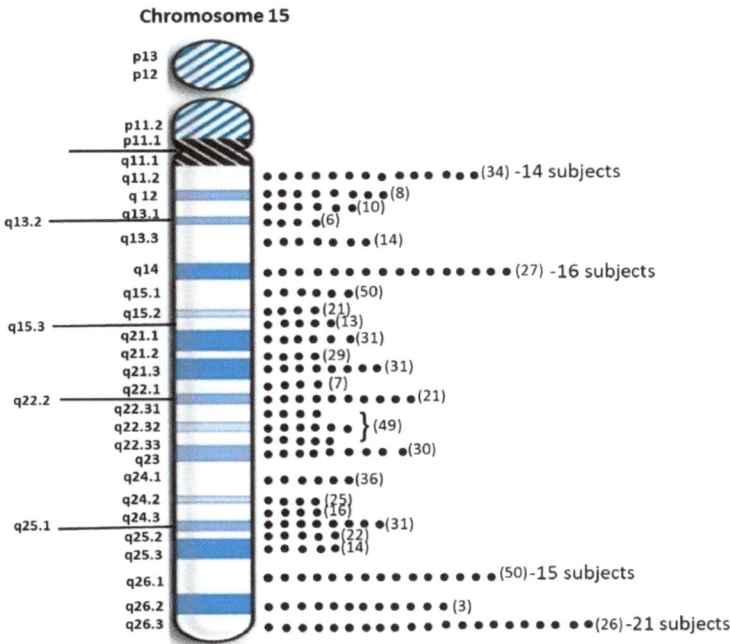

Figure 3. Distribution of chromosome 15 bands involved in segmental isodisomy 15 found by high-resolution microarray analysis and dense genotyping of chromosome 15 in our study of 154 PWS participants with maternal isodisomy 15 seen in 38 subjects. The number of protein coding genes in parentheses is noted per chromosome 15 band. The individual dots represent individual participants with that band involved in segmental or total maternal isodisomy 15. Chromosome 15q26.3 band was most often found in 21 PWS participants followed by 15q14 band in 16 participants.

One of these PWS subjects (ID #19-221457) with segmental isodisomy 15 also showed an extra X chromosome gain for the entire X chromosome consistent and an XXY male pattern or Klinefelter syndrome along with segmental isodisomy X; therefore, both chromosomes 15 and X were of maternal origin (see Figure 2). Klinefelter syndrome and PWS have also been reported previously as well as trisomy X and PWS indicative of a second female meiotic error during gametogenesis involving both chromosome 15s and the sex chromosome in these individuals [16].

Two PWS subjects (ID #20-068072 and ID #19-207448) had LOHs of 6.21 Mb and 5.57 Mb in size, respectively on chromosome 15. These patterns could support segmental isodisomy in the patients with clinical diagnosis of PWS where the homozygous regions can be smaller in size than 8 Mb without evidence of large ROHs elsewhere in the genome as seen in these two subjects and therefore no evidence of consanguinity which can account for increased number and size of areas of homozygosity [17]. Total isodisomy 15 was seen in four PWS individuals (ID #19-090094, #19-141589, #19-154156, #20-052607) representing an LOH of the entire long arm of chromosome 15 due to errors in female meiosis II.

Maternal heterodisomy 15 or non-deletion status was observed in 24 separate individuals with PWS whereby no cross-over events occurred in female meiosis I or due to a less likely or rare non-deletion (epimutation) involving the imprinting center (IC). Among these 24 heterodisomy/IC defect subjects, four (ID #18-093592, #19-143810, #19-148178, #19-193931) had LOHs of 3 Mb, 3.1 Mb, 4.9 Mb and 3.1 Mb in size, respectively. The other 20 cases showed no LOHs ≥8 Mb or chromosome 15q11-q13 deletions including the imprinting center. DNA microsatellite polymorphic probes from human chromosome 15 would be needed for those not having 15q11-q13 deletions or isodisomy 15 but potentially those with heterodisomy 15 which could resemble non-deletion imprinting center defects via chromosome microarray analysis alone. Therefore, to determine that both 15s are from the mother or maternal disomy 15, biparental (normal) inheritance would indicate an imprinting center defect when examining DNA samples from both parents and the PWS child.

Atypical PWS genetic findings were seen in five individuals with PWS. These included PWS subjects ID #18-085701 involving a pathogenic copy number change on chromosome 15. This small, atypical deletion of chromosome 15 occurred between proximal 15q11.2 breakpoint BP2 and distal 15q breakpoint BP3. The interpretation of this sample showed a female sex pattern by microarray analysis with a small, atypical deletion of approximately 2.3 Mb in size on the long arm of one chromosome 15 at cytogenetic band q11.2-q12 (chr15:23615768-25927232). This heterozygous deletion included the entire SNRPN gene and upstream imprinting centers. The deletion did not include the proximal TUBGCP5, CYFIP1, NIPA2 and NIPA1 genes or distal GABRB3, GABRA5, GABRG3 and OCA2 genes on chromosome 15. This type of deletion is associated with Prader-Willi syndrome when of paternal origin.

For PWS subject ID #18-140801, a pathogenic copy number change was detected on chromosome 15. This atypical deletion found in chromosome 15 included two genes (TUBGCP5 and CYFIP1) located in the 15q11.2 BP1-BP2 region but the two other genes (i.e., NIPA2 and NIPA1) in this region were not deleted. A second deletion was also found at genomic coordinates 23,290,786-28,560,269 involving the proximal long arm of chromosome 15 as typically seen in the 15q11-q13 deletion. Hence, this patient had an atypical deletion pattern not previously reported. Therefore, two different deletions were found, one approximately 195 kb in size involving TUBGCP5 and CYFIP1 genes at genomic coordinates 22,770,421-22,965,401 and a second deletion at 5.2 Mb in size at 15q11.2-q13.1 with coordinates 23,290,786-28,560,269. Due to the rarity of this chromosome deletion pattern, repeat microarray hybridization was undertaken, and the same result was found (see Figure 4).

For PWS subject ID #19-165349, a pathogenic copy number change was detected on chromosome 15. This atypical deletion in chromosome 15 included the 15q11-q14 region and involved a breakpoint distal to BP2 and included the very distal breakpoint BP5. Hence, the interpretation for this sample showed a male sex pattern by microarray analysis and a large, atypical deletion of approximately 9.42 Mb in size or about 50 percent larger than anticipated for a typical 15q11-q13 deletion. The deletion occurred at cytogenetic bands q11.2-q14 at genomic coordinates chr15:24263392-33680968. This deletion is distal to both the 15q11.2 breakpoint BP2 and the NDN gene, but proximal to the NPAP1 gene. This large deletion included the CHRNA7 gene. A separate atypical large interstitial deletion involving the 15q11-q14 region has been reported previously in a patient by one of the coauthors (i.e., MGB) having an expanded PWS phenotype with findings not typically seen in PWS such as congenital heart defects [18].

For PWS subject ID #19-171576, a loss of only one gene PWRN2 (611217) was detected in chromosome 15q11-q13 region. The MS-MLPA or methylation specific testing [19] was required to further confirm genetically the diagnosis of PWS not detectable with microarray analysis. The interpretation of this sample showed a female sex pattern, but no typical 15q11-q13 deletion or maternal segmental or total isodisomy 15. A deletion of approximately 154 kb in size on the long arm of chromosome 15 at cytogenetic band q11.2-q12(chr15:24350855-24504770) was detected. This region included only one gene (PWRN2-Prader-Willi Region Noncoding RNA2) which is poorly characterized and located between the NDN gene and C15orf2 as reported by Buiting et al. [20].

For PWS subject ID #19-191942, a pathogenic copy number change on chromosome 15 was seen with a small, atypical deletion including chromosome 15 between proximal 15q11.2 breakpoint BP2 and did not include the distal 15q breakpoint BP3. The interpretation of this sample showed a male sex pattern by microarray analysis and a deletion of approximately 187 kb on the long arm of a chromosome 15 at cytogenetic band q11.2-q12 (chr15:25178112-25365360). This heterozygous deletion included five genes or transcripts including SNRPN, SNHG14, PWAR5, SNORD116-1 and IPW located in the imprinting center region. The deletion did not include the proximal TUBGCP5, CYFIP1, NIPA2 and NIPA1 genes or distal GABRB3, GABRA5, GABRG3 and OCA2 genes on chromosome 15. This type of deletion is apparently associated with Prader-Willi syndrome and the imprinting center.

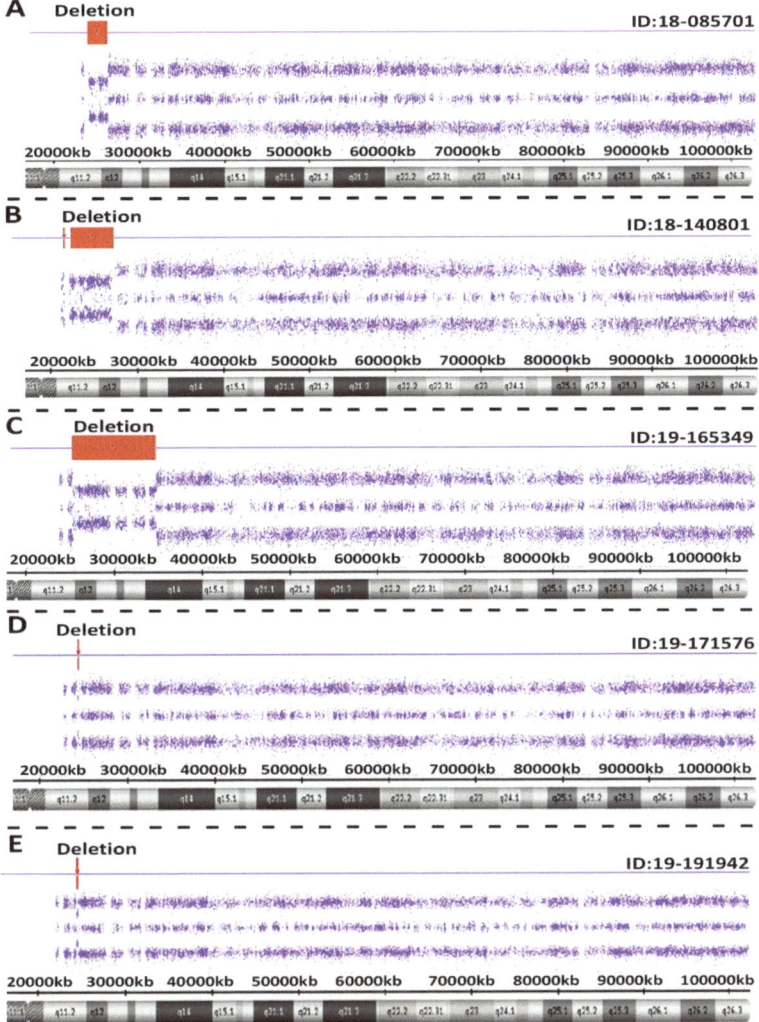

Figure 4. Atypical PWS deletion microarray results with red colored-bars representing the size and location of the deletion on chromosome 15 are shown in five separate PWS participants (**A–E**).

3. Discussion

A high-resolution chromosome microarray analysis was performed on 154 individuals (86 females, 68 males) with Prader-Willi syndrome and PWS molecular genetic classification was determined. Of these individuals 87 showed the typical 15q11-q13 deletion subtypes, 62 showed maternal disomy 15 subclasses and five individuals had an unusual high-resolution chromosome microarray result. One individual was identified having XXY or Klinefelter syndrome in addition to maternal disomy 15. Five individuals with PWS showed atypical chromosome 15 genetic defects including loss of single genes within or outside of the PWSCR, a microdeletion of the imprinting center or surrounding region. Our study is the first to use systematically advanced genetic testing in individuals with PWS clinically diagnosed and entered consecutively in a PWS-specific clinical trial internationally, the largest of its kind, useful for characterizing genetic lesions in a large PWS cohort and their frequencies. This study identified novel atypical genetic lesions of chromosome 15 in those with PWS. These findings will be useful in identifying underlying pathogenesis and disturbed biological pathways in PWS and stimulate further studies on gene-gene-protein interactions needed for development of therapeutic agents, disease surveillance and genetic counseling.

Maternal disomy 15 is thought to arise from an error in female gametogenesis with the egg containing two chromosome 15 s from the mother, and if fertilized by a normal sperm, then trisomy 15 results in the zygote. Trisomy 15 is lethal and is a relatively common cause of miscarriages in humans. However, if a trisomy 15 rescue event does occur with loss of a chromosome 15 then this leads to a normal 46 chromosome count and the embryo may survive. If the father's chromosome 15 is lost, then the two remaining chromosome 15s are from the mother leading to maternal disomy 15; hence, a PWS fetus is born. Segmental isodisomy 15 could also be impacted by the presence of centromeric interference preventing recombination near the centromere or mitotic recombination post-zygotically during early cell division in the embryo developing an abnormal clone. This could lead to mosaicism in the developing fetus, potentially impacting clinical involvement. In addition, a 15q11-q13 maternal deletion and uniparental disomy 15 of paternal origin leads to a second genomic imprinting disorder (Angelman syndrome).

Cytogenetic karyotyping to rule out Robertsonian translocations involving chromosome 15 may also be warranted to assess the chromosome origin and/or presence of marker chromosome 15 s and other rearranged chromosomes. These observations could impact on recurrence risk for subsequent pregnancies and is a limitation of a chromosome microarray analysis only. For example, if the unaffected mother has a 15/15 Robertsonian translocation, trisomy related rescue in the embryo could lead to maternal disomy 15 and PWS or if the unaffected father has this type of translocation and monosomy related rescue of the mother's chromosome 15 then could lead to PWS. These events may involve segregation in meiosis I and nullisomic events for chromosome 15 in the egg or sperm production.

The clinical differences occur in those patients with PWS having deletion subtypes when compared with maternal disomy 15 subclasses, particularly those with segmental or total isodisomy 15. They are at a greater risk for unusual or specific clinical findings potentially due to a second genetic disorder, if the unaffected mother is a carrier of a recessive or low penetrant dominant gene allele in the region. A large LOH having more genes in their isodisomic region would increase the likelihood of atypical features and having a second genetic condition.

There are approximately 600 protein-coding genes recognized on chromosome 15 with 454 annotated in OMIM (www.omim.org) (accessed on 30 August 2022) including 75 autosomal recessive, 44 autosomal dominant and 125 genes for causing clinical disorders. With about 80 Mb of DNA on chromosome 15 and with an average LOH size of 18 Mb in our study in those with maternal segmental isodisomy 15, one would anticipate about 20% of the 600 genes or about 120 would be located in the segmental region and at risk for a second genetic condition along with PWS. Fortunately, humans carry only a very small number of recessive alleles that are considered abnormal.

Those PWS patients with maternal isodisomy 15 may undergo surveillance depending on the disease-causing genes found in their isodisomic region or when a high index of suspicion arises due to an unexpected phenotype occurs and an altered evolution of the clinical course expected for a patient with PWS. Over 100 autosomal recessive genes have been recognized and localized on chromosome 15 (see Table 1). When dividing the recessive genes on chromosome 15 by chromosome 15 regions (i.e., proximal long arm of chromosome 15-chromosome bands 15q11.2 to 15q14; middle long arm of chromosome 15- chromosome bands 15q15.1 to 15q23 and distal long arm of chromosome 15- chromosome bands 15q24.1 to 15q26.3), there are 14 genes in the proximal long arm region, 57 genes in the middle long arm region with 17 involved with syndrome causation, and 42 genes in the distal long arm region with about 50 percent involved with syndrome causation. For example, Muthusamy et al. [21] summarized the literature regarding maternal disomy 15 and reported a second case of congenital ichthyosis in Prader-Willi syndrome with involvement of the ceramide synthase (*CERS3*) gene on chromosome 15 and two homozygous pathogenic variants in an adult female with PWS having maternal disomy 15. They also summarized the literature and found six reports in PWS patients with maternal disomy 15 with four other disorders with genes on chromosome 15 [Bloom syndrome (BLM gene at 15q26.1), Tay-Sachs disease (HEXA gene at 15q23), deafness-infertility (STRC gene at 15q15.3 and CATSPER2 gene at 15q15.3) and congenital ichthyosis (CERS3 gene at 15q26.3)]. Additionally, data from the ChromosOmics-Database http://cs.tl.de/DB/CA/UPD/0-Start.html [accessed on 14 December 2022] were summarized by L.B. Liehr from Jena, Germany regarding uniparental disomy (UPD) consisting of human case reports from nearly all chromosomes in the medical literature of over 1700 publications. There were greater than 1500 maternal disomy 15 cases with PWS reported with or without clear clinical correlation information in the literature but with normal karyotypes. Eleven of these PWS cases involved a second chromosome 15 gene disorder such as Bloom syndrome, congenital heart defects, congenital ichthyosis and CMT (POLG gene involvement) but no clinical features were characterized for six cases. There were six patients with PWS reported with maternal disomy 15 showing mosaicism ranging between 40% to 90%. There were 26 PWS cases with maternal disomy 15 with or without clear clinical correlation and having balanced karyotypes with 45 chromosomes: three showed der(13;15)(q10;q10)mat; four showed der(14;15)(q10;q10)mat; and 19 showed der(15;15)(q10;q10)mat. Twenty-four cases with PWS had an extra small marker chromosome 15, while 25 PWS cases with maternal disomy 15 involved other chromosome imbalances. These included four patients with PWS and maternal disomy 15 with a 47,XXX karyotype or trisomy X syndrome. Two patients with PWS with maternal disomy 15 also had a 47,XXY karyotype or Klinefelter syndrome. Three patients with PWS with maternal disomy 15 also had a 47,XYY karyotype. Eleven patients with PWS also had an extra chromosome 15 most often identified prenatally. The remaining PWS cases with maternal disomy 15 had other rare chromosomal anomalies or clinical phenotypes.

Table 1. Autosomal Recessive Genes and Location on Chromosome 15.

Cytogenetic Location	Genomic Coordinates	Gene Symbol	Phenotype
15q12-q13.1	15:27719008-28099315	OCA2	Albinism, brown oculocutaneous, Albinism, oculocutaneous, type II
15q13.1	15:28111040-28322179	HERC2	Intellectual developmental disorder
15q13.1	15:29264989-29269822	NSMCE3	Lung disease, immunodeficiency, chromosome breakage syndrome
15q13.1-q15.1	15:27800001-42500000	CILD4	Ciliary dyskinesia, primary, 4
15q13.3	15:30903852-30943108	FAN1	Interstitial nephritis, karyomegalic
15q14	15:34341719-34343136	NOP10	Dyskeratosis congenita
15q14	15:36579626-36810244	CDIN1	Dyserythropoietic anemia, congenital, type Ib
15q14	15:38488103-38564814	RASGRP1	Immunodeficiency 64
15q14	15:34229784-34338057	SLC12A6	Agenesis of the corpus callosum with peripheral neuropathy
15q14	15:33400001-39800000	EIG7	Epilepsy, juvenile myoclonic
15q15.1	15:40161069-40221123	BUB1B	Mosaic variegated aneuploidy syndrome 1
15q15.1	15:42359501-42412317	CAPN3	Muscular dystrophy, limb-girdle
15q15.1	15:40520993-40565042	CCDC32	Cardiofacioneurodevelopmental syndrome

Table 1. *Cont.*

Cytogenetic Location	Genomic Coordinates	Gene Symbol	Phenotype
15q15.1	15:41231268-41281887	CHP1	?Spastic ataxia 9, autosomal recessive
15q15.1	15:40470984-40473158	CHST14	Ehlers-Danlos syndrome, musculocontractural type 1
15q15.1	15:39934115-40035591	EIF2AK4	Pulmonary venoocclusive disease 2
15q15.1	15:40405795-40435947	IVD	Isovaleric acidemia
15q15.1	15:40594249-40664342	KNL1	Microcephaly 4, primary, autosomal recessive
15q15.1	15:41774484-41827855	MAPKBP1	Nephronophthisis 20
15q15.1	15:41387353-41403026	NDUFAF1	Mitochondrial complex I deficiency, nuclear type 11
15q15.1	15:40807089-40815084	ZFYVE19	Cholestasis, progressive familial intrahepatic, 9
15q15.2	15:42723544-42737128	CDAN1	Dyserythropoietic anemia, congenital, type Ia
15q15.2	15:43232590-43266928	TGM5	Peeling skin syndrome 2
15q15.2	15:42942897-43106038	UBR1	Johanson-Blizzard syndrome
15q15.3	15:43599563-43618800	STRC	Deafness, autosomal recessive 16
15q15.3	15:43371101-43409771	TUBGCP4	Microcephaly and chorioretinopathy
15q21.1	15:44711517-44718145	B2M	Immunodeficiency 43
15q21.1	15:45587123-45609716	BLOC1S6	?Hermansky-Pudlak syndrome 9
15q21.1	15:48729083-48811069	CEP152	Microcephaly 9, primary, autosomal recessive, Seckel syndrome 5
15q21.1	15:45092650-45114172	DUOX2	Thyroid dyshormonogenesis 6
15q21.1	15:45114326-45118421	DUOXA2	Thyroid dyshormonogenesis 5
15q21.1	15:45361124-45402227	GATM	Cerebral creatine deficiency syndrome 3
15q21.1	15:44665732-44711390	PATL2	Oocyte maturation defect 4
15q21.1	15:48206302-48304078	SLC12A1	Bartter syndrome, type 1
15q21.1	15:48120990-48142672	SLC24A5	Albinism, oculocutaneous, type VI, [Skin/hair/eye pigmentation 4, fair/dark skin]
15q21.1	15:45023195-45077185	SORD	Sorbitol dehydrogenase deficiency with peripheral neuropathy
15q21.1	15:45402336-45421415	SPATA5L1	Deafness, autosomal recessive 119, Neurodevelopmental disorder with hearing loss and spasticity
15q21.1	15:44562696-44663662	SPG11	Amyotrophic lateral sclerosis 5, juvenile, Charcot-Marie-Tooth disease, axonal, type 2X, Spastic paraplegia 11, autosomal recessive
15q21.1	15:45631148-45691281	SQOR	Sulfide:quinone oxidoreductase deficiency
15q21.1	15:44956687-44979229	TERB2	?Spermatogenic failure 59
15q21.2	15:50907492-51005895	AP4E1	Spastic paraplegia 51, autosomal recessive
15q21.2	15:51447791-51622771	DMXL2	?Polyendocrine-polyneuropathy syndrome, Developmental and epileptic encephalopathy 81
15q21.2	15:51341655-51413365	GLDN	Lethal congenital contracture syndrome 11
15q21.2	15:52115100-52191392	GNB5	Intellectual developmental disorder with cardiac arrhythmia, Language delay and ADHD/cognitive impairment with or without cardiac arrhythmia
15q21.2	15:52307283-52529050	MYO5A	Griscelli syndrome, type 1
15q21.2	15:50702266-50765706	SPPL2A	Immunodeficiency 86, mycobacteriosis
15q21.3	15:55417755-55508234	DNAAF4	Ciliary dyskinesia, primary, 25
15q21.3	15:58410554-58569844	LIPC	Hepatic lipase deficiency
15q21.3	15:56428724-56465137	MNS1	Heterotaxy, visceral, 9, autosomal, with male infertility
15q21.3	15:55319222-55355648	PIGB	Developmental and epileptic encephalopathy 80
15q21.3	15:55202966-55289813	RAB27A	Griscelli syndrome, type 2
15q21.3	15:53513741-53762878	WDR72	Amelogenesis imperfecta, type IIA3

Table 1. *Cont.*

Cytogenetic Location	Genomic Coordinates	Gene Symbol	Phenotype
15q22.2	15:63321378-63381846	CA12	Hyperchlorhidrosis, isolated
15q22.2	15:59132434-59372871	MYO1E	Glomerulosclerosis, focal segmental, 6
15q22.2	15:61852389-62060447	VPS13C	Parkinson disease 23, autosomal recessive, early onset
15q22.31	15:63608618-63833948	HERC1	Macrocephaly, dysmorphic facies, and psychomotor retardation
15q22.31	15:65001512-65029639	MTFMT	Combined oxidative phosphorylation deficiency 15, Mitochondrial complex I deficiency, nuclear type 27
15q22.31	15:64155817-64163022	PPIB	Osteogenesis imperfecta, type IX
15q22.31	15:65611350-65661002	SLC24A1	Night blindness, congenital stationary (complete), 1D, autosomal recessive
15q22.31	15:65045387-65053397	SLC51B	?Bile acid malabsorption, primary, 2
15q22.31	15:64963022-64989914	SPG21	MAST syndrome
15q22.31	15:64387836-64455303	TRIP4	?Muscular dystrophy, congenital, Davignon-Chauveau type, Spinal muscular atrophy with congenital bone fractures 1
15q23	15:68206992-68257215	CLN6	Ceroid lipofuscinosis, neuronal, 6A, Ceroid lipofuscinosis, neuronal, 6B (Kufs type)
15q23	15:72340924-72376014	HEXA	GM2-gangliosidosis, several forms, Tay-Sachs disease, [Hex A pseudo deficiency]
15q23	15:71822291-72118600	MYO9A	Myasthenic syndrome, congenital, 24, presynaptic
15q23	15:71810554-71818253	NR2E3	Enhanced S-cone syndrome
15q24.1	15:72686207-72738473	BBS4	Bardet-Biedl syndrome 4
15q24.1	15:74630558-74696024	EDC3	?Intellectual developmental disorder, autosomal recessive 50
15q24.1	15:73443164-73560013	REC114	Oocyte maturation defect 10
15q24.1	15:74409289-74433958	SEMA7A	?Cholestasis, progressive familial intrahepatic, 11
15q24.1	15:74179466-74212259	STRA6	Microphthalmia, isolated, with coloboma 8, Microphthalmia, syndromic 9
15q24.1-q24.2	15:74890042-74902219	MPI	Congenital disorder of glycosylation, type Ib
15q24.2	15:74919791-74938073	COX5A	?Mitochondrial complex IV deficiency, nuclear type 20
15q24.2	15:75355792-75368607	MAN2C1	Congenital disorder of deglycosylation 2
15q24.2-q24.3	15:76215353-76311469	ETFA	Glutaric acidemia IIA
15q24.3	15:77613027-77820900	LINGO1	Intellectual developmental disorder, autosomal recessive 64
15q24.3	15:76347904-76905340	SCAPER	Intellectual developmental disorder and retinitis pigmentosa
15q24.3-q25.1	15:77994985-78077711	TBC1D2B	Neurodevelopmental disorder with seizures and gingival overgrowth
15q24-q25	15:72400001-88500000	CILD8	Ciliary dyskinesia, primary, 8
15q25.1	15:80404382-80597933	ARNT2	?Webb-Dattani syndrome
15q25.1	15:78593052-78620996	CHRNA3	Bladder dysfunction, autonomic, with impaired pupillary reflex and secondary CAKUT
15q25.1	15:78104606-78131535	CIB2	Deafness, autosomal recessive 48, Usher syndrome, type IJ
15q25.1	15:80152789-80186949	FAH	Tyrosinemia, type I
15q25.1	15:78149362-78171945	IDH3A	Retinitis pigmentosa 90
15q25.1	15:78437431-78501453	IREB2	Neurodegeneration, early-onset, with choreoathetoid movements and microcytic anemia
15q25.1	15:80946289-80989819	MESD	Osteogenesis imperfecta, type XX
15q25.1	15:79843547-79897285	MTHFS	Neurodevelopmental disorder with microcephaly, epilepsy, and hypomyelination
15q25.2	15:82659281-82709875	AP3B2	Developmental and epileptic encephalopathy 48

Table 1. Cont.

Cytogenetic Location	Genomic Coordinates	Gene Symbol	Phenotype
15q25.2	15:82130233-82262734	EFL1	Shwachman-Diamond syndrome 2
15q25.2	15:84639285-84654283	WDR73	Galloway-Mowat syndrome 1
15q25.3	15:84817356-84873479	ALPK3	Cardiomyopathy, familial hypertrophic 27
15q25.3	15:84884662-84975649	SLC28A1	[Uridine-cytidineuria]
15q26.1	15:88803436-88875353	ACAN	Spondyloepimetaphyseal dysplasia, aggrecan type
15q26.1	15:90717346-90816166	BLM	Bloom syndrome
15q26.1	15:90229975-90265759	CIB1	Epidermodysplasia verruciformis 3
15q26.1	15:89243979-89317259	FANCI	Fanconi anemia, complementation group I
15q26.1	15:89617309-89663049	KIF7	?Al-Gazali-Bakalinova syndrome, ?Hydrolethalus syndrome 2, Acrocallosal syndrome, Joubert syndrome 12
15q26.1	15:89776332-89778754	MESP2	Spondylocostal dysostosis 2, autosomal recessive
15q26.1	15:89316320-89334824	POLG	Mitochondrial DNA depletion syndrome 4A (Alpers type), Mitochondrial DNA depletion syndrome 4B (MNGIE type), Mitochondrial recessive ataxia syndrome (includes SANDO and SCAE), Progressive external ophthalmoplegia, autosomal recessive 1
15q26.1	15:89209869-89221579	RLBP1	Bothnia retinal dystrophy
15q26.1	15:90930180-90954093	UNC45A	Osteo-oto-hepato-enteric syndrome
15q26.1	15:90998416-91022621	VPS33B	Arthrogryposis, renal dysfunction, and cholestasis 1, Cholestasis, progressive familial intrahepatic, 12, Keratoderma-ichthyosis-deafness syndrome, autosomal recessive
15q26.3	15:99971437-100341975	ADAMTS17	Weill-Marchesani 4 syndrome, recessive
15q26.3	15:100879831-100916626	ALDH1A3	Microphthalmia, isolated 8
15q26.3	15:100400395-100544683	CERS3	Ichthyosis, congenital, autosomal recessive 9
15q26.3	15:101175727-101252048	CHSY1	Temtamy preaxial brachydactyly syndrome
15q26.3	15:100566924-100602184	LINS1	Intellectual developmental disorder, autosomal recessive 27
15q26.3	15:100919357-101078257	LRRK1	Osteosclerotic metaphyseal dysplasia

Reference source 'Online Inheritance In Man' (www.omim.org)—reviewed online August 30, 2022.

A PWS child with segmental isodisomy 15, and particularly those with total isodisomy 15, may therefore need surveillance for disorders or phenotypes associated with disease-causing autosomal recessive genes on chromosome 15 within the isodisomic region as noted. Although the chance that the mother is a carrier of a recessive gene on chromosome 15 is unlikely, there is a chance and may be dependent on the family history. For example, about 2 percent of the general population are carriers of the POLG gene located at 15q26.1 band and leads to mitochondrial DNA depletion syndrome and related disorders [6]. Certain rare genetic disorders are more common in specific populations, e.g., Tay-Sachs disease with gene located at 15q23 and Ashkenazi-Jewish ancestry.

Another genetic phenomenon that can occur in females with PWS and maternal disomy 15 may involve the X chromosome. Females have two X chromosomes, while males have only one X chromosome, but the number of active X-linked genes remain constant in both sexes. This is due to gene dosage compensation as one of the X chromosomes becomes inactivated in females normally in early pregnancy and therefore only one set of X-linked genes are active. The X chromosome inactivation occurs at random and allows for an equal number of active X-linked genes in both sexes. The process of X chromosome inactivation occurs very early in pregnancy and occasionally this process is not random and skewness results. Butler et al. [22] characterized this phenomenon in females with PWS and maternal disomy 15 and showed an overabundance of extreme non-random X chromosome inactivation. Trisomy 15 rescue in early pregnancy of the developing PWS female may allow for a small number of cells to survive and populate embryo development. The small number cells rescued by the trisomic event may have the same X chromosome active leading to non-random X chromosome inactivation skewness in subsequent cell division and presence of an X-linked recessive condition such as colorblindness or hemophilia, if the mother is a carrier of this X-linked disorder but unaffected as a female. Therefore, this X-chromosome skewness can allow for expression of X-linked conditions in PWS females with maternal disomy 15 requiring disease surveillance.

4. Materials and Methods

The CytoScan HD array (hg19/GRCh37) consists of 750,000 genotype-able single nucleotides polymorphism (SNP) and 1.9 million non-polymorphic probes performed by Ambry Genetics (Aliso Viejo, CA, USA), a commercial CLIA/CAP genetics testing laboratory on people with PWS who were being screened for enrollment in the DESTINY PWS study. Chromosomal microarray testing was undertaken on buccal swab or peripheral blood samples. The electronic data files were sent to the University of Kansas Medical Center for computer generated data analysis and PWS molecular genetic classification and determination. The cutoff values to detect a deletion included 50 DNA probes occupying at least 20,000 base pairs and a duplication of 30,000 base pairs. Regions of homozygosity (ROH) was set at 3 Mb and loss of heterozygosity (LOH) for determination of the disomic status using ChAS version 3.3.0.139 (r10838) computer software to set at 8 Mb following established protocols or standards [5]. Consanguinity can present a diagnostic problem for detection of segmental uniparental disomy but consanguinity is associated with ROHs in multiple chromosomes and not usually found in abundance in terminal chromosome regions as seen in uniparental disomy [5,6,23]. The total sample in our study consisted of 154 individuals (86 females 68 males), mostly Caucasian with and average age of 13.95 years (range of 4 to 44 years). An image of the microarray data was generated for each participant and a report summarizing the microarray findings with the PWS molecular genetic class was produced.

5. Conclusions

In a clinical summary, individuals with PWS and segmental isodisomy 15 or total isodisomy 15 may require further evaluation for additional genetic disorders (e.g., recessive inheritance) where the disease genes would be present in the mother as a carrier status and both identical recessive gene alleles would be passed to the PWS child. Therefore, these PWS children would be at risk for hundreds of conditions where recessive genes are located on chromosome 15 and in the isodisomic region as summarized in Table 1. These children may need close surveillance for these genetic conditions (e.g., Tay-Sachs, Bloom, albinism, hearing loss, seizures, mitochondrial DNA depletion, and others) depending on the genes playing a role in disease causation located in the altered segmental or total isodisomic chromosome 15 regions with input on recurrence risk. In addition, PWS females with maternal disomy 15 may be at risk for X-linked disorders as trisomy 15 rescue occurs in early pregnancy of the disomic 15 female and the X chromosome may therefore be skewed in that PWS female allowing for the presence of X-linked conditions [6]. Healthcare providers may use this review with discussion and be alerted to potential genetic conditions which the PWS child may be at-risk based on their family history and genetic findings as described. More advanced genetic testing may be warranted such as next-generation sequencing of genes on chromosome 15 in both males and females with PWS having maternal segmental or total isodisomy 15 and females should also be screened for X chromosome disorders as noted.

Author Contributions: M.G.B. raised the question, designed the study and wrote original manuscript; W.A.H. analyzed the data and prepared the manuscript, M.G.B., N.C., A.B. and W.A.H. revised and edited the manuscript, reviewed and analyzed data; all authors agreed to the final version of the manuscript. All authors have read and agreed to the published version of the manuscript.

Funding: Funding and support from Soleno Therapeutics (ClinicalTrials.gov number NCT03440814) and the National Institute of Child Health and Human Development (NICHD), grant number HD 02528.

Institutional Review Board Statement: Participants were consented under IRB-approved protocol (IRB#00000533) undertaken by Soleno Therapeutics that allows research. All participants and/or guardians signed the IRB approved human subjects research forms prior to enrolling in the study.

Informed Consent Statement: All participants and/or guardians signed an IRB approved human subjects research forms prior to enrolling in study.

Data Availability Statement: Reasonable requests available from authors.

Acknowledgments: We thank the families and participants with PWS who enrolled in the study and the Prader-Willi Syndrome Association/USA.

Conflicts of Interest: The authors declare no conflict of interest in the data reported. A.B. and N.C. are employees of Soleno Therapeutics.

References

1. Ledbetter, D.H.; Riccardi, V.M.; Airhart, S.D.; Strobel, R.J.; Keenan, B.S.; Crawford, J.D. Deletions of chromosome 15 as a cause of the Prader-Willi syndrome. *N. Engl. J. Med.* **1981**, *5*, 325–329. [CrossRef]
2. Delach, J.A.; Rosengren, S.; Kaplan, L.; Greenstein, R.M.; Cassidy, S.B.; Benn, P.A. Comparison of high- resolution chromosome banding and fluorescence in situ hybridization (FISH) for the laboratory evaluation of Prader-Willi syndrome and Angelman syndrome. *Am. J. Med. Genet.* **1994**, *52*, 85–91. [CrossRef]
3. Butler, M.G.; Fischer, W.; Kibiryeva, N.; Bittel, D.C. Array comparative genomic hybridization (aCGH) analysis in Prader-Willi syndrome. *Am. J. Med. Genet. A* **2008**, *146A*, 854–860. [CrossRef] [PubMed]
4. Butler, M.G.; Duis, J. Chromosome 15 Imprinting Disorders: Genetic Laboratory Methodology and Approaches. *Front. Pediatr.* **2020**, *12*, 154. [CrossRef] [PubMed]
5. Papenhausen, P.; Schwartz, S.; Risheg, H.; Keitges, E.; Gadi, I.; Burnside, R.D.; Jaswaney, V.; Pappas, J.; Pasion, R.; Friedman, K.; et al. UPD detection using homozygosity profiling with a SNP genotyping microarray. *Am. J. Med. Genet. A* **2011**, *155A*, 757–768. [CrossRef] [PubMed]
6. Butler, M.G. Single Gene and Syndromic Causes of Obesity: Illustrative Examples. *Prog. Mol. Biol. Transl. Sci.* **2016**, *140*, 1–45. [CrossRef] [PubMed]
7. Butler, M.G.; Lee, P.D.K.; Whitman, B.Y. Management of Prader-Willi Syndrome. In *Management of Prader-Willi Syndrome*, 3rd ed.; Springer: Berlin/Heidelberg, Germany, 2006; pp. 1–550.
8. Butler, M.G.; Thompson, T. Prader-Willi Syndrome: Clinical and Genetic Findings. *Endocrinologist.* **2000**, *10* (Suppl. 1), 3S–16S. [CrossRef]
9. Bittel, D.C.; Butler, M.G. Prader-Willi syndrome: Clinical genetics, cytogenetics and molecular biology. *Expert. Rev. Mol. Med.* **2005**, *25*, 1–20. [CrossRef]
10. Butler, M.G.; Hartin, S.N.; Hossain, W.A.; Manzardo, A.M.; Kimonis, V.; Dykens, E.; Gold, J.A.; Kim, S.J.; Weisensel, N.; Tamura, R.; et al. Molecular genetic classification in Prader-Willi syndrome: A multisite cohort study. *J. Med. Genet.* **2019**, *56*, 149–153. [CrossRef]
11. Butler, M.G.; Bittel, D.C.; Kibiryeva, N.; Talebizadeh, Z.; Thompson, T. Behavioral differences among subjects with Prader-Willi syndrome and type I or type II deletion and maternal disomy. *Pediatrics* **2004**, *113 Pt 1*, 565–573. [CrossRef]
12. Zarcone, J.; Napolitano, D.; Peterson, C.; Breidbord, J.; Ferraioli, S.; Caruso-Anderson, M.; Holsen, L.; Butler, M.G.; Thompson, T. The relationship between compulsive behaviour and academic achievement across the three genetic subtypes of Prader-Willi syndrome. *J. Intellect. Disabil. Res.* **2007**, *51 Pt 6*, 478–487. [CrossRef]
13. Roof, E.; Stone, W.; MacLean, W.; Feurer, I.D.; Thompson, T.; Butler, M.G. Intellectual characteristics of Prader-Willi syndrome: Comparison of genetic subtypes. *J. Intellect. Disabil. Res.* **2000**, *44*, 25–30. [CrossRef] [PubMed]
14. Butler, M.G.; Matthews, N.A.; Pate, N.; Surampalli, A.; Gold, J.A.; Khare, M.; Thompson, T.; Cassidy, S.B.; Kimonis, V.E. Impact of genetic subtypes of Prader-Willi syndrome with growth hormone therapy on intelligence and body mass index. *Am. J. Med. Genet. A* **2019**, *179*, 1826–1835. [CrossRef] [PubMed]
15. Miller, J.L.; Yanovski, J.; Bird, L.; Salehi, P.; Abuzzahab, J.; Shoemaker, A.; Fleishman, A.; Stevenson, D.; Angulo, M.; Viskochil, D.; et al. Long-term Ssfety and efficacy evaluation of diazoxide choline Eetended-release (DCCR) tablets in patients with Prader-Willi syndrome. In Proceedings of the 11th International Prader-Willi Syndrome Organisation Conference, Limerick, Ireland, 6–10 July 2022.
16. Butler, M.G.; Hedges, L.K.; Rogan, P.K.; Seip, J.R.; Cassidy, S.B.; Moeschler, J.B. Klinefelter and trisomy X syndromes in patients with Prader-Willi syndrome and uniparental maternal disomy of chromosome 15–a coincidence? *Am. J. Med. Genet.* **1997**, *72*, 111. [CrossRef]
17. Kearney, H.M.; Kearney, J.B.; Conlin, L.K. Diagnostic implications of excessive homozygosity detected by SNP-based microarrays: Consanguinity, uniparental disomy, and recessive single-gene mutations. *Clin. Lab. Med.* **2011**, *4*, 595–613. [CrossRef]

18. Butler, M.G.; Bittel, D.C.; Kibiryeva, N.; Cooley, L.D.; Yu, S. An interstitial 15q11-q14 deletion: Expanded Prader-Willi syndrome phenotype. *Am. J. Med. Genet. A* **2010**, *152A*, 404–408, Erratum in: *Am. J. Med. Genet. A* **2010**, *152A*, 1331–1332. [CrossRef] [PubMed]
19. Henkhaus, R.S.; Kim, S.J.; Kimonis, V.E.; Gold, J.A.; Dykens, E.M.; Driscoll, D.J.; Butler, M.G. Methylation-specific multiplex ligation-dependent probe amplification and identification of deletion genetic subtypes in Prader-Willi syndrome. *Genet. Test Mol. Biomark.* **2012**, *16*, 178–186. [CrossRef]
20. Buiting, K.; Nazlican, H.; Galetzka, D.; Wawrzik, M.; Gross, S.; Horsthemke, B. C15orf2 and a novel noncoding transcript from the Prader-Willi/Angelman syndrome region show monoallelic expression in fetal brain. *Genomics* **2007**, *89*, 588–595. [CrossRef]
21. Multhusamy, K.; Macke, E.L.; Klee, E.W.; Tebben, P.J.; Hand, J.L.; Hasadsri, L.; Marcou, C.A.; Schimmenti, L.A. Congenital ichthyosis in Prader-Willi syndrome associated with maternal chromosome 15 uniparental disomy: Case report and review of autosomal recessive conditions unmasked by UPD. *Am. J. Med. Genet. A* **2020**, *182*, 2442–2449. [CrossRef]
22. Butler, M.G.; Theodoro, M.F.; Bittel, D.C.; Kuipers, P.J.; Driscoll, D.J.; Talebizadeh, Z. X-chromosome inactivation patterns in females with Prader-Willi syndrome. *Am. J. Med. Genet. A* **2007**, *143A*, 469–475. [CrossRef]
23. Del Gaudio, D.; Shinawi, M.; Astbury, C.; Tayeh, M.K.; Deak, L.; Raca, G. ACMG Laboratory Quality Assurance Committee. Diagnostic testing for uniparental disomy: A point to consider statement from the American College of Medical Genetics and Genomics (ACMG). *Genet. Med.* **2020**, *22*, 1133–1141. [CrossRef] [PubMed]

Disclaimer/Publisher's Note: The statements, opinions and data contained in all publications are solely those of the individual author(s) and contributor(s) and not of MDPI and/or the editor(s). MDPI and/or the editor(s) disclaim responsibility for any injury to people or property resulting from any ideas, methods, instructions or products referred to in the content.

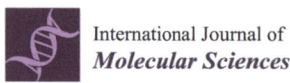 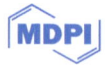

Case Report

Mowat–Wilson Syndrome: Case Report and Review of *ZEB2* Gene Variant Types, Protein Defects and Molecular Interactions

Caroline St. Peter [1], Waheeda A. Hossain [1], Scott Lovell [2], Syed K. Rafi [1] and Merlin G. Butler [1,*]

[1] Departments of Psychiatry & Behavioral Sciences and Pediatrics, University of Kansas Medical Center, 3901 Rainbow Blvd. MS 4015, Kansas City, KS 66160, USA; c527s208@kumc.edu (C.S.P.); whossain@kumc.edu (W.A.H.); rafigene@yahoo.com (S.K.R.)

[2] Protein Structure Laboratory, University of Kansas, Lawrence, KS 66047, USA; swlovell@ku.edu

* Correspondence: mbutler4@kumc.edu; Tel.: +1-(913)-588-1300; Fax: +1-(913)-588-1305

Abstract: Mowat–Wilson syndrome (MWS) is a rare genetic neurodevelopmental congenital disorder associated with various defects of the zinc finger E-box binding homeobox 2 (*ZEB2*) gene. The *ZEB2* gene is autosomal dominant and encodes six protein domains including the SMAD-binding protein, which functions as a transcriptional corepressor involved in the conversion of neuroepithelial cells in early brain development and as a mediator of trophoblast differentiation. This review summarizes reported *ZEB2* gene variants, their types, and frequencies among the 10 exons of *ZEB2*. Additionally, we summarized their corresponding encoded protein defects including the most common variant, c.2083 C>T in exon 8, which directly impacts the homeodomain (HD) protein domain. This single defect was found in 11% of the 298 reported patients with MWS. This review demonstrates that exon 8 encodes at least three of the six protein domains and accounts for 66% (198/298) of the variants identified. More than 90% of the defects were due to nonsense or frameshift changes. We show examples of protein modeling changes that occurred as a result of *ZEB2* gene defects. We also report a novel pathogenic variant in exon 8 in a 5-year-old female proband with MWS. This review further explores other genes predicted to be interacting with the *ZEB2* gene and their predicted gene–gene molecular interactions with protein binding effects on embryonic multi-system development such as craniofacial, spine, brain, kidney, cardiovascular, and hematopoiesis.

Keywords: Mowat–Wilson syndrome (MWS); case report; review; *ZEB2* gene variants; ZEB2 protein domains and defects; ZEB2 functional molecular interactions

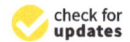

Citation: St. Peter, C.; Hossain, W.A.; Lovell, S.; Rafi, S.K.; Butler, M.G. Mowat–Wilson Syndrome: Case Report and Review of *ZEB2* Gene Variant Types, Protein Defects and Molecular Interactions. *Int. J. Mol. Sci.* **2024**, *25*, 2838. https://doi.org/10.3390/ijms25052838

Academic Editor: Mario Costa

Received: 21 November 2023
Revised: 12 January 2024
Accepted: 23 February 2024
Published: 29 February 2024

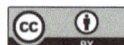

Copyright: © 2024 by the authors. Licensee MDPI, Basel, Switzerland. This article is an open access article distributed under the terms and conditions of the Creative Commons Attribution (CC BY) license (https://creativecommons.org/licenses/by/4.0/).

1. Introduction

Rare genetic disorders have been estimated to affect up to 10% of the population [1]. Advances in genomic technologies such as exome sequencing are becoming more widely used to gain insight into the cause and diagnosis of these rare disorders by identifying specific molecular defects and outcomes in patients with Mendelian or non-Mendelian disorders. Exome sequencing studies have shown underlying causative genes in approximately 25% of cases [2]. A growing number of gene variants and types involved in protein production have not been well characterized in rare disorders, including Mowat–Wilson syndrome.

Mowat–Wilson syndrome (MWS) is an example of a rare genetic disorder with intellectual disabilities with multiple congenital anomalies and multi-system involvement. This disorder was first reported in 1998 [3] and now about 300 patients have been found in the medical literature or databases. Chromosome 2q22-2q23 deletions were reported in the first patients with this disorder and the zinc finger E-box binding homeobox 2 (*ZEB2*; NM_014795.4) gene was found in this region. Other patients with MWS with overlapping features having *ZEB2* gene deletions or duplications of different sizes and intragenic variants have been identified [4–6].

Mowat–Wilson syndrome shows clinical variability and is recognized as a multiple congenital anomaly disorder involving several organ systems. Clinical facial features include a square-shaped face with a prominent and triangular chin, high forehead, large eyebrows with medial flaring, hypertelorism, deep-set and large eyes, broad and depressed nasal bridge, rounded nasal tip, prominent columella, open mouth, and M-shaped upper lip. The ears are posteriorly rotated with large, uplifted earlobes with a central depression reminiscent of a red blood corpuscle. The face lengthens with age and the chin becomes more prominent with the appearance of broad-appearing eyebrows. Individuals with this disorder often have severe intellectual disability with a mean age of walking at four years and a wide-based gait with a tendency for flexed arms in resting position [7–10]. Most individuals with MWS have seizures (84%) and an abnormal EEG. Short stature and microcephaly are often present with cerebral anomalies including corpus callosum and hippocampal defects, enlargement of cerebral ventricles, white matter abnormalities, large basal ganglia, and cortical and cerebellar malformations. Gastrointestinal problems such as chronic constipation are present and are most often related to lack of innervation causing Hirschsprung disease of either the short or long segment variety and are documented in about 50% of patients. Congenital heart disease is reported in 58% of patients including patent ductus arteriosus, atrial septal or ventricular septal defects, pulmonary stenosis, aortic coarctation, Tetralogy of Fallot, aortic valve abnormalities, and a pulmonary artery sling with or without tracheal stenosis/hypoplasia. Genitourinary and kidney anomalies are common including hypospadias, bifid scrotum, cryptorchidism, pelvic or duplex kidneys, and hydronephrosis [7,8]. The wide range of clinical findings may relate to different *ZEB2* gene variants and therefore additional research is needed to identify the type and frequency of gene variants and their impact on protein structure and function.

The *ZEB2* gene is located on chromosome 2q22.3 and expressed in the human nervous system throughout development, exemplifying its importance in gliogenic and neurogenic processes. ZEB2 has been documented to play roles in the induction of the neuroectoderm and neural crest. It acts to direct neural crest cells and regulates the development of cerebral regions, along with development of the spinal cord, cardiac, and enteric systems [8,9]. Hence, individuals with MWS can present with a combination of multi-system deficits with variable penetrance [10–12].

In searching the medical literature and unreported databases, we found a total of 298 patients with MWS and *ZEB2* variants. We tabulated these variants in the *ZEB2* gene and protein and summarized the frequency of gene variants within each of the 10 exons and their relationship to protein structure and function. We also obtained the predicted *ZEB2* gene interactions with other genes implicated and molecular pathways pertaining to neurodevelopmental multi-system involvement. Additionally, we described a new patient with MWS having a novel pathogenic variant due to a heterozygous c.2471_2475del5 in exon 8 of the *ZEB2* gene.

2. Detailed Case Description
2.1. Clinical Case Report

Our proband was prenatally diagnosed with a complex cardiovascular single ventricular disorder and subsequent amniocentesis genetic testing was normal. She was delivered at 37 weeks' gestation with a double outlet right ventricle, subaortic and anterior muscular ventricular septal defects, and hypoplastic mitral and tricuspid valves with a hypoplastic left heart. The family initially took her home for palliative care, but upon further evaluation, underwent multiple cardiac and surgical procedures, including Fontan and Glenn procedures. These surgical interventions, which took place between one and six months of age, led to a partial recovery of cardiac function.

Our proband has two healthy siblings without cardiac or other disorders. The family history was also unremarkable for birth defects and no consanguinity was noted. The patient required G-tube feedings and close health monitoring with multiple evaluations and hospitalizations throughout infancy. She had a normal karyotype and chromosomal microarray studies during infancy.

Around one year of age, a comprehensive connective tissue genetic test including the autosomal dominant *ZEB2* gene (NM_014795) was ordered via a commercially approved genetic testing laboratory (Connective Tissue Gene Tests (CTGT)). The DNA sequencing revealed a heterozygous c.2471_2475del5 in exon 8 of the *ZEB2* gene. These five base pair deletions resulted in a frameshift, causing aberrant mRNA transcription and the defective protein causing MWS. All coding exons and exon boundaries of the gene were amplified by PCR and ABI 3730 sequencers, as standard genetic testing at the time. Additionally, coding exons and exon boundaries were analyzed for copy number variation using a high-density targeted array. The genetic defect was considered de novo in view of the negative family history, including two unaffected siblings for birth defects or features of MWS. *ZEB2* is an autosomal dominant gene and parental DNA testing was not undertaken.

At about three years of age her height was 87.3 cm (6%ile), weight was 11.7 kg (7%ile), and body mass index was 15.35 kg/m^2 (36%ile). At that age, her heart rate was 120, respiration was 20, oxygen saturation was 80%, blood pressure (right arm) was 85/33, and blood pressure (right leg) was 107/54. At five years and four months of age, her height was 102.1 cm (3%ile), weight was 14.3 kg (3%ile), and body mass index was 13.72 kg/m^2 (15%ile). She was able to write, recognize a few written words, and perform several preschool-appropriate skills. She spoke at the level of a two-and-a-half-year-old and communicated her wants and needs, both verbally and with sign language. She had severe cardiac defects, including, but not limited to hypoplastic left heart syndrome (HLHS), ventricular septal defects (VSDs), left pulmonary artery (LPA) sling causing tracheomalacia, dysplastic tricuspid valve causing severe tricuspid regurgitation (TR), and partial anomalous pulmonary venous connection (PAPVR). She presented with typical MWS facial features, a duplex kidney and VUR, visual deficits, tooth abnormalities, hypotonia, global delays, secondary kidney and liver issues, high intracranial pressure (pseudotumor cerebri), and GI issues. She was not able to eat food, as she would develop severe abdominal pain, intractable vomiting, GI bleeding, and colitis, often requiring hospitalization for several weeks requiring IV fluids and/or TPN after ingestion of any amount of food. She was treated with diuretics. She was G-tube dependent and fed neonate infant formula (an elemental formula), with some GI bleeding, vomiting, and discomfort noted at baseline. Although Hirschsprung disease was ruled out based on rectal biopsy studies, she had gastroparesis and chronic constipation. Her EEG studies on more than one occasion were normal. She had no documented seizures/epilepsy (see Figure 1). Her overall health status, function, and quality of life continued to decline in spite of continuous care and monitoring. Her parents made the ultimate decision to enroll her in hospice care where she passed away at about 5 years of age.

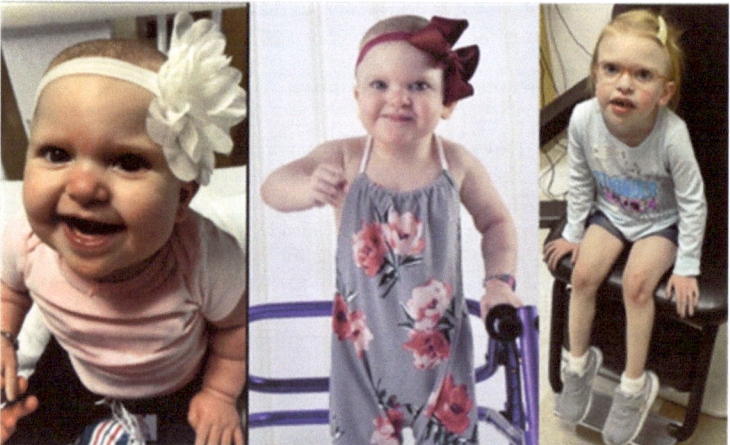

Figure 1. Our proband with typical craniofacial features and phenotype of MWS. She had a pathogenic heterozygous c.2471_2475del5 in exon 8 of the *ZEB2* gene. Photos were obtained with consent during infancy, early childhood, and before her death at about five years of age.

2.2. Genetic and Protein Domain Data Collection of Patients with Mowat-Wilson Syndrome

Computer literature and unreported databases were searched for keywords such as Mowat–Wilson, *ZEB2* gene and protein defects or variants, or clinical features using PUBMED (www.pubmed.com; accessed on 1 October 2022) and performed from 2001 to the present (2023). About 180 published reports were found with the most useful data obtained from approximately 20 articles, as summarized in Table 1. From this study, we analyzed 266 cases of Mowat–Wilson syndrome and an additional 32 deidentified unpublished patients accessed from the Mowat–Wilson Syndrome Foundation for a total of 298 patients. These sources were used to collect data regarding *ZEB2* gene variants, types, frequencies, and protein defects along with domain locations and functions. We found that exon 8 encodes at least three of the six protein domains of the *ZEB2* gene and accounts for 66% (198/298) of the variants identified.

Table 1. Review of Mowat–Wilson syndrome with *ZEB2* gene and protein variants.

Our Study ID	Publication ID/ (Patient Number)	ZEB2 Exon	ZEB2 Gene Variant or Defect	Protein Defect	Type of Genetic Defect	ZEB2 Protein Domain
1	Mowat–Wilson Syndrome Foundation [MWSF]/(P1)	-	c.2180del	p.Leu727Tyrfs*7	Frameshift	-
2	MWSF/(P2)	8	c.2083C>T	p.Arg695Ter	Nonsense	HD
3	MWSF/(P3)	9	c.3002del	p.Cys1001LeufsX74	Frameshift	C-ZFa
4	MWSF/(P4)	8	c.2761C>T	p.Arg921*	Nonsense	-
5	MWSF/(P5)	9	c.3095G>A	p.Cys1032Tyr	Missense	C-ZFb
6	MWSF/(P6)	10	c.3213dup	p.Q1072AfsX52	Frameshift	C-ZFb
7	MWSF/(P7)	6	c.696C>G	p.Tyr232*	Nonsense	N-ZFa
8	MWSF/(P8)	6	c.805C>T	p.Q269X	Nonsense	N-ZFb
9	MWSF/(P9)	8	c.2061del	p.Phe687Leufs*2	Frameshift	HD
10	MWSF/(P10)	10	-	p.Tyr999*	Nonsense	C-ZFa
11	MWSF/(P11)	3	c.108del	p.E37fsX74	Frameshift	-
12	MWSF/(P12)	8	c.2721del	p.Thr908LeufsTer22	Frameshift	-
13	MWSF/(P13)	2	c.81_84dup	p.Asp29Leufs*2	Frameshift	-
14	MWSF/(P14)	8	c.2094C>A	p.Y698X	Nonsense	HD
15	MWSF/(P15)	6	c.763C>T	p.Q255X	Nonsense	N-ZFa
16	MWSF/(P16)	intron 3	c.331+1_331+2dup	-	Splicing	-
17	MWSF/(P17)	10	c.3533del	-	Deletion	-
18	MWSF/(P18)	10	c.3196C>T	p.His1066Tyr	Missense	C-ZFb
19	MWSF/(P19)	8	c.2083C>T	p.R695X	Nonsense	HD
20	MWSF/(P20)	8	c.2083C>T	p.R695X	Nonsense	HD
21	MWSF/(P21)	8	c.2367del	-	Frameshift	CID
22	MWSF/(P22)	6	c.674C>A	p.S225X	Nonsense	N-ZFa
23	MWSF/(P23)	8	c.909_910ins	p.H304Ffs*5	Frameshift	N-ZFc
24	MWSF/(P24)	8	c.1795del	p.His599MetfsX8	Frameshift	-
25	MWSF/(P25)	2	c.31del	p.Arg11Glyfs*16	Frameshift	-
26	MWSF/(P26)	8	c.1571_1572ins	p.Ser524Argfs*4	Frameshift	-
27	MWSF/(P27)	1–10	6.2 Mb deletion Ch2q22.1-q22.3	-	Chromosome deletion	-

Table 1. Cont.

Our Study ID	Publication ID/ (Patient Number)	ZEB2 Exon	ZEB2 Gene Variant or Defect	Protein Defect	Type of Genetic Defect	ZEB2 Protein Domain
28	MWSF/(P28)	8	c.1956C>A	p.Y652X	Nonsense	HD
29	MWSF/(P29)	1–10	6.9 Mb deletion Ch2q22.1-q22.3	-	Chromosome deletion	-
30	MWSF/(P30)	4	c.357_358del	p.Met120GlyfsX11	Frameshift	-
31	MWSF/(P31)	-	144 kb deletion Ch2q22.3	-	Chromosome deletion	-
32	MWSF/(P32)	10	c.3212_3215dup	p.Gln1072HisfsTer53	Frameshift	C-ZFb
33	[13] Zou et al., 2020/(P1)	3	c.290G>A	p.Trp97X	Nonsense	-
34	Zou et al., 2020/(P2)	8	c.1067_1068ins	p.Val357Aspfs*15	Frameshift	-
35	Zou et al., 2020/(P3)	8	c.2761C>T	p.Arg921X	Nonsense	-
36	Zou et al., 2020/(P4)	8	c.3214C>T	p.Gln1072X	Nonsense	C-ZFb
37	[14] Hu et al., 2020/(P1)	3	c.250G>T	p.E84*	Nonsense	-
38	[15] Ho et al., 2020/(P1)	8&9	ZEB2 gene Exons 8 and 9 deletion	-	Deletion	-
39	Ho et al., 2020/(P2)	8	c.1472_c.1473ins	p.Met491Ilefs*9	Small insertion, Frameshift	-
40	Ho et al., 2020/(P3)	8	c.2083C>T	p.Arg695*	Nonsense	HD
41	Ho et al., 2020/(P4)	8	c.1387del	p.Val463Phefs*24	Frameshift	SMD
42	Ho et al., 2020/(P5)	8	c.2646del	p.Val883Cysfs*4	Small deletion, Frameshift	-
43	Ho et al., 2020/(P6)	3	c.189del	p.Ser64Valfs*11	Small deletion, Frameshift	-
44	Ho et al., 2020/(P7)	3	c.189del	p.Ser64Valfs*11	Small deletion, Frameshift	-
45	Ho et al., 2020/(P8)	1–10	ZEB2 gene Exons 1-10 deletion	-	Deletion	-
46	Ho et al., 2020/(P9)	9	c1297C>T	p.Gln433*	Nonsense	-
47	Ho et al., 2020/(P10)	10	c.3335del	p.Tyr1112Cysfs*128	Small deletion, Frameshift	-
48	Ho et al., 2020/(P11)	1–10	ZEB2 gene Exons 1-10 deletion	-	Deletion	-
49	Ho et al., 2020/(P12)	7	c.857_858del	p.Glu286Valfs*8	Small deletion, Frameshift	N-ZFb
50	Ho et al., 2020/(P13)	3	c.291G>A	p.Trp97*	Nonsense	-
51	Ho et al., 2020/(P14)	8	c.2865C>A	p.Tyr955*	Nonsense	-
52	Ho et al., 2020/(P15)	9	c.169delins	p.Leu565*	Small indel, Frameshift	-
53	[16] Wenger et al., 2014/(P1)	8	-	p.R695X	Nonsense	HD
54	Wenger et al., 2014/(P2)	8	-	p.Q384X	Nonsense	-

Table 1. *Cont.*

Our Study ID	Publication ID/ (Patient Number)	ZEB2 Exon	ZEB2 Gene Variant or Defect	Protein Defect	Type of Genetic Defect	ZEB2 Protein Domain
55	Wenger et al., 2014/(P3)	8	-	p.G1182KfsX59	Frameshift	-
56	Wenger et al., 2014/(P4)	5	-	p.E181RfsX211X	Frameshift	-
57	Wenger et al., 2014/(P5)	9	-	p.F1008C	Missense	C-ZFa
58	Wenger et al., 2014/(P6)	7	c.808-1G>T	-	Splicing	N-ZF
59	Wenger et al., 2014/(P7)	10	-	p.Ser1071Pro	Missense	C-ZFb
60	Wenger et al., 2014/(P8)	8	-	p.L894FfsX53	Frameshift	-
61	Wenger et al., 2014/(P9)	8	-	p.S434Vfs7X	Frameshift	-
62	Wenger et al., 2014/(P10)	8	-	p.R695X	Nonsense	HD
63	Wenger et al., 2014/(P11)	8	-	p.R695X	Nonsense	HD
64	Wenger et al., 2014/(P12)	8	-	p.R695X	Nonsense	HD
65	Wenger et al., 2014/(P13)	8	-	p.M476WfsX11	Frameshift	-
66	Wenger et al., 2014/(P14)	8	-	p.P906LfsX24	Frameshift	-
67	Wenger et al., 2014/(P15)	6	-	p.Q209X	Nonsense	-
68	Wenger et al., 2014/(P16)	8	-	p.V627SfsX4	Frameshift	-
69	Wenger et al., 2014/(P17)	9	-	p.S1011AfsX53	Frameshift	C-ZFa
70	Wenger et al., 2014/(P18)	6	-	p.R218RfsX21	Frameshift	-
71	Wenger et al., 2014/(P19)	8	-	p.V621AfsX25	Frameshift	-
72	Wenger et al., 2014/(P20)	1–10	-	-	Whole gene deletion	-
73	Wenger et al., 2014/(P21)	8	-	p.S359TfsX3	Frameshift	-
74	Wenger et al., 2014/(P22)	8	-	p.R695X	Nonsense	HD
75	Wenger et al., 2014/(P23)	8	-	p.Q962X	Nonsense	-
76	Wenger et al., 2014/(P24)	8	-	p.A907LfsX23	Frameshift	-
77	Wenger et al., 2014/(P25)	8	-	p.G351VfsX19	Frameshift	-
78	Wenger et al., 2014/(P26)	5	-	p.E181RfsX211	Frameshift	-
79	Wenger et al., 2014/(P27)	8	c.1224del	-	Deletion	-
80	Wenger et al., 2014/(P28)	8	-	p.I390LfsX6 & p.L388F	Frameshift	-
81	[6] Baxter et al., 2017/(P1)	1&2	-	-	Partial duplication	-
82	[17] Mundhofir et al., 2012/(P1)	8	c.1965C>G	p.Tyr652*	Nonsense	HD
83	[18] Murray et al., 2015/(P1)	8	c.2083C>T	p.R695X	Nonsense	HD
84	[19] Wang et al., 2019/(P1)	7	c.904C>T	p.R302X	Nonsense	N-ZFc
85	Wang et al., 2019/(P2)	6	c.756C>A	p.Y252X	Nonsense	N-ZFa
86	Wang et al., 2019/(P3)	8	c.2761C>T	p.R921X	Nonsense	-
87	[20] Yamada et al., 2014/(P1)	3	c.259G>T	p.E87X	Nonsense	-

Table 1. Cont.

Our Study ID	Publication ID/ (Patient Number)	ZEB2 Exon	ZEB2 Gene Variant or Defect	Protein Defect	Type of Genetic Defect	ZEB2 Protein Domain
88	Yamada et al., 2014/(P2)	3	c.259G>T	p.E87X	Nonsense	-
89	Yamada et al., 2014/(P3)	3	c.259G>T	p.E87X	Nonsense	-
90	Yamada et al., 2014 (P4)	7	c.811C>T	p.Q271X	Nonsense	N-ZFb
91	Yamada et al., 2014/(P5)	7	c.904C>T	p.R302X	Nonsense	N-ZFc
92	Yamada et al., 2014/(P6)	8	c.936C>A	p.C312X	Nonsense	N-ZFc
93	Yamada et al., 2014/(P7)	8	c.1027C>T	p.R343X	Nonsense	-
94	Yamada et al., 2014/(P8)	8	c.1027C>T	p.R343X	Nonsense	-
95	Yamada et al., 2014/(P9)	8	c.1027C>T	p.R343X	Nonsense	-
96	Yamada et al., 2014/(P10)	8	c.1298C>T	p.Q433X	Nonsense	-
97	Yamada et al., 2014/(P11)	8	c.1489C>T	p.Q497X	Nonsense	-
98	Yamada et al., 2014/(P12)	8	c.1645A>T	p.R549X	Nonsense	-
99	Yamada et al., 2014/(P13)	8	c.1825G>T	p.E609X	Nonsense	-
100	Yamada et al., 2014/(P14)	8	c.2083C>T	p.R695X	Nonsense	HD
101	Yamada et al., 2014/(P15)	8	c.2083C>T	p.R695X	Nonsense	HD
102	Yamada et al., 2014/(P16)	8	c.2083C>T	p.R695X	Nonsense	HD
103	Yamada et al., 2014/(P17)	8	c.2083C>T	p.R695X	Nonsense	HD
104	Yamada et al., 2014/(P18)	8	c.2083C>T	p.R695X	Nonsense	HD
105	Yamada et al., 2014/(P19)	8	c.2083C>T	p.R695X	Nonsense	HD
106	Yamada et al., 2014/(P20)	8	c.2083C>T	p.R695X	Nonsense	HD
107	Yamada et al., 2014/(P21)	8	c.2083C>T	p.R695X	Nonsense	HD
108	Yamada et al., 2014/(P22)	8	c.2083C>T	p.R695X	Nonsense	HD
109	Yamada et al., 2014/(P23)	8	c.2083C>T	p.R695X	Nonsense	HD
110	Yamada et al., 2014/(P24)	8	c.2083C>T	p.R695X	Nonsense	HD
111	Yamada et al., 2014/(P25)	8	c.2083C>T	p.R695X	Nonsense	HD
112	Yamada et al., 2014/(P26)	8	c.2399C>G	p.S800X	Nonsense	CID
113	Yamada et al., 2014/(P27)	8	c.2615C>G	p.S872X	Nonsense	-
114	Yamada et al., 2014/(P28)	8	c.2761C>T	p.R921X	Nonsense	-
115	Yamada et al., 2014/(P29)	8	c.2761C>T	p.R921X	Nonsense	-
116	Yamada et al., 2014/(P1)	3	c.162_164del	p.P55Lfs*20	Frameshift	-
117	Yamada et al., 2014/(P2)	3	c.175_182del	p.T60Sfs*3	Frameshift	-
118	Yamada et al., 2014/(P3)	3	c270_272del	p.G91Vfs*17	Frameshift	-
119	Yamada et al., 2014/(P4)	3	c.311_312dup	p.A105Sfs*16	Frameshift	-
120	Yamada et al., 2014/(P5)	5	c.459_460del	p.E154Rfs*58	Frameshift	-
121	Yamada et al., 2014/(P6)	6	c.635_638dup	p.P214Lfs*26	Frameshift	-
122	Yamada et al., 2014/(P7)	6	c.647del	p.C216Sfs*8	Frameshift	-
123	Yamada et al., 2014/(P8)	6	c.759_760dup	p.Q255Pfs*8	Frameshift	N-ZFa
124	Yamada et al., 2014/(P9)	7	c.852_855del	p.T285Rfs*9	Frameshift	N-ZFb
125	Yamada et al., 2014/(P10)	7	c.855_858del	p.E286Vfs*8	Frameshift	N-ZFb
126	Yamada et al., 2014/(P11)	7	c.862_863del	p.G288Afs*10	Frameshift	N-ZFb

Table 1. Cont.

Our Study ID	Publication ID/ (Patient Number)	ZEB2 Exon	ZEB2 Gene Variant or Defect	Protein Defect	Type of Genetic Defect	ZEB2 Protein Domain
127	Yamada et al., 2014/(P12)	8	c.1169ins	p.I390Tfs*41	Frameshift	-
128	Yamada et al., 2014/(P13)	8	c.1169_1170del	p.T392Qfs*4	Frameshift	-
129	Yamada et al., 2014/(P14)	8	c.1174_1178del	p.T392Nfs*3	Frameshift	-
130	Yamada et al., 2014/(P15)	8	c.1176del	p.E393Nfs*3	Frameshift	-
131	Yamada et al., 2014/(P16)	8	c.1212_1213del	p.A405Lfs*12	Frameshift	-
132	Yamada et al., 2014/(P17)	8	c.1268_1273del	p.S424Lfs*2	Frameshift	-
133	Yamada et al., 2014/(P18)	8	c.1280_1286del7ins	p.G427Dfs*2	Frameshift	-
134	Yamada et al., 2014/(P19)	8	c.1334_1337dup	p.L447Ffs*9	Frameshift	SMD
135	Yamada et al., 2014/(P20)	8	c.1395_1408del14ins	p.Q465Hfs*9	Frameshift	SMD
136	Yamada et al., 2014/(P21)	8	c.1417del	p.R473Gfs*14	Frameshift	SMD
137	Yamada et al., 2014/(P22)	8	c.1417del	p.R473Gfs*14	Frameshift	SMD
138	Yamada et al., 2014/(P23)	8	c.1421_1426dup	p.M476Nfs*6	Frameshift	SMD
139	Yamada et al., 2014/(P24)	8	c.1492_1493del	p.P498Lfs*18	Frameshift	-
140	Yamada et al., 2014/(P25)	8	c.1534_1535del	p.G512Vfs*4	Frameshift	-
141	Yamada et al., 2014/(P26)	8	c.1822del	p.E608Kfs*13	Frameshift	-
142	Yamada et al., 2014/(P27)	8	c.1966_1967del	p.M656Vfs*17	Frameshift	HD
143	Yamada et al., 2014/(P28)	8	c.2178_2180del	p.L727Ifs*28	Frameshift	-
144	Yamada et al., 2014/(P29)	8	c.2254dup	p.T752Nfs*4	Frameshift	-
145	Yamada et al., 2014/(P30)	8	c. 2282del	p.T761Kfs*26	Frameshift	CID
146	Yamada et al., 2014/(P31)	8	c.2349_2351dup	p.S784Ffs*11	Frameshift	CID
147	Yamada et al., 2014/(P32)	8	c.2579del	p.L860Rfs*3	Frameshift	CID
148	Yamada et al., 2014/(P33)	8	c.2740_2743dup	p.S916Dfs*34	Frameshift	-
149	Yamada et al., 2014/(P34)	10	c.3608_3614del	p.D1204Rfs*29	Frameshift	-
150	[21] Tronina et al., 2023/(P1)	6	-	p.Gln694Ter	Missense	HD
151	[22] Jakubiak et al., 2021/(P1)	8	c.1027C > T	p.R343*	Nonsense	-
152	Jakubiak et al., 2021/(P2)	1–10	-	-	Deletion	-
153	Jakubiak et al., 2021/(P3)	6	c.648C > A	p.C216*	Nonsense	-
154	Jakubiak et al., 2021/(P4)	10	ZEB2 gene Exon 10 deletion	-	Deletion	-
155	Jakubiak et al., 2021/(P5)	8	c.1946del	p.I649Tfs*17	Frameshift	HD
156	Jakubiak et al., 2021/(P6)	6	c.607ins	p.Thr203IlefsTer37	Frameshift	-
157	Jakubiak et al., 2021/(P7)	4	c.399_400dup	p.Thr134IlefsTer3	Frameshift	-
158	Jakubiak et al., 2021/(P8)	8	c.1276T > A	p.Leu426Ile	Missense	-
159	Jakubiak et al., 2021/(P9)	6	c.696C > G	p.Y232*	Nonsense	N-ZFa
160	Jakubiak et al., 2021/(P10)	-	8 Mb deletion 2q22.3q23.3	-	Chromosome deletion	-
161	Jakubiak et al., 2021/(P11)	1–10	-	-	Deletion	-
162	Jakubiak et al., 2021/(P12)	3–10	-	-	Deletion	-

Table 1. Cont.

Our Study ID	Publication ID/ (Patient Number)	ZEB2 Exon	ZEB2 Gene Variant or Defect	Protein Defect	Type of Genetic Defect	ZEB2 Protein Domain
163	Jakubiak et al., 2021/(P13)	7	c.857-858del	p.Glu286ValfsTer8	Frameshift	N-ZFb
164	Jakubiak et al., 2021/(P14)	6	c.607ins	p.Thr203IlefsTer37	Frameshift	-
165	Jakubiak et al., 2021/(P15)	8	c.1445T>G	p.Leu482*	Nonsense	SMD
166	Jakubiak et al., 2021/(P16)	3	c.84T>G	p.Tyr28*	Nonsense	-
167	Jakubiak et al., 2021/(P17)	8	c.1421-1426del	p.Gln474_Met476delins	Insertion, deletion	SMD
168	Jakubiak et al., 2021/(P18)	8	c.2230A>G	p.Ile744Val	Missense	-
169	Jakubiak et al., 2021/(P19)	10	c.3202G>T	p.Gly1068Cys	Missense	C-ZFb
170	Jakubiak et al., 2021/(P20)	8	c.2087_2088del	Lys696Serfs*24	Frameshift	HD
171	Jakubiak et al., 2021/(P21)	8	c.2073G>A	p.Trp691Ter	Nonsense	HD
172	Jakubiak et al.,2021/(P22)	-	-	-	Deletion	-
173	Jakubiak et al., 2021/(P23)	8	c.2562_2564del	p.N855Lfs*3	Frameshift	CID
174	Jakubiak et al., 2021/(P24)	8	c.1177dup	p.E393Gfs*7	Frameshift	-
175	Jakubiak et al., 2021/(P25)	8	c.1437_1440del	p.H304Qfs*3	Frameshift	N-ZFc
176	Jakubiak et al., 2021/(P26)	8	c.2083C>T	p.Arg695Ter	Nonsense	HD
177	Jakubiak et al., 2021/(P27)	8	c.2083C>T	p.Arg695Ter	Nonsense	HD
178	Jakubiak et al., 2021/(P28)	3–10	258.2 kb deletion	-	Chromosome deletion	-
179	[23] Refaat et al., 2021/(P1)	-	2.27 Mb deletion	-	Chromosome deletion	-
180	[24] Musaad et al., 2022/(P1)	-	Chr2:145161574del	-	Frameshift	-
181	[25] Pachajoa et al., 2022/(P1)	8	c.2761C>T	p.Arg921Ter	Nonsense	-
182	[26] Wu et al., 2022/(P1)	8	c.2417del	p.Phe807Serfs*11	Frameshift	CID
183	Wu et al., 2022/(P2)	8	c.1200T>A	p.Tyr400X	Nonsense	-
184	Wu et al., 2022/(P3)	8	c.1027C>T	p.Arg343X	Nonsense	-
185	Wu et al., 2022/(P4)	8	c.2621del	p.Asn874Ilefs*12	Frameshift	-
186	Wu et al., 2022/(P5)	8	c.2456C>G	p.Ser819X	Nonsense	CID
187	Wu et al., 2022/(P6)	8	c.2002del	p.Glu668Serfs*8	Frameshift	HD
188	Wu et al., 2022/(P7)	2–10	Chr2:145147017-145274917del	-	Large deletion	-
189	Wu et al., 2022/(P8)	5	c.492_517del	p.Glu164Aspfs*9	Frameshift	-
190	Wu et al., 2022/(P9)	6	c.779dup	p.Met260Ilefs*19	Frameshift	N-ZFa
191	Wu et al., 2022/(P10)	1–10	chr2:141213978-148010654del	-	Large deletion	-
192	Wu et al., 2022/(P11)	8	c.2083C>T	p.Arg695X	Nonsense	HD
193	Wu et al., 2022/(P12)	1–10	chr2:145000000-145351228 del	-	Large deletion	-
194	Wu et al., 2022/(P13)	7	c.904C>T	p.Arg302X	Nonsense	N-ZFc
195	Wu et al., 2022/(P14)	8	c.2712del	p.Pro906Leufs*24	Frameshift	-
196	Wu et al., 2022/(P15)	8	c.2670_2677del	p.Ala891Phefs*55	Frameshift	-

Table 1. Cont.

Our Study ID	Publication ID/ (Patient Number)	ZEB2 Exon	ZEB2 Gene Variant or Defect	Protein Defect	Type of Genetic Defect	ZEB2 Protein Domain
197	Wu et al., 2022/(P16)	8	c.2177_2180del	p.Ser726Tyrfs*7	Frameshift	-
198	Wu et al., 2022/(P17)	1–10	chr2:138434153-145285163 del	-	Large Deletion	-
199	Wu et al., 2022/(P18)	8	c.2851C>T	p.Gln951X	Nonsense	-
200	Wu et al., 2022/(P19)	8	c.1426dup	p.Met476Asnfs*5	Frameshift	SMD
201	Wu et al., 2022/(P20)	8	c.2761C>T	p.Arg921X	Nonsense	-
202	Wu et al., 2022/(P21)	8	c.1027C>T	p.Arg343X	Nonsense	-
203	Wu et al., 2022/(P22)	8	c.1106_1115delins	p.Leu369X	Nonsense	-
204	[27] Fu et al., 2022/(P1)	8	c.2136del	p.Lys713Serfs*3	Frameshift	-
205	Fu et al., 2022/(P2)	8	c.2740del	p. Gln914Argfs*16	Frameshift	-
206	Fu et al., 2022/(P3)	7	c.808-2del	-	Splicing	N-ZFb
207	[28] Wei et al., 2021/(P1)	8	c.1137_1146del	p.S380Nfs*13	Deletion	-
208	[29] Şenbil et al., 2021/(P1)	6	c.646dup	p.Cys216LeufsTer23	Frameshift	-
209	[30] Ivanoski et al., 2018/(P1)	6	c.805C>T	p.Q269*	Nonsense	N-ZFb
210	Ivanoski et al., 2018/(P2)	1–10	ZEB2 gene deletion	-	Large deletion	-
211	Ivanoski et al., 2018/(P3)	1–10	7.3 Mb deletion Ch2q22.1q22.3	-	Large deletion	-
212	Ivanoski et al., 2018/(P4)	8	c.1381C>T	p.Q461*	Nonsense	SMD
213	Ivanoski et al., 2018/(P5)	8	c.1052_1057delins	p.G351Vfs*19	Small deletion, Frameshift	-
214	Ivanoski et al., 2018/(P6)	6	c.696C>G	p.Y232*	Nonsense	N-ZFa
215	Ivanoski et al., 2018/(P7)	8	c.1073_1122delins	p.S359Tfs*3	Small indel, Frameshift	-
216	Ivanoski et al., 2018/(P8)	3	c.310C>T	p.Q104*	Nonsense	-
217	Ivanoski et al., 2018/(P9)	1–10	2.6 Mb deletion Ch2q22.2q22.3	-	Large deletion	-
218	Ivanoski et al., 2018/(P10)	8	c.2718del	p.A907Lfs*23	Small deletion, Frameshift	-
219	Ivanoski et al., 2018/(P11)	8	c.2180T>A	p.L727*	Nonsense	-
220	Ivanoski et al., 2018/(P12)	1–10	ZEB2 gene deletion	-	Large deletion	-
221	Ivanoski et al., 2018/(P13)	8	c.1381C>T	p.Q461*	Nonsense	SMD
222	Ivanoski et al., 2018/(P14)	8	c.2083C>T	p.R695*	Nonsense	HD
223	Ivanoski et al., 2018/(P15)	5	c.460G>T	p.E154*	Nonsense	-
224	Ivanoski et al., 2018/(P16)	8	c.2083C>T	p.R695*	Nonsense	HD
225	Ivanoski et al., 2018/(P17)	8	c.1426dup	p.M476Nfs*6	Small insertion, Frameshift	SMD
226	Ivanoski et al., 2018/(P18)	1–10	4.6 Mb deletion Ch2q22q22.3	-	Large deletion	-
227	Ivanoski et al., 2018/(P19)	8	c.2682_2687delins	p.L894Ffs*36	Small indel, Frameshift	-
228	Ivanoski et al., 2018/(P20)	3	c.274G>T	p.G92*	Nonsense	-

Table 1. *Cont.*

Our Study ID	Publication ID/ (Patient Number)	ZEB2 Exon	ZEB2 Gene Variant or Defect	Protein Defect	Type of Genetic Defect	ZEB2 Protein Domain
229	Ivanoski et al., 2018/(P21)	8	c.2053C>T	p.Q685*	Nonsense	HD
230	Ivanoski et al., 2018/(P23)	9	c.3031del	p.S1011Afs*64	Small deletion, Frameshift	C-ZFa
231	Ivanoski et al., 2018/(P24)	8	c.2227del	p.S743Lfs*2	Small deletion, Frameshift	-
232	Ivanoski et al., 2018/(P25)	5	c.460del	p.E154Rfs*58	Small deletion, Frameshift	-
233	Ivanoski et al., 2018/(P26)	6	c.625C>T	p.Q209*	Nonsense	-
234	Ivanoski et al., 2018/(P27)	7	c.817del	p.L273*	Nonsense	N-ZFb
235	Ivanoski et al., 2018/(P28)	8	c.1635_1636ins	p.D546Lfs*11	Small insertion, Frameshift	-
236	Ivanoski et al., 2018/(P29)	3	c.310C>T	p.Q104*	Nonsense	-
237	Ivanoski et al., 2018/(P30)	3	c.310C>T	p.Q104*	Nonsense	-
238	Ivanoski et al., 2018/(P31)	8	c.2701C>T	p.Q901*	Nonsense	-
239	Ivanoski et al., 2018/(P32)	8	c.2083C>T	p.R695*	Nonsense	HD
240	Ivanoski et al., 2018/(P34)	8	c.2718del	p.A907Lfs*23	Small deletion, Frameshift	-
241	Ivanoski et al., 2018/(P35)	8	c.2317_2318del	p.E773Kfs*8	Small deletion, Frameshift	CID
242	Ivanoski et al., 2018/(P36)	1–10	0.6 Mb deletion Ch2q22.2	-	Large deletion	-
243	Ivanoski et al., 2018/(P37)	3	c.264_267del	p.I88Mfs*19	Small deletion, Frameshift	-
244	Ivanoski et al., 2018/(P38)	8	c.1541del	p.P414Rfs*2	Small deletion, Frameshift	-
245	Ivanoski et al., 2018/(P39)	8	c.2856del	p.R953Efs*24	Small deletion, Frameshift	-
246	Ivanoski et al., 2018/(P40)	8	c.2254dup	p.Y752Nfs*4	Small insertion, Frameshift	-
247	Ivanoski et al., 2018/(P41)	8	c.930C>A	p.Y310*	Nonsense	N-ZFc
248	Ivanoski et al., 2018/(P42)	8&9	c.917_3067del	p.E307_G1023del	Deletion, in-frame	N-ZFc C-ZFa
249	Ivanoski et al., 2018/(P43)	8	c.975C>A	p.Y325*	Nonsense	N-ZFc
250	Ivanoski et al., 2018/(P44)	8	c.2083C>T	p.R695*	Nonsense	HD
251	Ivanoski et al., 2018/(P45)	6	c.691dup	p.Y232Vfs*7	Frameshift	N-ZFa
252	Ivanoski et al., 2018/(P46)	8	c.2083C>T	p.R695*	Nonsense	HD
253	Ivanoski et al., 2018/(P47)	7	c.901del	p.L301Cfs*37	Small deletion, Frameshift	N-ZFc
254	Ivanoski et al., 2018/(P48)	1–10	ZEB2 gene deletion	-	Large deletion	-
255	Ivanoski et al., 2018/(P49)	3	c.81_84dup	p.D29Lfs*2	Small insertion, Frameshift	-
256	Ivanoski et al., 2018/(P50)	8	c.1202dup	p.K401Ifs*17	Small insertion, Frameshift	-
257	Ivanoski et al., 2018/(P51)	6	c.648C>A	p.C216*	Nonsense	-

Table 1. Cont.

Our Study ID	Publication ID/ (Patient Number)	ZEB2 Exon	ZEB2 Gene Variant or Defect	Protein Defect	Type of Genetic Defect	ZEB2 Protein Domain
258	Ivanoski et al., 2018/(P52)	8	c.1910C>G	p.S637*	Nonsense	-
259	Ivanoski et al., 2018/(P53)	8	c.2713del	p.P906Lfs*24	Small deletion, Frameshift	-
260	Ivanoski et al., 2018/(P54)	8	c.2083C>T	p.R695*	Nonsense	HD
261	Ivanoski et al., 2018/(P55)	5	c.540del	p.E181Rfs*31	Small deletion, Frameshift	-
262	Ivanoski et al., 2018/(P56)	6	c.609del	p.P204Qfs*9	Small deletion, Frameshift	-
263	Ivanoski et al., 2018/(P57)	5	c.477_484del	p.H159Qfs*10	Small deletion, Frameshift	-
264	Ivanoski et al., 2018/(P58)	8	c.2083C>T	p.R695*	Nonsense	HD
265	Ivanoski et al., 2018/(P59)	5–8	c.403_2887del	p.V135Gfs*5	Frameshift	-
266	Ivanoski et al., 2018/(P60)	8	c.2083C>T	p.R695*	Nonsense	HD
267	Ivanoski et al., 2018/(P61)	1–10	16.7 Mb deletion Ch2q21.1q22.3	-	Large deletion	-
268	Ivanoski et al., 2018/(P62)	6	c.653_654ins	p.G219Pfs*21	Small insertion, Frameshift	-
269	Ivanoski et al., 2018/(P63)	8	c.1851del	p.H617Qfs*4	Small deletion, Frameshift	-
270	Ivanoski et al., 2018/(P64)	4	c.389_390dup	p.T134Lfs*3	Small insertion, Frameshift	-
271	Ivanoski et al., 2018/(P65)	8	c.2076del	p.F692Lfs*24	Small deletion, Frameshift	HD
272	Ivanoski et al., 2018/(P66)	8	c.2083C>T	p.R695*	Nonsense	HD
273	Ivanoski et al., 2018/(P67)	7	c.823C>T	p.Q275*	Nonsense	N-ZFb
274	Ivanoski et al., 2018/(P68)	8	c.1313del	p.H438Pfs*2	Small deletion, Frameshift	SMD
275	Ivanoski et al., 2018/(P69)	1&2	ZEB2 gene Exons 1 and 2 deletion	-	Large deletion	-
276	Ivanoski et al., 2018/(P70)	8	c.1027C>T	p.R343*	Nonsense	-
277	Ivanoski et al., 2018/(P71)	6	c.648C>A	p.C216*	Nonsense	-
278	Ivanoski et al., 2018/(P72)	1–10	ZEB2 gene deletion	-	Large deletion	-
279	Ivanoski et al., 2018/(P73)	8	c.1381C>T	p.Q461*	Nonsense	SMD
280	Ivanoski et al., 2018/(P74)	10	ZEB2 gene Exon 10 deletion (3'UTR c.3642+750)	-	Large deletion	-
281	Ivanoski et al., 2018/(P75)	8	c.1946del	p.I649Tfs*17	Small deletion, Frameshift	HD
282	Ivanoski et al., 2018/(P76)	2	c.32dup	p.R11Pfs*9	Small insertion, Frameshift	-
283	Ivanoski et al., 2018/(P77)	6	c.761del	p.Q255Sfs*7	Small deletion, Frameshift	N-ZFa
284	Ivanoski et al., 2018/(P78)	8	c.1553del	p.H518Lfs*26	Small deletion, Frameshift	-

Table 1. *Cont.*

Our Study ID	Publication ID/ (Patient Number)	ZEB2 Exon	ZEB2 Gene Variant or Defect	Protein Defect	Type of Genetic Defect	ZEB2 Protein Domain
285	Ivanoski et al., 2018/(P79)	8	c.936C>A	p.C312*	Nonsense	N-ZFc
286	Ivanoski et al., 2018/(P80)	3	c.187_228dup	p.A77Lfs*13	Small insertion, Frameshift	-
287	Ivanoski et al., 2018/(P81)	8	c.1150C>T	p.Q384*	Nonsense	-
288	Ivanoski et al., 2018/(P82)	5	c.553_554ins	p.R185Lfs*28	Small insertion, Frameshift	-
289	Ivanoski et al., 2018/(P83)	7	c.857_858del	p.E286Vfs*8	Small deletion, Frameshift	N-ZFb
290	Ivanoski et al., 2018/(P84)	10	c.3567_3568ins	p.M1190Pfs*52	Small insertion, Frameshift	-
291	Ivanoski et al., 2018/(P85)	8	c.2677del	p.P893Lfs*37	Small deletion, Frameshift	-
292	Ivanoski et al., 2018/(P86)	8	c.2372del	p.T791Nfs*26	Small deletion, Frameshift	CID
293	Ivanoski et al., 2018/(P87)	6	c.715del	p.E239Rfs*23	Small deletion, Frameshift	N-ZFa
294	Ivanoski et al., 2018/(P88)	IVS1	c.-69-2A>C	p.M1_N24delins	Splicing	-
295	Ivanoski et al., 2018/(P89)	8	c.1578_1579delins	p.D527Tfs*17	Small indel, Frameshift	-
296	[12] Ghoumid et al., 2013/(P1)	10	c.3134A>G	p.His1045Arg	Missense	C-ZFb
297	Ghoumid et al., 2013/(P2)	10	c.3164A>G	p.Tyr1055Cys	Missense	C-ZFb
298	Ghoumid et al., 2013/(P3)	10	c.3211T>C	p.Ser1071Pro	Missense	C-ZFb

Ter, X or * represent stop codons at the time of publication; N-ZF = N-terminal zinc finger clusters domain (221–334); SMD = SMAD-binding domain (437–482); IVS1 = intervening sequence; HD = homeodomain-like domain (644–703); CID = CtBP-interacting domain (757–868); C-ZF = C-terminal zinc finger clusters domain (998–1078). Protein domain regions coded by exons are represented based on codon location within the domains (e.g., exon 9 codes for C-ZFa and exon 10 codes for C-ZFb). References are listed in brackets [6,12–30].

2.3. ZEB2 Gene Variant Types and Frequencies

ZEB2 gene variants, types, and frequencies were analyzed from 298 studied individuals with MWS and summarized in Figure 2. The most prevalent variant type was frameshift (134 patients; 45%) followed by nonsense (112 patients; 38%).

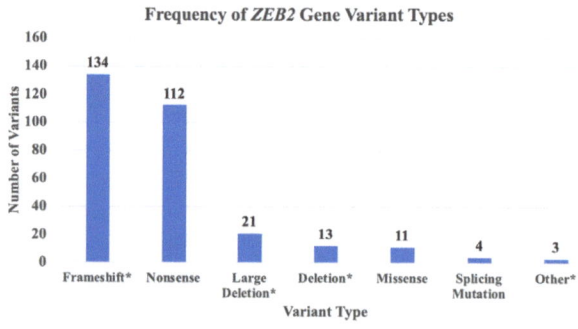

Figure 2. Frequency of ZEB2 gene variants identified by variant type in 298 reported patients with MWS. The frequencies of ZEB2 gene variants were identified and grouped. Frameshift* represents a

combination of frameshift alone (N = 88), and frameshift plus variants such as frameshift with small deletion (N = 29), frameshift with small insertion (N = 13), or frameshift with small indel (N = 4). Large deletion* represents a combination of large deletions (N = 15) and chromosome deletions (N = 6). Deletion* represents a combination of deletions involving DNA (N = 9) or whole exome based (N = 4). Other* represents a combination of in-frame defects with intragenic deletion (N = 1), partial duplication (N = 1) or insertion deletion (N = 1).

Of the 298 patients with MWS, 262 had sufficient information to determine the *ZEB2* exon variant type and to analyze the distribution and frequency of *ZEB2* variants within a specific exon. Figure 3 represents the exons within the gene, along with the frequency and type of variants within each exon. The most common variant site or location was c.2083C>T within exon 8 of the *ZEB2* gene. This variant was found in 11 percent of all patients reported with MWS.

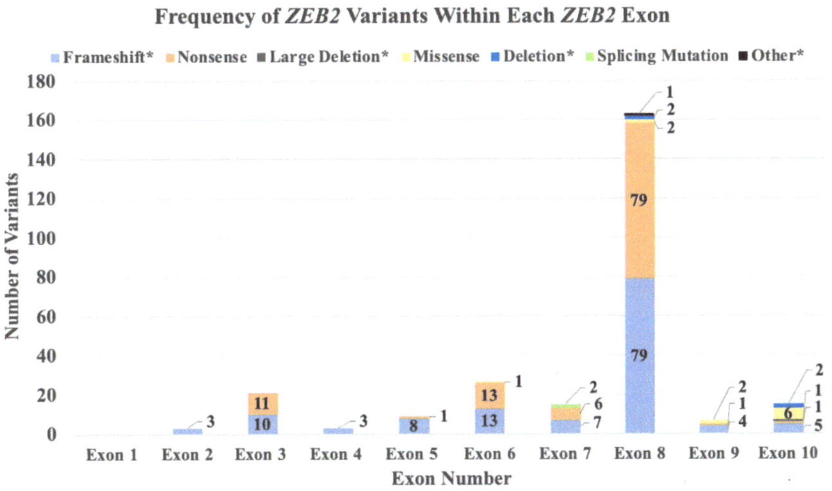

Figure 3. Number of *ZEB2* gene variants and types identified in each exon.

2.4. ZEB2 Gene–Gene or Protein Interactions

The protein–protein interaction networks for the *ZEB2* gene were obtained as shown in Figure 4. ZEB2 interacts with 24 other proteins and these interactions are predicted to impact gene expression and the binding of encoded proteins (see Figure 4). Seventeen of the twenty-four genes are predicted to show co-expression with ZEB2 protein binding, while ten genes are predicted to interact via protein binding. The two SMAD proteins, SMAD1 and SMAD3, which are shown to interact with ZEB2 via co-expression and binding, are main signal transducers for receptors of the transforming growth factor beta superfamily, critical for regulating cell development and growth. The encoded ZEB2 protein contains a SMD protein domain. Additionally, the ZEB2 protein is predicted to interact with four PAX proteins, two POU3F proteins, and two GATA proteins. These interactions have the potential to impact the ZEB2 protein's functional pathways and interactions related to the TGF receptor for which ZEB1, ZEB2, and SMAD are major players.

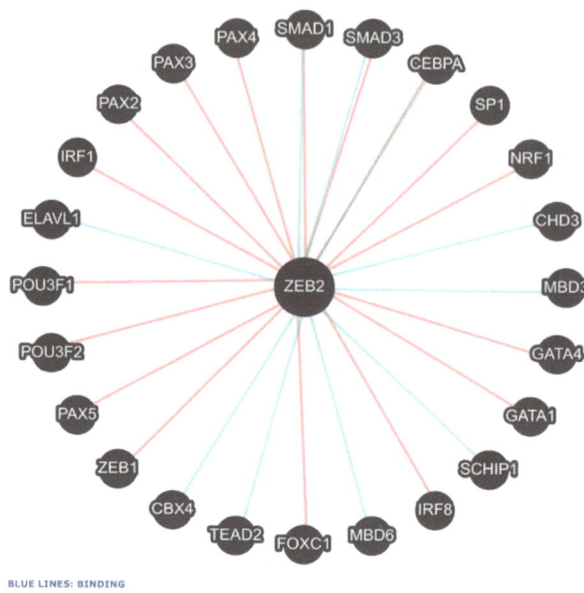

Figure 4. *ZEB2* gene–gene functional interactions are identified via binding (blue lines) and co-expression (red lines) [http://pathwaycommons.org/pc12/Pathway_751ce7ccec6e191682a33d7252aac8] (accessed on 1 November 2023). These gene interactions relate to TGF receptor pathways in which ZEB1, ZEB2, and SMAD are major players.

2.5. ZEB2 Structural Protein Domains, Functions and Models

The ZEB2 protein domains and their corresponding exons are represented in Figure 5. As illustrated in this figure, the *ZEB2* gene consists of 10 exons, each of varying size, and encodes for six protein domains with specific functions and domain relationships described below.

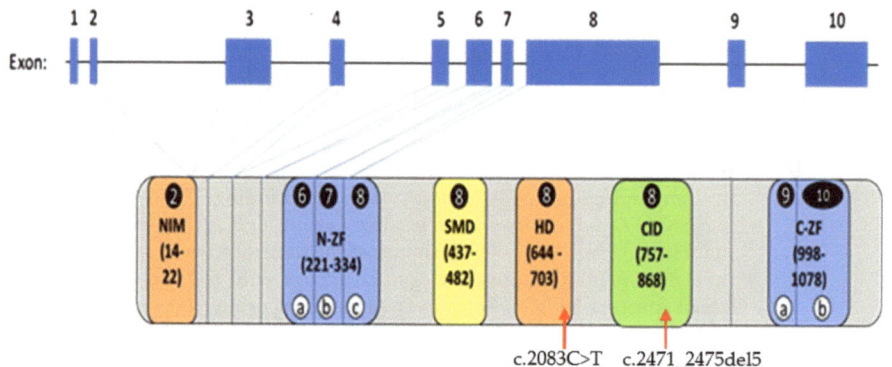

Figure 5. Schematic representation of *ZEB2* gene structure, exons, and codons listed and incorporated into each of the six protein domains. The protein domains and their corresponding exons are illustrated and modified from Zou et al. [13] such as NIM (nucleosome remodeling and deacetylase-interaction motif), N-ZF (N-terminal zinc finger cluster), SMD (SMAD-binding domain), HD (homeodomain), CID (CtBP-interacting domain), and C-ZF (C-terminal zinc finger cluster) modified from reference [13]. Exons coding the individual protein domains and domain regions are circled. The circled lowercase letters (a/b/c) found in both the N-ZF and C-ZF domains represent the regions coded by different exons

(exon numbers circled). The most common gene variant (c.2083C>T) found in our study of 298 patients with MWS and the pathogenetic variant (c.2471_2475del5) found in our 5-year-old proband along with their locations in the HD and CID domains, respectively, are indicated by red arrows.

A predicted model from a computer-based Alphafold2 program (Uniprot:O60315) was used to generate an altered ZEB2 protein structure from a truncated protein, while haploinsufficiency leads to a lower amount of protein resulting from non-sense mediated decay (NMD) of mRNA containing the abnormal gene defect. As shown below in Figure 6A, the ZEB2 protein is composed of many flexible/disordered regions that contain well-structured ZF domains. Residues after R695, the most common protein defect/site found in our studied MWS population, generated a stop codon in exon 8, which may result in a polypeptide lacking the C-terminal zinc finger (C-ZF) domain due to a truncated protein as shown in Figure 6B. Additionally, the N-ZF contains ZF domains predicted to coordinate zinc ions by the residues shown in Figure 6C.

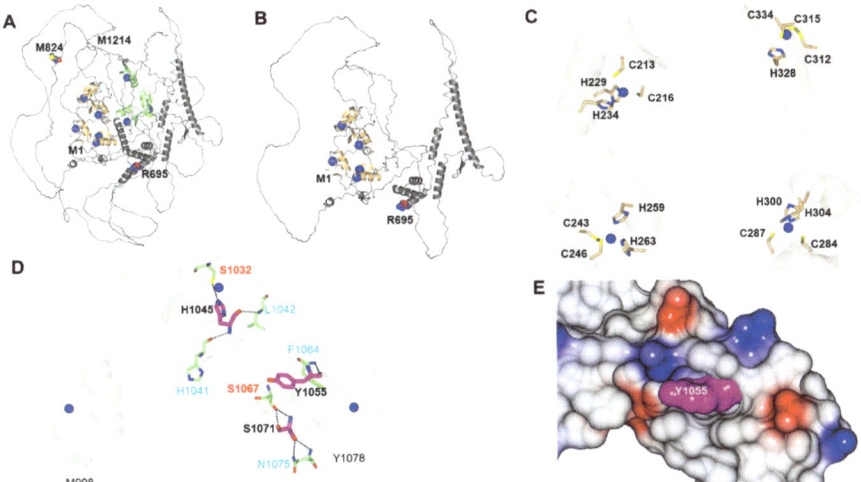

Figure 6. Predicted AlphaFold2 structure of ZEB2 (www.uniprot.org/uniprotkb/O60315/entry; accessed on 29 September 2023). (**A**) Full-length structure showing the N-terminal zinc finger domain (tan, L211-C334) and the C-terminal zinc finger domain (green, M998-Y1078) with codon positions at R695 and M824 with their predicted zinc ion binding sites drawn as blue spheres. M824 is a codon that is deleted in our case report of a 5-year-old female with a pathogenic variant c.2472_2475del5 in exon 8, while the R695 protein variant was the most common protein defect found in the 298 reported patients with MWS summarized in Table 1. (**B**) Same view as panel A but with residues after R695 omitted, resulting in a polypeptide lacking the C-terminal zinc finger domain. (**C**) N-terminal zinc finger domain shows the predicted zinc binding sites and coordination with ZEB2 residues. (**D**) C-terminal zinc finger domain shows predicted side chain hydrogen bond interactions (dashed lines) between H1045, Y1055, and S1071 missense ZEB2 changes reported by Ghoumid et al. [12] and other ZEB2 residues (red). Y1055 does not form interactions with the side chain -OH but does form a backbone hydrogen bond interaction with the backbone N-atom of F1064. Other backbone interactions with H1045 and Y1055 are indicated with blue text. (**E**) Electrostatic surface representation shows packing of Y1055 within a cleft of the ZEB2 C-terminal zinc finger domain.

The depicted H1045R, Y1055C, and S1071P variants in three patients with MWS were reported in 2013 by Ghoumid et al. [12] as missense mutations within the C-ZF protein domain. Interestingly, the H1045R and S1071P variants would likely result in the breakage of hydrogen bonds between the side chains and residues of S1032 and S1067 which could destabilize the ZF domains (Figure 6D). Although the side chain of Y1055 does not form hydrogen bond interactions with its side chain, this residue is tightly packed within a cleft and mutations would likely affect this interaction (Figure 6E).

The five base pair ZEB2 deletion in exon 8 at c.2471_2475del5 at the M824 residue in our proband would potentially impact codons of four of the six domains (about one-third of the N-ZF domain and all of the SMD, HD, and CID domains). Hence, this novel ZEB2 deletion variant could not be predicted or modeled due to a lack of computer protein access data information for modeling purposes with the involvement of such a large proportion of the ZEB2 protein. The Met824 residue is predicted to be absent leading to disruption of the Lys825 residue upstream of the C-ZF protein domain. This predicted mistranslated string of residues would result in the removal of the C-ZF domain. Therefore, the ZEB2 protein would be altered and/or presumably degraded in our proband, potentially impacting 24 other interacting genes found in gene–gene interaction and protein binding studies, as noted in Figure 4.

3. Discussion

3.1. Mowat–Wilson Syndrome (MWS) and Clinical Findings

Mowat–Wilson syndrome (MWS) is a rare autosomal dominant disorder caused by pathogenic variants in the ZEB2 gene, located at chromosome 2q22.3. We identified about 300 known cases of MWS in the literature or unpublished databases. Most cases of MWS are sporadic heterozygous de novo occurrences with a low recurrence risk in siblings. We analyzed and summarized a wide range of ZEB2 defects including frameshift, nonsense, missense, and deletions or duplications. Those with the larger deletions tend to have more clinical severity.

Mowat–Wilson syndrome was first reported in 1998 [3,7] with multi-organ system involvement along with moderate-to-severe intellectual disability, speech delay, and microcephaly with brain anomalies. Seizures are often found with onset between several months to over 10 years of age. Specific facial dysmorphisms exist with a wide range of cardiac anomalies requiring intervention. Genitourinary and kidney anomalies are also present in about 50% of cases including undescended testicles, penile malformations, hydronephrosis, and kidney defects. Gastrointestinal problems include Hirschsprung disease in nearly one-half of reported patients accompanied by constipation. Other occasional abnormalities include long tapering toes and fingers, pes planus, nystagmus, cleft lip/palate, and pigmentary changes [3,7–10].

3.2. ZEB2 Gene Structure and Variants

The ZEB2 gene consists of ten exons of different lengths and codes for six protein domains of variable sizes and functions. Exon 8 showed the largest number of variants and comprised 162 of the cases in our study population, followed by exon 6 with 27 variants. The large exon 8 accounts for about one-half of the ZEB2 coding sequence and encodes the last zinc finger region of the N-ZF domain along with SMD, HD, and CID protein domains; hence, about 60% of the ZEB2 protein is coded by this exon, representing a similar proportion of the reported ZEB2 gene defects. Exon 8 is also involved in our 5-year-old proband with MWS.

Frameshift mutations or premature termination codons (PTCs) do lead to non-sense mediated decay (NMD), impacting protein production. NMD is a process that typically affects the mRNA of most genes with PTCs before the last exon, which leads to mRNA degradation with haploinsufficiency. It is likely that NMD does occur, affecting the amount of protein produced and causing the truncated protein to alter protein function in MWS as well as other genetic disorders. However, it is predicted that mutated transcripts of ZEB2 may not undergo non-sense mediated decay in MWS, but more research is needed [31].

We studied ZEB2 variant types and their locations within each exon. Nine of the ten exons, except exon 1, harbored damaging frameshift variants. Frameshift mutations occur when one or two bases are either inserted or deleted from a strand of DNA. This results in an aberrant protein impacting the protein function. This aligns with the fact that a frameshift defect was the most identified variant seen in our study, followed by nonsense mutations present in 6 of the 10 exons. A frameshift defect was seen in 134 of the 298 individuals [45%] reported with MWS. The second most frequent variant in our patient population was a nonsense defect seen in 112 patients [38%]. The third most frequent variant found was a large deletion in 21 individuals [7%]. These patients had a complete absence or deletion of the chromosome 2 region where the ZEB2 gene is located. This was followed by missense variants in 11 individuals [4%]. Collectively, MWS is caused by haploinsufficiency of the autosomal dominant ZEB2 gene function due to the heterozygous variants and copy number variations. Further studies to elucidate the precise molecular mechanisms for the pathogenicity of MWS are needed.

3.3. ZEB2 Gene Functions and Interactions

Recognized cellular components impacted by the ZEB2 gene include the chromatin, cytosol, nucleolus, nucleus, and nucleoplasm, and impacted processes include the molecular function and disturbances of DNA-binding transcription factor activity via RNA polymerase and transcription repression, metal ion binding for zinc, and phosphatase regulatory activity. These derangements of the ZEB 2 protein may play a role in clinical outcomes, variability, and severity with early multi-organ development in MWS (www.uniprot.org/uniprotkb/O60315/entry, accessed on 1 November 2023). As described in our review, the ZEB2 gene, when disturbed, could impact other interacting developmental genes by leading to a cascade of early perturbed biological processes and abnormal embryogenesis, requiring more research. The ZEB2 gene functions as a transcriptional inhibitor by binding to specific DNA structure (5′-CACCT-3′) at gene promoters. It represses the transcription of cadherin 1 (*CDH1*; NM_004360.5) gene and cell adhesion required for the establishment and maintenance of epithelial cells during embryogenesis and adulthood which are important for brain and other organ development and function [32]. The mesenchyme homeobox 2 (*MEOX2*; NM_005924.5) gene [33] also interacts with ZEB2 as a homeobox gene involved in the regulation of anatomical development such as morphogenesis. Moreover, homeodomain proteins regulate gene expression and cell differentiation during early embryonic development and organogenesis including the heart, brain, and gut [34], which are involved in Mowat–Wilson syndrome. Gene functions and outcomes may also be altered by gene–gene or protein interactions or epistasis, whereby a single gene function may be impacted by interactions with other genes and disease processes [35].

3.4. Genes That Interact with ZEB2 and Potential Relationship with Mowat–Wilson Syndrome

The 24 genes recognized to interact with ZEB2 are shown in Figure 4. These gene–gene or protein interactions may play important roles in the derangement of multi-system embryogenesis and organogenesis. Among the interactive genes are five gene families (*SMAD, GATA, IRF, PAX*, and *POU3F*) represented with the ZEB1 gene, presumably contributing to clinical findings seen in MWS. One of the interacting genes is a member of the *SMAD* gene family, *SMAD1* (*SMAD1*; NM_005900.3). The SMAD-related protein domain is one of the six domains found in the ZEB2 protein. The SMAD1 encoded protein is Involved in the downstream signaling pathway for bone morphogenic protein (BMP) subfamily members [36]. BMPs are known to play vital roles during the formation and maintenance of various organs disturbed in MWS, are members of TGF-β receptor signaling and are involved in skeletal dysplasia, DNA-binding transcription factor activity, and protein kinase binding. *SMAD3* (*SMAD*; NM_005902.4) targets genes involved in epithelial cells including cyclin-dependent kinase (CDK) inhibitors that generate a cytostatic response important for the regulation of muscle-specific genes [8]. The GATA-binding protein 1 (GATA1) interactive gene is X-linked and encodes the zinc finger DNA-binding transcription factor, which plays a critical role in the normal development of hematopoietic cells and is associated with thrombocytopenia, beta thalassemia, and dyserythropoietic anemia. The *GATA4* (*GATA4*; NM_001308093.3) interactive gene is associated with congenital heart disease, as seen in our 5-year-old female, and cardiac conduction, testicular development, and chromatin binding [37,38].

Other interactive genes include interferon regulatory factor 1 (*IRF1*: NM_002198.3) which is highly regulated in human vascular lesions and exhibits a growth inhibitory function in coronary artery smooth muscle, nitric oxide production, endothelial tissue, vascular intimal growth with healing, and pathophysiology of primary atherosclerosis [39]. The *IRF8* (*IRF8*; NM_002163.4) gene codes transcriptional agents of the interferon regulatory factor (IRF) family involved with conserved DNA-binding domains in the N-terminal regions and divergent C-terminal regions serving as regulatory sites, and in immunodeficiency [40].

The paired box 2 (*PAX2*; NM_000278.5) gene and other *PAX* family members are involved with mesenchyme to epithelium transition in renal development and related pathways for neural stem cells, lineage-specific markers, and Wnt/Hedgehog/Notch signaling [8]. For example, defects of the *PAX3* (*PAX3*: NM_181458.4) gene cause Waardenburg syndrome, involved with chromatin organization and binding, ectoderm differentiation, and craniofacial-spinal development with myogenesis, which are possibly important in MWS, as well [41]. The *PAX4* (*PAX4*; NM_001366110.1) gene encodes transcription factors that are essential for the formation of several tissues representing all germ layers and induced pluripotent stem cells with lineage-specific markers [42]. *PAX5* (*PAX5*; NM_016734.3) is a transcription factor gene essential for B-cell differentiation and other hematopoietic lineages and diseases [43]. The POU domain, class 3, transcription factor 1 (*POU3F1*; NM_002699.4) gene is associated with related pathways involved with nervous system development, mammalian neurogenesis, and myelination [8,44,45]; *POU3F2* (*POU3F2*; NM_005604.4) is involved with microphthalmia and melanoma, and *MECP2* (*MECP2*; NM_001110792.2) activity that is disturbed in Rett syndrome [8].

The STRING database (STRING.org) was used to study predicted protein–protein associations, networks, and functional enrichment analysis [46]. In this database, there are 10 significantly associated proteins with ZEB2 including CTBP1, CHURC1, ARHGAP31, TWIST1, TWIST2, SMAD3, CDH1, CDH2, HDAC1, and ZEB1. Only ZEB1 and SMAD3 are in common between this database and the Pathwayscommons.org database [32] depicted in Figure 4.

The C-terminal binding protein 1 (CTBP1) which interacts with the ZEB2 protein in the STRING database involves dehydrogenase activity and functions in brown adipose tissue differentiation [47]. The Churchill domain-containing 1 (CHURC1) protein is involved in the positive regulation of transcription with ubiquitous expression in multiple tissues [8]. The Rho GTPase-activating protein 31 (ARHGAP31) functions as a GTPase-activating protein (GAP) for RAC1 and CDC42 required for cell spreading, polarized lamellipodia formation, and cell migration. The Twist family transcription factor 1 or twist-related protein 1 (TWIST1) also acts as a transcriptional regulator, inhibits myogenesis, and represses the expression of pro-inflammatory cytokines such as TNFA and IL1B. It also regulates cranial suture patterning and fusion. The Twist-related protein 2 (TWIST2) binds to the E-box consensus sequence 5′-CANNTG-3′ and represses the expression of proinflammatory cytokines involved with glycogen storage and energy metabolism as well as inhibiting the premature differentiation of pre-osteoblasts during osteogenesis. The Mothers against decapentaplegic homolog 3, receptor-regulated (SMAD3) binds to the TRE element of the promotor of many genes regulated by TGF-β, working with the *SMAD4* (*SMAD4*: NM_005359.6) gene, playing a role in multiple organ development and wound healing. Both cadherin-1 (CDH1) and cadherin-2 (CDH2) are calcium-dependent cell adhesion proteins, specifically for neural stem cells, and mediate anchorage to ependymocytes during maturation. Histone deacetylase 1 (HDAC1) is responsible for the deacetylation of lysine residues on the N-terminal part of the core histones and is involved in epigenetic repression with an important role in transcriptional regulation, cell cycle progression, and developmental events. Lastly, the zinc finger E-box-binding homeobox 1 (*ZEB1*; NM_001174096.2) is directly related to the *ZEB2* gene causing Mowat–Wilson syndrome and acts as a transcriptional repressor by inhibiting interleukin-2 (*IL-2*; NM_000586.4) gene expression. It also represses the E-cadherin promoter and induces an epithelial mesenchymal transition that positively regulates neuronal differentiation and plays a role in neurogenesis, as similarly seen with ZEB2 [47,48].

3.5. ZEB2 Protein Domains and Functions

There are six protein domains within the ZEB2 gene, and these negatively impact ZEB2 function, if altered by gene variants. The NIM (nucleosome remodeling and deacetylase interaction motif) protein domain functions as one of the major chromatin remodeling complexes. The N-ZF (N-terminal zinc finger cluster) and C-ZF (C-terminal zinc finger cluster) are significant players in gene regulation and function [49]. Moreover, in Xenopus, the N-ZF domain was also found to have an important role in early stages of neural induction [50]. These two zinc finger clusters are responsible for functions such as ZEB2 binding to DNA. These DNA-binding proteins often work to pack and modify DNA or regulate gene expression and are therefore crucial for proper functioning for DNA binding in vitro [51]. The SMD (SMAD-binding domain) functions to mediate TGF-β signaling in metazoan embryo development and adult tissue regeneration and homeostasis [52], while HD (homeodomain) regulates the expression of other genes in development [53]. The CID (CtBP-interacting domain) functions to regulate transcription, predominantly as a corepressor in the nucleus [54] impeding transcription and translation. The CtBP-interacting domain (CID) is responsible for the direct interaction of ZEB2 with CtBPs found at repeated PLDLS-like motifs thought to make ZEB2 more efficient at transcriptional suppression. CtBPs on their own do not necessarily have the ability to bind DNA in a gene/promoter specific context but rely on the recruitment of DNA-binding transcription factors such as ZEB2 to function [48]. Additional research is required to further understand the role of these protein domains and their function in causing clinical variability among patients diagnosed with MWS. This research would impact diagnosis, clinical care, treatment, and surveillance as well as genetic counseling of first-degree family members.

4. Conclusions

In our study, we report on a 5-year-old female with features commonly seen in MWS and with a novel pathogenic heterozygous c.2471_2475del5 in exon 8 of the ZEB2 gene. This frameshift defect presumably disrupts ZEB2 protein production, quantity, and quality, as the five base pair deletion in exon 8 would impact the coding of three protein domains (CID, HD, and SMD) and about one-third of the N-ZF domain. The novel defect directly affects the encoding of the CID domain. The CID domain plays a role as a transcriptional corepressor, the HD domain regulates the expression of developmental genes, the SMD domain regulates signaling protein and embryo development, while the N-ZF domain is involved in gene regulation.

Computer literature and unreported databases were searched for keywords such as Mowat–Wilson, ZEB2 gene and protein defects or variants, or clinical features and about 180 published reports were found including 298 patients. These sources were used to collect data regarding ZEB2 gene variants, types, frequencies, and protein defects along with domain locations and functions. Frameshift variants followed by nonsense variants accounted for more than 90% of the ZEB2 gene defects. We found that exon 8, as the largest exon, encodes at least three of the six protein domains of the ZEB2 gene and accounts for 66% (198/298) of the variants identified. ZEB2 gene-gene or protein interactions were studied, and 24 separate proteins were predicted to share molecular functions with protein binding effects on embryo development impacting craniofacial, spine, brain, cardiovascular, kidney and hematopoiesis. ZEB2 also plays a role in the conversion of neuroepithelial cells in early brain formation and as a mediator of trophoblast differentiation.

Author Contributions: Research design conceptualization, M.G.B. and W.A.H.; methodology, validation, investigation, formal analysis, data curation: M.G.B., W.A.H., C.S.P., S.L. and S.K.R.; writing—original draft preparation: C.S.P., W.A.H. and M.G.B.; writing—review and editing, C.S.P., W.A.H., M.G.B., S.L. and S.K.R.; and funding acquisition: M.G.B. All authors have read and agreed to the published version of the manuscript.

Funding: This research is supported by the Mowat–Wilson Syndrome Foundation, grant number KU Endowment 41149 and the National Institute of Child Health and Human Development (NICHD), grant number U54 HD061222.

Institutional Review Board Statement: The participant consented under an IRB-approved protocol (IRB# 11608) for research at the University of Kansas Medical Center (KUMC). The IRB-approved form was signed by the guardian prior to the study.

Informed Consent Statement: Written informed consent and photo permit forms were obtained from the parents as the patient was a minor.

Data Availability Statement: Data are contained within the article.

Acknowledgments: We thank the parents of the child with Mowat–Wilson syndrome for allowing us to describe the clinical findings in this report and thank the Mowat–Wilson Syndrome Foundation for their support and encouragement.

Conflicts of Interest: The authors declare no conflicts of interest.

References

1. Haendel, M.; Vasilevsky, N.; Unni, D.; Bologa, C.; Harris, N.; Rehm, H.; Hamosh, A.; Baynam, G.; Groza, T.; McMurry, J.; et al. How many rare diseases are there? *Nat. Rev. Drug Discov.* **2020**, *19*, 77–78. [CrossRef]
2. Yang, Y.; Muzny, D.M.; Reid, J.G.; Bainbridge, M.N.; Willis, A.; Ward, P.A.; Braxton, A.; Beuten, J.; Xia, F.; Niu, Z.; et al. Clinical whole-exome sequencing for the diagnosis of Mendelian Disorders. *N. Engl. J. Med.* **2013**, *369*, 1502–1511. [CrossRef]
3. Mowat, D.R.; Croaker, G.D.; Cass, D.T.; Kerr, B.A.; Chaitow, J.; Adès, L.C.; Chia, N.L.; Wilson, M.J. Hirschsprung disease, microcephaly, mental retardation, and characteristic facial features: Delineation of a new syndrome and identification of a locus at chromosome 2q22-q23. *J. Med. Genet.* **1998**, *8*, 617–623. [CrossRef] [PubMed]
4. Wakamatsu, N.; Yamada, Y.; Yamada, K.; Ono, T.; Nomura, N.; Taniguchi, H.; Kitoh, H.; Mutoh, N.; Yamanaka, T.; Mushiake, K.; et al. Mutations in SIP1, encoding Smad interacting protein-1, cause a form of Hirschsprung disease. *Nat. Genet.* **2001**, *4*, 369–370. [CrossRef]
5. Cacheux, V.; Dastot-Le Moal, F.; Kääriäinen, H.; Bondurand, N.; Rintala, R.; Boissier, B.; Wilson, M.; Mowat, D.; Goossens, M. Loss-of-function mutations in SIP1 Smad interacting protein 1 result in a syndromic Hirschsprung disease. *Hum. Mol. Genet.* **2001**, *14*, 1503–1510. [CrossRef] [PubMed]
6. Baxter, A.L.; Vivian, J.L.; Hagelstrom, R.T.; Hossain, W.A.; Golden, W.L.; Wassman, E.R.; Vanzo, R.J.; Butler, M.G. A Novel Partial Duplication of ZEB2 and Review of ZEB2 Involvement in Mowat-Wilson Syndrome. *Mol. Syndromol.* **2017**, *4*, 211–218. [CrossRef] [PubMed]
7. Mowat, D.R.; Wilson, M.J.; Goossens, M. Mowat-Wilson syndrome. *J. Med. Genet.* **2003**, *5*, 305–310. [CrossRef] [PubMed]
8. Adam, M.P.; Feldman, J.; Mirzaa, F.M.; Pagon, R.A.; Wallace, S.E.; Bean, L.J.H.; Gripp, K.W.; Amemiya, A. (Eds.) *GeneReviews [Internet]*; University of Washington, Seattle: Seattle, WA, USA, 2023.
9. Hegarty, S.V.; Sullivan, A.M.; O'Keeffe, G.W. Zeb2: A multifunctional regulator of nervous system development. *Prog. Neurobiol.* **2015**, *132*, 81–95. [CrossRef] [PubMed]
10. Zweier, C.; Thiel, C.T.; Dufke, A.; Crow, Y.J.; Meinecke, P.; Suri, M.; Ala-Mello, S.; Beemer, F.; Bernasconi, S.; Bianchi, P.; et al. Clinical and mutational spectrum of Mowat–Wilson syndrome. *Eur. J. Med. Genet.* **2005**, *2*, 97–111. [CrossRef]
11. Saunders, C.J.; Zhao, W.; Ardinger, H.H. Comprehensive ZEB2 gene analysis for Mowat-Wilson syndrome in a North American cohort: A suggested approach to molecular diagnostics. *Am. J. Med. Genet. A* **2009**, *11*, 2527–2531. [CrossRef]
12. Ghoumid, J.; Drevillon, L.; Alavi-Naini, S.M.; Bondurand, N.; Rio, M.; Briand-Suleau, A.; Nasser, M.; Goodwin, L.; Raymond, P.; Yanicostas, C.; et al. ZEB2 zinc-finger missense mutations lead to hypomorphic alleles and a mild Mowat-Wilson syndrome. *Hum. Mol. Genet.* **2013**, *22*, 2652–2661. [CrossRef]
13. Zou, D.; Wang, L.; Wen, F.; Xiao, H.; Duan, J.; Zhang, T.; Yin, Z.; Dong, Q.; Guo, J.; Liao, J. Genotype-phenotype analysis in Mowat-Wilson syndrome associated with two novel and two recurrent ZEB2 variants. *Exp. Ther. Med.* **2020**, *6*, 263. [CrossRef] [PubMed]
14. Hu, Y.; Peng, Q.; Ma, K.; Li, S.; Rao, C.; Zhong, B.; Lu, X. A novel nonsense mutation of ZEB2 gene in a Chinese patient with Mowat-Wilson syndrome. *J. Clin. Lab. Anal.* **2020**, *9*, e23413. [CrossRef] [PubMed]
15. Ho, S.; Luk, H.M.; Chung, B.H.; Fung, J.L.; Mak, H.H.; Lo, I.F.M. Mowat-Wilson syndrome in a Chinese population: A case series. *Am. J. Med. Genet. A* **2020**, *182*, 1336–1341. [CrossRef] [PubMed]
16. Wenger, T.L.; Harr, M.; Ricciardi, S.; Bhoj, E.; Santani, A.; Adam, M.P.; Barnett, S.S.; Ganetzky, R.; McDonald-McGinn, D.M.; Battaglia, D. CHARGE-like presentation, craniosynostosis and mild Mowat-Wilson Syndrome diagnosed by recognition of the distinctive facial gestalt in a cohort of 28 new cases. *Am. J. Med. Genet. A* **2014**, *164A*, 2557–2566, Erratum in *Am. J. Med. Genet. A* **2015**, *167*, 1682–1683. [CrossRef] [PubMed]
17. Mundhofir, F.E.; Yntema, H.G.; van der Burgt, I.; Hame, B.C.; Faradz, S.M.; van Bon, B.W. Mowat-Wilson syndrome: The first clinical and molecular report of an indonesian patient. *Case Rep. Genet.* **2012**, *2012*, 949507. [CrossRef]

18. Murray, S.B.; Spangler, B.B.; Helm, B.M.; Vergano, S.S. Polymicrogyria in a 10-month-old boy with Mowat-Wilson syndrome. *Am. J. Med. Genet. A* **2015**, *167A*, 2402–2405. [CrossRef] [PubMed]
19. Wang, H.; Yan, Y.C.; Li, Q.; Zhang, Z.; Xiao, P.; Yuan, X.Y.; Li, L.; Jiang, Q. Clinical and genetic features of Mowat-Wilson syndrome: An analysis of 3 cases. *Zhongguo Dang Dai Er Ke Za Zhi* **2019**, *21*, 468–473. (In Chinese) [CrossRef]
20. Yamada, Y.; Nomura, N.; Yamada, K.; Matsuo, M.; Suzuki, Y.; Sameshima, K.; Kimura, R.; Yamamoto, Y.; Fukushi, D.; Fukuhara, Y.; et al. The spectrum of ZEB2 mutations causing the Mowat-Wilson syndrome in Japanese populations. *Am. J. Med. Genet. A* **2014**, *164A*, 1899–1908, Erratum in *Am. J. Med. Genet. A* **2015**, *167*, 1428. [CrossRef] [PubMed]
21. Tronina, A.; Świerczyńska, M.; Filipek, E. First Case Report of Developmental Bilateral Cataract with a Novel Mutation in the ZEB2 Gene Observed in Mowat-Wilson Syndrome. *Medicina* **2023**, *59*, 101. [CrossRef]
22. Jakubiak, A.; Szczałuba, K.; Badura-Stronka, M.; Kutkowska-Kaźmierczak, A.; Jakubiuk-Tomaszuk, A.; Chilarska, T.; Pilch, J.; Braun-Walicka, N.; Castaneda, J.; Wołyńska, K.; et al. Clinical characteristics of Polish patients with molecularly confirmed Mowat-Wilson syndrome. *J. Appl. Genet.* **2021**, *62*, 477–485. [CrossRef]
23. Refaat, K.; Helmy, N.; Elawady, M.; El Ruby, M.; Kamel, A.; Mekkawy, M.; Ashaat, E.; Eid, O.; Mohamed, A.; Rady, M. Interstitial Deletion of 2q22.2q22.3 Involving the Entire ZEB2 Gene in a Case of Mowat-Wilson Syndrome. *Mol. Syndromol.* **2021**, *12*, 87–95. [CrossRef]
24. Musaad, W.; Lyons, A.; Allen, N.; Letshwiti, J. Mowat-Wilson syndrome presenting with Shone's complex cardiac anomaly. *BMJ Case Rep.* **2022**, *15*, e246913. [CrossRef]
25. Pachajoa, H.; Gomez-Pineda, E.; Giraldo-Ocampo, S.; Lores, J. Mowat-Wilson Syndrome as a Differential Diagnosis in Patients with Congenital Heart Defects and Dysmorphic Facies. *Pharmgenom. Pers. Med.* **2022**, *15*, 913–918. [CrossRef]
26. Wu, L.; Wang, J.; Wang, L.; Xu, Q.; Zhou, B.; Zhang, Z.; Li, Q.; Wang, H.; Han, L.; Jiang, Q.; et al. Physical, language, neurodevelopment and phenotype-genotype correlation of Chinese patients with Mowat-Wilson syndrome. *Front. Genet.* **2022**, *13*, 1016677. [CrossRef] [PubMed]
27. Fu, Y.; Xu, W.; Wang, Q.; Lin, Y.; He, P.; Liu, Y.; Yuan, H. Three Novel *De Novo* ZEB2 Variants Identified in Three Unrelated Chinese Patients With Mowat-Wilson Syndrome and A Systematic Review. *Front. Genet.* **2022**, *13*, 853183. [CrossRef]
28. Wei, L.; Han, X.; Li, X.; Han, B.; Nie, W. A Chinese Boy with Mowat-Wilson Syndrome Caused by a 10 bp Deletion in the ZEB2 Gene. *Pharmgenom. Pers. Med.* **2021**, *14*, 1041–1045. [CrossRef]
29. Şenbil, N.; Arslan, Z.; Sayın Kocakap, D.B.; Bilgili, Y. A Case Report of a Prenatally Missed Mowat-Wilson Syndrome With Isolated Corpus Callosum Agenesis. *Child. Neurol. Open.* **2021**, *8*, 2329048X211006511. [CrossRef] [PubMed]
30. Ivanovski, I.; Djuric, O.; Caraffi, S.G.; Santodirocco, D.; Pollazzon, M.; Rosato, S.; Cordelli, D.M.; Abdalla, E.; Accorsi, P.; Adam, M.P.; et al. Phenotype and genotype of 87 patients with Mowat-Wilson syndrome and recommendations for care. *Genet. Med.* **2018**, *20*, 965–975. [CrossRef] [PubMed]
31. Available online: http://pathwaycommons.org/pc12/Pathway_751ce7c7ccec6e191682a33d7252aac8 (accessed on 1 December 2023).
32. Long, J.; Zuo, D.; Park, M. Pc2-mediated sumoylation of Smad-interacting protein 1 attenuates transcriptional repression of E-cadherin. *J. Biol. Chem.* **2005**, *280*, 35477–35489. [CrossRef]
33. Chen, Y.; Banda, M.; Speyer, C.L.; Smith, J.S.; Rabson, A.B.; Gorski, D.H. Regulation of the expression and activity of the antiangiogenic homeobox gene GAX/MEOX2 by ZEB2 and microRNA-221. *Mol. Cell. Biol.* **2010**, *15*, 3902–3913. [CrossRef]
34. Holland, W. Evolution of homeobox genes. *Wiley Interdiscip. Rev. Dev. Biol.* **2013**, *2*, 31–45. [CrossRef]
35. Chen, Y.; Wu, X.; Jiang, R. Integrating human omics data to prioritize candidate genes. *BMC Med. Genom.* **2013**, *6*, 57. [CrossRef]
36. Han, C.; Hong, K.-H.; Kim, Y.H.; Kim, M.-J.; Song, C.; Kim, M.J.; Kim, S.-J.; Raizada, M.K.; Oh, S.P. SMAD1 deficiency in either endothelial or smooth muscle cells can predispose mice to pulmonary hypertension. *Hypertension* **2013**, *61*, 1044–1052. [CrossRef]
37. Calligaris, R.; Bottardi, S.; Cogoi, S.; Apezteguia, I.; Santoro, C. Alternative translation initiation site usage results in two functionally distinct forms of the GATA-1 transcription factor. *Proc. Nat. Acad. Sci. USA* **1995**, *92*, 11598–11602. [CrossRef] [PubMed]
38. Cirillo, L.A.; Lin, F.R.; Cuesta, I.; Friedman, D.; Jarnik, M.; Zaret, K.S. Opening of compacted chromatin by early developmental transcription factors HNF3(FoxA) and GATA-4. *Mol. Cell* **2002**, *2*, 279–289. [CrossRef] [PubMed]
39. Zhang, J.; Wang, S.; Wesley, R.A.; Danner, R.L. Adjacent sequence controls the response polarity of nitric oxide-sensitive Sp factor binding sites. *J. Biol. Chem.* **2003**, *278*, 29192–29200. [CrossRef]
40. Holtschke, T.; Löhler, J.; Kanno, Y.; Fehr, T.; Giese, N.; Rosenbauer, F.; Lou, J.; Knobeloch, K.P.; Gabriele, L.; Waring, J.F.; et al. Immunodeficiency and chronic myelogenous leukemia-like syndrome in mice with a targeted mutation of the ICSBP gene. *Cell* **1996**, *87*, 307–317. [CrossRef] [PubMed]
41. Buckingham, M.; Rigby, P.W. Gene regulatory networks and transcriptional mechanisms that control myogenesis. *Dev. Cell* **2014**, *28*, 225–238. [CrossRef]
42. Mansouri, A.; St-Onge, L.; Gruss, P. Role of Pax genes in endoderm-derived organs. *Trends Endocr. Metab.* **1999**, *10*, 164–167. [CrossRef]
43. Kawamata, N.; Pennella, M.A.; Woo, J.L.; Berk, A.J.; Koffler, H.P. Dominant-negative mechanism of leukemogenic PAX5 fusions. *Oncogene* **2012**, *31*, 966–977. [CrossRef]
44. Schreiber, E.; Tobler, A.; Malipiero, U.; Schaffner, W.; Fontana, A. cDNA cloning of human N-Oct 3, a nervous-system specific POU domain transcription factor binding to the octamer DNA motif. *Nucleic Acids Res.* **1993**, *21*, 253–258. [CrossRef]

45. Atanasoski, S.; Toldo, S.S.; Malipiero, U.; Schreiber, E.; Fries, R.; Fontana, A. Isolation of the human genomic brain-2/N-Oct 3 gene (POUF3) and assignment to chromosome 6q16. *Genomics* **1995**, *26*, 272–280. [CrossRef] [PubMed]
46. Szklarczyk, D.; Kirsch, R.; Koutrouli, M.; Nastou, K.; Mehryary, F.; Hachilif, R.; Gable, A.L.; Fang, T.; Doncheva, N.T.; Pyysalo, S.; et al. The STRING database in 2023: Protein-protein association networks and functional enrichment analyses for any sequenced genome of interest. *Nucleic Acids Res.* **2023**, *51*, D638–D646. [CrossRef]
47. Wang, J.; Lee, S.; The, C.E.; Bunting, K.; Ma, L.; Shannon, M.F. The transcription repressor, ZEB1, cooperates with CtBP2 and HDAC1 to suppress IL-2 gene activation in T cells. *Int. Immunol.* **2009**, *3*, 227–235. [CrossRef]
48. Wang, H.; Xiao, Z.; Zheng, J.; Wu, J.; Hu, X.L.; Yang, X.; Shen, Q. ZEB1 Represses Neural Differentiation and Cooperates with CTBP2 to Dynamically Regulate Cell Migration during Neocortex Development. *Cell Rep.* **2019**, *27*, 2335–2353.e6. [CrossRef]
49. Güleray Lafcı, N.; Karaosmanoglu, B.; Taskiran, E.Z.; Simsek-Kiper, P.O.; Utine, G.E. Mutated Transcripts of *ZEB2* Do Not Undergo Nonsense-Mediated Decay in Mowat-Wilson Syndrome. *Mol. Syndromol.* **2023**, *14*, 258–265. [CrossRef]
50. Chinnadurai, G. CtBP Family Proteins: Unique Transcriptional Regulators in the Nucleus with Diverse Cytosolic Functions. In *Madame Curie Bioscience Database [Internet]*; Landes Bioscience: Austin, TX, USA, 2007. Available online: https://www.ncbi.nlm.nih.gov/books/NBK6557/ (accessed on 1 November 2023).
51. Li, X.; Han, M.; Zhang, H.; Liu, F.; Pan, Y.; Zhu, J.; Liao, Z.; Chen, X.; Zhang, B. Structures and biological functions of zinc finger proteins and their roles in hepatocellular carcinoma. *Biomark. Res.* **2022**, *10*, 2. [CrossRef] [PubMed]
52. Birkhoff, J.C.; Huylebroeck, D.; Conidi, A. ZEB2, the Mowat-Wilson Syndrome Transcription Factor: Confirmations, Novel Functions, and Continuing Surprises. *Genes* **2021**, *12*, 1037. [CrossRef] [PubMed]
53. Macias, M.J.; Martin-Malpartida, P.; Massagué, J. Structural determinants of Smad function in TGF-β signaling. *Trends Biochem. Sci.* **2015**, *40*, 296–308. [CrossRef]
54. Bürglin, T.R. Homeodomain subtypes and functional diversity. *Subcell. Biochem.* **2011**, *52*, 95–122. [CrossRef] [PubMed]

Disclaimer/Publisher's Note: The statements, opinions and data contained in all publications are solely those of the individual author(s) and contributor(s) and not of MDPI and/or the editor(s). MDPI and/or the editor(s) disclaim responsibility for any injury to people or property resulting from any ideas, methods, instructions or products referred to in the content.

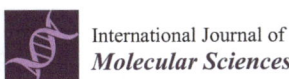

Review

Genetics of Obesity in Humans: A Clinical Review

Ranim Mahmoud [1,2], Virginia Kimonis [1,3,4,*] and Merlin G. Butler [5]

1. Department of Pediatrics, University of California, Irvine, CA 92697, USA
2. Department of Pediatrics, Faculty of Medicine, Mansoura University, Mansoura 35516, Egypt
3. Departments of Neurology and Pathology, University of California, Irvine, CA 92697, USA
4. Children's Hospital of Orange County, Orange, CA 92868, USA
5. Departments of Psychiatry & Behavioral Sciences and Pediatrics, University of Kansas Medical Center, Kansas City, KS 66160, USA
* Correspondence: vkimonis@uci.edu

Abstract: Obesity is a complex multifactorial disorder with genetic and environmental factors. There is an increase in the worldwide prevalence of obesity in both developed and developing countries. The development of genome-wide association studies (GWAS) and next-generation sequencing (NGS) has increased the discovery of genetic associations and awareness of monogenic and polygenic causes of obesity. The genetics of obesity could be classified into syndromic and non-syndromic obesity. Prader–Willi, fragile X, Bardet–Biedl, Cohen, and Albright Hereditary Osteodystrophy (AHO) syndromes are examples of syndromic obesity, which are associated with developmental delay and early onset obesity. Non-syndromic obesity could be monogenic, polygenic, or chromosomal in origin. Monogenic obesity is caused by variants of single genes while polygenic obesity includes several genes with the involvement of members of gene families. New advances in genetic testing have led to the identification of obesity-related genes. Leptin (*LEP*), the leptin receptor (*LEPR*), proopiomelanocortin (*POMC*), prohormone convertase 1 (*PCSK1*), the melanocortin 4 receptor (*MC4R*), single-minded homolog 1 (*SIM1*), brain-derived neurotrophic factor (*BDNF*), and the neurotrophic tyrosine kinase receptor type 2 gene (*NTRK2*) have been reported as causative genes for obesity. NGS is now in use and emerging as a useful tool to search for candidate genes for obesity in clinical settings.

Keywords: obesity; genetics; monogenic; polygenic; Prader-Willi; syndrome

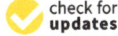

Citation: Mahmoud, R.; Kimonis, V.; Butler, M.G. Genetics of Obesity in Humans: A Clinical Review. *Int. J. Mol. Sci.* **2022**, *23*, 11005. https://doi.org/10.3390/ijms231911005

Academic Editor: Ahmed Bettaieb

Received: 31 July 2022
Accepted: 10 September 2022
Published: 20 September 2022

Publisher's Note: MDPI stays neutral with regard to jurisdictional claims in published maps and institutional affiliations.

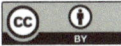

Copyright: © 2022 by the authors. Licensee MDPI, Basel, Switzerland. This article is an open access article distributed under the terms and conditions of the Creative Commons Attribution (CC BY) license (https://creativecommons.org/licenses/by/4.0/).

1. Introduction

Obesity is a major health problem worldwide. It is more common in established countries but is on the increase in developing countries. The worldwide prevalence of obesity [body mass index (BMI) $\geq$ 30 kg m^2] has doubled between 1980 and 2008, with a prevalence of 13% in the adult population reported in 2014. In 2013, there were 42 million obese children below the age of five years [1]. BMI, according to the World Health Organization (WHO), is classified in adults as overweight at 25–29.9 kg/m^2, obese at 30–39 kg/m^2, and morbidly obese at 40 kg/m^2 and above [2].

Obesity is a complex multifactorial disorder with genetic and environmental factors. The increased prevalence of obesity is impacted by the environment as high caloric food sources with a sedentary lifestyle has decreased energy expenditure. Twin and family studies have documented the role of genetic factors in obesity, with the risk of childhood obesity increasing with a positive family history of obesity. There is a high concordance rate for obesity in monozygotic twins vs dizygotic twins and an estimated heritability for obesity at between 40% and 75% in twin studies [3].

The recognition of obesity and inheritance with associated genes has been impeded by a limited knowledge and understanding of genetics at the human genome level and with the biological pathways involved in obesity. However, the development of genome-wide association studies (GWAS) and next-generation sequencing (NGS) has increased the discovery of genetic associations and awareness of monogenic and polygenic causes of obesity. About 127 informative sites in the human genome have been reported to show linkage with obesity by GWAS [4] and over 500 obesity-related genes recognized in humans [5]. There are approximately 30 neuro-endocrine peptides in humans that are known to inhibit eating behavior, but only ghrelin increases eating with an important role in appetite regulation and energy balance [6]. This balance is in response to changes in peripheral circulating signals from adipose tissue, stomach, and endocrine organs. Regions of the brain and neurons help with energy balance and homeostasis by sensing and processing various metabolic signals with major activity observed in the hypothalamus. Many monogenic neuroendocrine disorders involving the leptin pathway are recognized and associated with early onset obesity in childhood. The genetics of obesity could be classified into syndromic and non-syndromic obesity with or without congenital defects and developmental delay. For example, Prader–Willi, fragile X, Bardet–Biedl, Cohen, and Albright Hereditary Osteodystrophy (AHO) syndromes are associated with developmental delay and early onset obesity [7]. Non-syndromic obesity could be monogenic, polygenic, or chromosomal in origin. Monogenic obesity is caused by variants of single genes while polygenic obesity includes several genes with the involvement of members of gene families with or without syndromic findings but accompanied with obesity and recognized phenotypes.

New advances in genetic evaluation and analysis have led to the identification of obesity-related genes. For example, eight genes have been reported as causes for obesity, including leptin (*LEP*), the leptin receptor (*LEPR*), proopiomelanocortin (*POMC*), prohormone convertase 1 (*PCSK1*), the melanocortin 4 receptor (*MC4R*), single-minded homolog 1 (*SIM1*), brain-derived neurotrophic factor (*BDNF*), and the neurotrophic tyrosine kinase receptor type 2 gene (*NTRK2*) [8,9], from over 500 obesity-related genes [5]. One important method is termed GWAS, which incorporates hundreds, or thousands, of polymorphic DNA markers and single nucleotide polymorphisms (SNPs) located throughout the human genome with the ability to search for markers for new genes with no previous evidence of disease involvement. In the past decade, close to 1000 published GWAS results have been reported and 165 traits found in humans with a number of SNPs from obese and nonobese individuals marked gene loci and potential candidate obesity genes [10]. Hence, genetic factors can be divided into the following three categories: Mendelian (monogenic) syndromic obesity, Mendelian non-syndromic obesity, and polygenic obesity. Meanwhile, NGS is now in use and emerging as a useful tool to search for candidate genes for obesity in clinical settings [5,11]. The results of these recent investigations need to be replicated to warrant further consideration.

2. Obesity-Related Genes and Defects

2.1. Leptin

Leptin is a protein secreted by white adipose tissue and encoded by a gene on chromosome 7 in humans. Leptin crosses the blood–brain barrier to bind to the presynaptic GABAergic neurons of the hypothalamus and decreases appetite and increases energy expenditure [12]. In the arcuate nucleus of the hypothalamus, leptin binds to its receptor and inhibits the neuropeptide Y (NPY)/agouti-related protein (AgRP) pathway [13]. The role of leptin and the leptin receptor gene in human obesity is now emerging but not well understood [14]. Farooqi (2005) reported that inherited human leptin deficiency in patients caused severe early-onset obesity (e.g., 8 years and 86 kg, or 2 years and 29 kg) due to a frame-shift mutation in the homozygous obesity leptin gene (deletion of G133) and a truncated protein [7]. Other studies reported a high level of leptin in obese patients, but it was associated with a decrease in the level of soluble leptin receptors, which contributed directly to leptin function. Another study on 110 patients including 55 obese and 55 healthy controls showed significantly higher levels of leptin in the obese group than in controls [4]. This phenomenon is known as leptin resistance. These receptors are not only found in the

CNS but are also present in peripheral organs, such as the liver, skeletal muscles, pancreatic beta cells, and even adipose cells, thereby playing an important role in energy regulation.

2.2. Proopiomelanocortin (POMC) Deficiency

POMC is an appetite inhibitory gene found on chromosome 2 in humans. It influences the leptin–melanocortin system as a deficiency of the POMC protein causes an absence of ACTH and alpha-MSH, which are cleaved from the POMC protein [15]. Hence, a deficiency of POMC leads to hyperphagia, lower resting metabolic rate, and resultant severe obesity with red hair and pale skin [16]. Errors in the cleavage of master proteins such as *POMC* require pro-hormone convertase, which cleaves this large protein into smaller functional peptides and as noted, interacts with appetite control, pigment, and obesity [17].

2.3. Melanocortin-4 Receptor

The melanocortin-4 receptor *(MC4R)* gene is now considered the most common associated gene for childhood obesity and found in about 4% of affected cases prior to advanced genetic testing and next generation sequencing (NGS) [9]. It was first discovered to be related to body weight in 1998 and now multiple studies have investigated its mechanism and the function of different mutations [18]. The *MC4R* gene codes for the MC4R protein, which plays an important role in energy homeostasis and food intake behavior [19]. The central melanocortin pathway regulates energy balance and homeostasis by activating or inhibiting leptin and its receptor is mediated by two subsets of neurons as well as MC3R and MC4R in the arcuate nucleus of the hypothalamus.

2.4. FTO (Fat Mass and Obesity Associated Gene)

FTO was the first obesity-susceptibility gene discovered through GWAS in European patients with type 2 diabetes [20]. Multiple single nucleotide polymorphisms (SNPs) in the first intron of the gene have shown a significant association with type 2 diabetes. However, after controlling for BMI, there was no association with type 2 diabetes, thereby suggesting that the FTO and type 2 diabetes association was mediated through FTO's effect on BMI. Another study was conducted in Sardinian patients and confirmed the same results. The rs9939609 and rs9930506 SNPs were identified in *FTO* with significant association with BMI [21,22]. Other GWAS studies in European populations have reported several other SNPs located in the same chromosomal location. In addition, significant association between *FTO* SNPs (rs9939609, rs17817449, rs12149832) and BMI was reported in three large studies conducted in Asian populations [23–25].

Kalantari et al. (2018) reported that the role of *FTO* gene polymorphisms, a haplotype not a SNP, are close to each other so that they can affect other gene expression through a sequence of the first intron region [26]. The association between *FTO* SNPs with food intake and physical activity was investigated in many studies, which revealed the associations between *FTO* SNPs and increased intake of dietary fat, protein, energy, increased appetite, but decreased satiety. However, *FTO* SNPs were not associated with the level of physical activity. This finding highlighted the importance of physical activity in the modulation of body weight even in those with genetic susceptibility to obesity [27].

Additional studies by Castro et al. on four obesity-related genes (*PPARG*-rs1801282; *PPARGC1A*-rs8192678; *FTO*-rs9939609; *MC4R*-rs17782313) showed that three of the four genes (*PPARG, FTO, MC4R*) had a combined effect on overweight and obesity at an odds ratio of 1.65 ($p = 0.008$) in a large case-control study in the Brazilian population [28]. The same *MC4R* variant (rs17782313) and an *FTO* variant (rs9930506) were significantly associated with obesity in children, reported in multiple separate studies involving thousands of individual subjects, particularly Caucasians and Asians [29]. Further studies in children and adolescents with the same genes (*FTO* and *MC4R*) and variants were reported by Resende et al. in a systematic review of the literature with an association with overweight and obesity [30].

Dastgheib et al. performed a metanalysis involving 13 studies with 9565 cases and 11,956 controls on *MC4R* rs17782313 and 18 studies with 4789 cases and 15,918 controls on *FTO* rs9939609. They found that odds ratios showed significant results indicating that these variants were associated with a higher risk of obesity [29].

Many forms of obesity are thought to be polygenic with variants involved in the same or different genes that act synergistically per individual affecting body weight, composition, and size quantitatively. Polycystic ovary syndrome (PCOS) is a common polygenic metabolic disorder affecting 5–8% of women in the childbearing period. PCOS is defined according to the Rotterdam consensus based on diagnostic criteria to include at least two of the following features: (1) clinical or biochemical hyperandrogenism; (2) oligo-anovulation; and (3) polycystic ovaries (PCO) and excluding similar endocrinopathies. Most women with PCOS are overweight or obese. Many studies investigated the role of genetic contribution for obesity in patients with PCOS [31,32]. Ewens et al. reported five SNPs in *FTO* and two in *MC4R* with significant association with BMI in the PCOS families [33]. Another study by Tu et al. reported association between *LEPR* Lys109Arg (rs1137100) and PCOS susceptibility in 326 Han Chinese patients with PCOS [34].

2.5. Chromosomal Defects and Obesity

Syndromic childhood obesity is a rare form of obesity that is part of multiple clinical manifestations. Advanced genetic testing has helped in the detection of structural defects of the chromosome and at the DNA level and has led to the diagnosis of rare and common forms of obesity. The determination of genetic causes of obesity could be helpful for genetic counselling and the selection of appropriate treatment. In addition, Dasouki et al. and Cheon et al. each summarized chromosomal abnormalities with syndromic obesity [35,36]. Kaur et al. reported 79 obesity syndromes described in the literature, with obesity considered to be a cardinal feature in 55 of them, while the prevalence of obesity in the other 24 syndromes was higher than that in the general population. Forty-nine syndromes have been mapped to specific chromosome regions or locations including a causative gene [1]. Some examples of syndromic obesity due to chromosomal defects will be discussed in this review such as Prader–Willi syndrome (PWS), Down syndrome, Bardet–Biedl syndrome, fragile X syndrome, Alstrom syndrome, and Cornelia de Lange syndrome. Table 1 highlights other common causes of obesity syndromes and their clinical and genetic findings.

Table 1. Other obesity-related disorders with reported clinical and genetic findings.

Syndrome	Gene	Mode of Inheritance	Clinical Features	Reference
Borjeson–Forssman–Lehmann syndrome	PHF6	X-linked	Developmental delay Obesity Seizure Skeletal anomalies Large ears Hypogonadism Gynecomastia Distinctive facial features	[37]
Carpenter syndrome	RAB23	Autosomal recessive	Peculiar facies Brachydactyly of the hands Syndactyly Preaxial polydactyly Congenital heart defects Intellectual disability Hypogenitalism Obesity	[38]

Table 1. Cont.

Syndrome	Gene	Mode of Inheritance	Clinical Features	Reference
Cornelia de Lange syndrome	NIPBL-CdLS, RAD21-CdLS, SMC3-CdLS, BRD4-CdLS, HDAC8-CdLS, SMC1A-CdLS	Autosomal dominant X-linked	Microcephaly Synophrys Short nasal bridge Long and/or smooth philtrum Highly arched palate with or without cleft palate Behavioral problems Micrognathia Hearing loss Tendency to overweight	[39]
CHOPS syndrome	AFF4	Autosomal dominant	Cognitive impairment Coarse facies Heart defects Obesity Short stature, and Skeletal dysplasia.	[40]
Chudley-Lowry syndrome	ATRX	X-linked	Intellectual disability Short stature Macrosomia Obesity Hypogonadism Distinctive facial features	[41]
Coffin–Lowry syndrome	RPS6KA3	X-linked	Severe intellectual disability Kyphoscoliosis, Behavioral problems, Progressive spasticity, Paraplegia, Sleep apnea Stroke	[42]
Kleefstra syndrome	EHMT1	9q34.3 deletion Autosomal dominant	Intellectual disability Obesity Hypotonia Congenital heart defects Genitourinary anomalies Seizures Distinctive facial features	[43]
Rubinstein–Taybi syndrome	CREBBP, EP300	Autosomal dominant	Distinctive facial features, Broad thumbs and hallluces Short stature Intellectual disability Obesity in childhood or adolescence	[44]
Temple syndrome	Aberrations at the 14q32.2 imprinted region	Maternal disomy 14	Feeding difficulties Hypotonia Motor developmental delay Childhood-onset central obesity Mild facial dysmorphism	[45]

3. Obesity-Related Syndromes

3.1. Prader–Willi Syndrome

Prader–Willi syndrome (PWS) is a complex genetic disorder affecting multiple body systems. It occurs in 1 in 10,000 to 1 in 29,000 people, affecting both males and females equally and in all races [6,46]. PWS is characterized by hypotonia, decreased muscle tone, and extreme floppiness as an infant, which leads to feeding difficulty and poor weight gain in the newborn or in infancy. Then, completely on the other end of the spectrum, it progresses after infancy to hyperphagia or excessive food drive, which can lead to obesity in childhood and beyond [47]. PWS is a chromosomal disorder with the region associated with PWS located on the chromosome 15q11.2-q13. Typically, people have two different copies of chromosome 15, one inherited from their mother and one from their father. The paternal copy is important for typical development; if a person has not inherited a copy of this region from their father, such as a paternal 15q11-q13 deletion, PWS occurs. Most genes in the 15q11.2-q13 region include imprinted genes and snoRNAs, which are involved in RNA and protein processing of neuroregulators and hormones. When altered, neuronal development and endocrine function are impacted [48].

There are three different genetic mechanisms by which PWS can occur. The most common genetic etiology of PWS is due to the loss of paternal gene expression in the 15q11.2-q13 region, which accounts for about 70% of all PWS cases, caused by a de novo paternally derived chromosome 15q11.2-q13 deletion [48]. The less common form of PWS, occurring in about 30% of all PWS cases, is caused when an individual inherits both copies of chromosome 15 from the mother, known as maternal uniparental disomy (UPD) [6]. A rare form, occurring in about 3% of PWS cases, is a mutation or defect of the imprinting control center in chromosome 15. Therefore, PWS is due to genomic imprinting errors and disturbances of an epigenetic phenomenon resulting in parent-of-origin gene expression, involving methylation and histone modifications and causing monoallelic expression of specific genes [49].

As PWS is characterized by severe hypotonia in the newborn period causing severe floppiness and difficulty in feeding, it can eventually lead to the placement of a feeding gastric tube (G-tube) directly into the stomach or nasogastric tube for feeding assistance in early infancy. A study in France of 19 infants, who were diagnosed with PWS before two months of age, concluded that hospitalization time and duration of tube feeding were reduced due to very early diagnosis. They also found that multidisciplinary care provided (which included growth hormone treatment given between ages 6 months to just under 2 years old) resulted in only 1 infant becoming obese at age 2.5 years [50]. A cross-sectional study of 42 children with PWS and 9 controls, aged 7 months–5 years, investigated differences in appetite hormones that may explain the development of abnormal eating behavior. They found no significant relationship between eating behavior in PWS and the level of any hormone or insulin resistance, independent of age [51]. Oldzej et al. reported that PWS patients with deletion were significantly heavier than those with UPD [52]. Further, Mahmoud et al. in 2021 concluded from a large cohort of PWS patients that higher BMI scores were present in patients with the deletion subtype compared to UPD [53].

PWS has been classically described as having two clinical stages: poor feeding, with failure to thrive (FTT) in infancy (Stage 1), followed by hyperphagia leading to obesity in later childhood (Stage 2). The identification of these phases has assisted in the diagnosis of individuals affected with PWS. Additionally, a study identified a total of seven different nutritional phases, with five main phases and sub-phases in phases 1 and 2 and concluded the progression of nutritional phases in PWS is more complex than previously recognized [54]. An awareness of the various nutritional phases for parents of newly diagnosed infants with PWS may prevent or possibly slow the early onset of obesity. Those affected with PWS are characterized in later infancy or early childhood with hyperphagia or excessive eating with hyperphagia as a difficult symptom to cope with because of the constant desire to eat, even though the individual may have just eaten. (See Figure 1 of an individual with Prader–Willi syndrome as an example of syndromic obesity).

The source of hyperphagia is believed to be located deep in the brain structure in the hypothalamus, a small gland that has multiple roles. It is both an endocrine gland and a key center for a wide variety of behaviors related to survival. The hypothalamus signals to its close neighbor, the pituitary gland, which acts as a master gland with secretions controlling many other glands to release hormones necessary for growth, metabolism, learning, and memory. The hypothalamus also contains key centers for controlling aggression, body temperature, sexual activity, and food and water intake as well as hunger [55]. For people with PWS, the hypothalamus does not regulate emotions and appetite normally as the brain does not receive/process signals of feeling "full or satisfied" and drives the individual to consume more food or eat as much as possible [56]. The brain of an individual with PWS sends signals that the body is starving, lowers the metabolic rate to conserve energy, and drives the individual to find food and eat as much as possible. This excessive food drive, plus the slowed metabolic rate, leads to rapid weight gain and morbid obesity [57]. Obesity often changes the body structure, causing a shorter torso and larger mid-section appearance. Obesity is a major cause of morbidity due to respiratory disease and non-insulin dependent (type 2) diabetes mellitus with comorbidities [57,58].

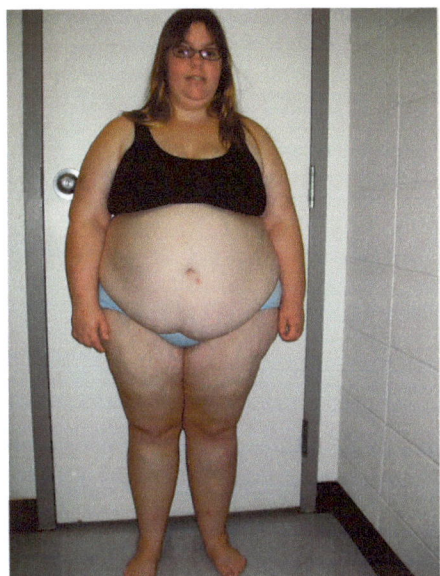 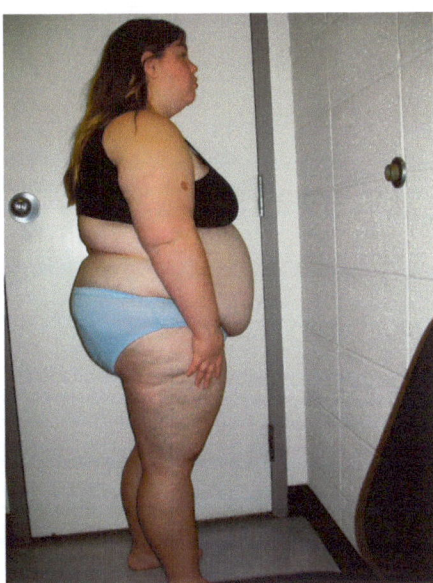

Figure 1. Frontal and profile views of a 16-year-old female with Prader–Willi syndrome due to maternal disomy 15, showing the classical features observed in this obesity-related syndrome.

3.2. Alstrom Syndrome

Alstrom syndrome is a rare obesity-related single gene disorder inherited in an autosomal recessive pattern. The estimated range is from 1 in 500,000 to 1 in 1,000,000 and is due to mutations in the *ALMS1* gene located on chromosome 2p13. The ALMS1 protein has an important role in ciliary function, energy metabolism, and cell cycle control. Li et al. (2007) suggested that the absence of the ALMS1 protein leads to abnormal ciliary formation with Alstrom syndrome classified as one of the ciliopathies due to abnormal ciliary function [59].

More than one hundred different mutations have been reported in the literature in the *ALMS1* gene. The symptoms usually start in infancy and progress during childhood with expanded variability in presentation, which makes the diagnosis challenging. The first clinical manifestations are visual problems, nystagmus, and early blindness due to cone-rod dystrophy. Many endocrine abnormalities are reported to occur in Alstrom syndrome including hypothyroidism, hypogonadotropic hypogonadism in males, hyperandrogenism in females, childhood truncal obesity, hypertriglyceridemia, and insulin resistance with type 2 diabetes mellitus. More than 70% of patients with Alstrom syndrome have congestive heart failure due to cardiomyopathy along with short stature, neurodevelopmental delay, scoliosis and kyphosis, and progressive pulmonary, hepatic, and renal dysfunction with associated complications [60].

3.3. Fragile X Syndrome (FXS)

FXS is the most common cause of intellectual disability in males. It affects about 1 in 4000 males in the general population and occurs due to the triplet repeat expansion of

CGG repeats greater than 200 in size in the 5' untranslated region of the *FMR1* gene at chromosome Xq27.3 [61]. The carrier state or the premutation form of this gene occurs when the number of CGG repeats is between 50 and 200. Premutation occurs in females and could expand to a full mutation in the subsequent generation. This mutation leads to the loss of fragile X mental retardation protein (FMRP), a protein that plays an important role in protein translation for neuronal synaptic connections [62].

The common clinical features include intellectual disability, large ears, a narrow head, long face, and prognathism. Joint laxity, mitral valve prolapse, and macroorchidism are also common. Behavioral problems in FXS include anxiety, autistic behavior, self-injury, and compulsive disorders. About 10% of individuals with FXS will have severe obesity, hyperphagia, hypogonadism, or delayed puberty as observed in PWS. This type of FXS patient is termed the Prader–Willi phenotype (PWP) [63]. A large survey of families with FXS reported that the prevalence of obesity in adults with FXS was similar to the general population [64]. Another study conducted by the Fragile X Clinical and Research Consortium reported that patients with FXS had higher weights than in the general population [65]. Choo et al. conducted a longitudinal study on 1223 patients with FXS in different age groups and found an increasing BMI with age and higher BMI Z-scores in adulthood, further supporting obesity as a feature [66].

3.4. Down Syndrome

Down syndrome (DS) is one of the most common chromosomal disorders in humans [67]. It occurs in 1:600–700 newborns. The most common cause of DS is the presence of an extra copy of chromosome 21. The other causes are Robertsonian translocations and mosaicism involving chromosome 21. In Robertsonian translocations, the long arm of chromosome 21 is translocated and attached to another acrocentric chromosome. In mosaicism, the meiotic non-division occurs after fertilization and at some point during cell division, a chromosome 21 is lost so that the patient has mosaic DS or now has two cell lineages (one with the normal number of chromosomes, and other one with an extra number 21) [68].

Many reviews have examined obesity in children with developmental disabilities specifically targeting children with physical disabilities, coordination disorder, and intellectual disability [69–71]. Many mechanisms have been proposed for the development of obesity in DS including increased serum leptin levels associated with increased appetite as the leptin hormone affects the hunger and satiety centers in the brain, decreases energy expenditure, and decreases physical activity [72,73].

The high risk of obesity in DS could be linked to many factors such as genetic predisposition, hypothyroidism, decreased physical activity, high serum cholesterol and triglycerides, and an abnormal diet. In addition, hypotonia, increased susceptibility to systemic inflammation, decreased metabolic rate, depression, and absence of social and financial support could play a role. Decreased cognitive function could be one of the precipitating factors for obesity as it could affect food choice and level of physical activity. Nordstrom et al. in 2020 compared DS patients with mild and moderate intellectual disability along with their nutritional status and found no significant correlation [74]. Fructuoso et al. in 2018 reported an increase in the level of obesity-associated inflammatory biomarkers galectin-3 and HSP72 in a mouse model of DS [75]. This suggested that increased levels in the adipose tissue leading to low-grade inflammation are important risk factors for the development of obesity in DS.

3.5. Bardet–Biedl Syndrome

Bardet–Biedl syndrome is a rare form of syndromic obesity that is inherited in an autosomal recessive pattern. The main clinical manifestations are central obesity, retinal cone-rod dystrophy, postaxial polydactyly, learning difficulties, hearing loss, hypogonadism, and genitourinary abnormalities with renal problems such as polycystic kidney disease.

BBS is associated with high genetic heterogeneity, variable expressivity, and pleiotropy. Twenty-four loci are involved with different types of mutations or variants, which could explain different clinical presentations and findings [67]. The different types of mutations include missense, nonsense, deletions, and insertions/duplications of genes causing Bardet–Biedl syndrome. Bardet–Biedl syndrome is a multisubunit complex with involvement of eight proteins coded by *BBS1*, *BBS2*, *BBS4*, *BBS5*, *BBS7*, *TTC8*, *BBS9*, and *BBIP* genes. Most of the Bardet–Biedl syndrome cases in Europe and North America present with mutations in either *BBS1* or *BBS10* genes. Obesity is a common feature as it affects 89% of BBS cases with an early age onset of 2 to 3 years. Obesity occurs in BBS due to gene mutations that lead to a decrease in the number of cilia and altered neuroendocrine signaling from ciliated neurons to fat storage tissues. These disturbances lead to the dysregulation of appetite with changes in leptin resistance and impaired leptin receptor signaling [76].

3.6. Albright Hereditary Osteodystrophy

Albright hereditary osteodystrophy (AHO) is an autosomal dominant genetic disorder due to mutations in the *GNAS1* gene. The clinical manifestations include short stature, brachydactyly, developmental delay, pseudo-hypoparathyroidism, a round face, and early onset obesity [77]. *GNAS* is a complex imprinted locus on chromosome 20q13.11. and many transcripts are produced using alternative promoters and splice sites. Alteration in these transcripts can lead to many clinical disorders or presentations. The GNAS1 gene coding Gα_s (stimulatory G-protein alpha subunit) mediates signaling by hormones and ligands that bind to G protein–coupled receptors (GPCRs) for generating cyclic AMP. When mutations occur on the maternally inherited alleles expressed in the thyroid or pituitary glands and the renal proximal tubule, a resistance develops to parathyroid hormone (PTH) and other hormones that signal through the Gα_s-coupled receptors generating disease (pseudohypoparathyroidism type 1A). When mutations occur on the paternally inherited alleles, the patients develop Albright hereditary osteodystrophy without hormone resistance. The role of genomic imprinting is involved in the development of this genetic disorder [78,79].

The etiology of obesity in AHO is not well known but different theories exist including mutations in *MC4R*, which is transduced by Gsα, and mediated anorexigenic signals from hormones and other neurotransmitters. The loss of such anorexigenic signals through MC4R could produce hyperphagia, but this hypothesis has not been widely studied in AHO individuals with obesity [80,81].

3.7. WAGR Syndrome

WAGR syndrome occurs due to deletion at chromosome 11p13 (location of the *WT1* and *PAX6* genes). This syndrome is characterized by predisposition to Wilms tumor aniridia, ambiguous genitalia, and mental retardation (WAGR). Many behavioral and psychiatric disorders have been reported in this syndrome including autism spectrum disorders, attention-deficit disorder, obsessive-compulsive disorder, other anxiety disorders, and depression. WAGR syndrome has been associated with a deletion in the brain-derived neurotrophic factor (*BDNF*) gene in the chromosome 11p13 region, which leads to the obesity phenotype. Although persons with WAGR syndrome typically have low-normal birth weight, marked obesity subsequently develops in a substantial subgroup of patients [82,83]. Many case reports have been described with severe hyperphagia, obesity, and cytogenetic deletions of chromosome 11p *BDNF* gene locus [84–86]. Han et al. (2008) conducted a study on 33 patients with WAGR and reported that patients with *BDNF* haploinsufficiency had significantly higher BMIs during childhood, with a 100% prevalence of childhood-onset obesity [87].

3.8. Cohen Syndrome

Cohen syndrome is caused by a mutation of the vacuolar protein sorting 13 homolog B (*VPS13B*) gene on chromosome 8q22.2. VPS13B is a transmembrane protein that plays an important role in the development and function of the eye, hematological system, and central nervous system via vesicle-mediated transport and the sorting of proteins within the cells [88]. Cohen syndrome has variable clinical manifestations including progressive retinochoroidal dystrophy and myopia, acquired microcephaly, developmental delay, hypotonia, joint laxity, characteristic facial features with prominent central incisors, truncal obesity, cheerful disposition, and neutropenia. Patients with Cohen syndrome usually suffer from failure to gain weight in infancy and early childhood, but later become significantly overweight in their teenage years with mainly truncal fat accumulation. This change usually occurs very rapidly, with a weight gain of 10–15 kg observed over a short period of time from four to six months [89]. Functional studies have shown that the increased fat accumulation in patients with Cohen syndrome is due to an increased propensity of pre-adipocytes lacking the VPS13B protein to differentiate into fat-storing cells [90].

3.9. Smith–Magenis Syndrome

Smith–Magenis syndrome is a genetic condition due to an interstitial deletion of chromosome 17p11.2, which is inherited in an autosomal dominant pattern. Patients with Smith–Magenis syndrome are characterized by mental retardation, developmental delay, renal anomalies, sleep disturbances, dysmorphic features, and behavioral problems including maladaptive/self-injurious, aggressive, and food seeking behaviors like patients with PWS. More than 90% of patients with Smith–Magenis syndrome are overweight or obese after 10 years of age [91].

3.10. Kallmann Syndrome

Kallmann syndrome is a rare genetic condition of gonadotropin-releasing hormone deficiency and anosmia. Some patients have some additional anomalies including abnormal eye movements, ptosis, hearing loss, unilateral renal agenesis, cleft lip or palate, and obesity. It occurs due to mutations in *KAL1*, *FGFR1*, *FGF8*, *PROKR2*, and *PROK2* genes and most of the cases are inherited in an X-linked recessive pattern and autosomal recessive or dominant pattern with incomplete penetrance [92].

4. Management of Genetic Obesity

There are three therapeutic categories to treat obesity: lifestyle modification, medical treatment, and bariatric surgery. The role of genetic factors in obesity is not only a risk factor but also affects the response to therapeutic options for losing weight based on pharmacogenetics and precision medicine with a multidisciplinary approach. Since hyperphagia is a main clinical feature of monogenic obesity, the most effective management is food restriction. This will need adequate training and involvement of the parents and care providers to prevent early onset obesity. Environmental factors such as physical activity, socioeconomic state, and type of diet could modulate the penetrance of obesity associated with pathogenic mutations to avoid unhealthy environments for these patients [9].

Setmelanotide (Imcivree) is a melanocortin-4 (MC4) receptor agonist used for the treatment of obesity due to proopiomelanocortin (POMC), proprotein convertase subtilisin/keying type 1 (PCSK1), or leptin receptor (LEPR) deficiency. The US Food and Drug Administration approved the drug for chronic weight management in patients 6 years and older with obesity caused by POMC, PCSK1, and LEPR deficiency. Setmelanotide is under consideration for other rare genetic disorders associated with obesity including Bardet–Biedl syndrome, Alstrom syndrome, POMC, and other MC4R pathway heterozygous deficiency obesities. Setmelanotide activates areas in the brain that regulate appetite and fullness, causing patients with specific defects in these areas of the brain not to eat as much and helps to lose weight. It also may increase resting metabolism that can contribute to weight loss. Setmelanotide may lead to weight loss in patients with obesity associated with these conditions but does not treat the genetic defects that cause the condition or other symptoms or signs [93].

The management of adrenal insufficiency is very important with the maintenance of physiologic hydrocortisone replacement in POMC deficiency. Patients with congenital leptin deficiency could be treated by daily injections of recombinant human leptin, which decreases obesity and associated phenotypic abnormalities. Leptin treatment may reduce food intake, fat mass, hyperinsulinemia, and hyperlipidemia in humans, and restores normal pubertal development, endocrine, and immune function [94].

Growth hormone treatment is beneficial in the management of PWS. One of the first comprehensive studies to measure the benefits of growth and body composition with the use of growth hormone on individuals with Prader–Willi syndrome was completed in 1997 by Lindgren et al. This study included 27 affected individuals: 15 with growth hormone treatment for 2 years and 12 with growth hormone treatment for 1 year [95]. They reported that all 27 enrolled individuals showed an increase in height velocity and muscle mass and a decrease in body fat percentage, regardless of time on growth hormone. This study also suggested measurable benefits with growth hormone treatment in regard to a decline in adverse behavioral and psychiatric issues that are associated with PWS [95].

A follow-up study to the aforementioned study was completed by Lindgren et al. in 1998. The intent of this study was to measure and compare the growth and body composition in affected individuals with Prader–Willi syndrome treated with growth hormone in comparison to those not treated. Lindgren et al. found in this study that those treated with growth hormone had an increase in height and a decrease in fat mass and BMI in comparison to those not treated [96].

Another comprehensive study to measure the benefits of growth hormone treatment in affected individuals was completed in 1998 by Eiholzer et al. Twelve affected individuals with Prader–Willi syndrome were enrolled in this study and were grouped and compared based on three different groups: (1) overweight and pre-pubertal, (2) underweight and pre-pubertal, and (3) pubertal. After 12 months of growth hormone treatment within all groups, this study showed a marked increase in growth including height, foot and hand length, and arm span and an increase in lean body mass, muscle mass, and physical performance with increased energy expenditure. They also showed a marked decrease in weight for height, BMI, skin fold thickness, and body fat. Finally, individuals in this study reported to be more active and had increased energy [97].

Whitman et al. also documented similar changes in behavior and physical characteristics with the use of growth hormone treatment in PWS individuals. They noted that the benefits of growth hormone treatment in these patients included having more energy and being more physically fit and demonstrated improvement in memory, sleeping patterns, and social skills [98].

Goldstone et al. in 2008 determined that the highest level of benefit with the treatment of growth hormone to all patients with PWS is similar to those with isolated growth hormone deficiency, including improvement in growth, body composition, and behavior [99]. Festen et al. in 2008 also noted improvement in body composition as one of the most appreciable benefits of growth hormone treatment in affected individuals [100]. Because studies show significant benefits with treatment of growth hormone in individuals with Prader–Willi syndrome, the Food and Drug Administration in 2000 approved injectable somatropin (growth hormone) as a treatment and thus the standard of care for PWS [101]. Similar positive impacts of GH treatment in previously untreated adults with PWS on weight, fat mass, and physical activity levels were also noted by Butler et al. in 2013 [102].

Author Contributions: Writing—original draft preparation, R.M.; writing—review and editing, V.K. and M.G.B.; supervision, V.K. and M.G.B. All authors have read and agreed to the published version of the manuscript.

Funding: National Institutes of Health (NIH) grant number U54 HD061222 and RR019478, as well as the Prader–Willi Syndrome Association USA.

Informed Consent Statement: Written informed consent for publication of the photograph was obtained from the patient.

Data Availability Statement: The data supporting reported material can be obtained upon request from the co-authors.

Conflicts of Interest: The authors declare no conflict of interest.

References

1. Kaur, Y.; de Souza, R.J.; Gibson, W.T.; Meyre, D. A systematic review of genetic syndromes with obesity. *Obes. Rev.* **2017**, *18*, 603–634. [CrossRef] [PubMed]
2. Purnell, J.Q. Definitions, Classification, and Epidemiology of Obesity. In *Endotext*; Feingold, K.R., Anawalt, B., Boyce, A., Chrousos, G., de Herder, W.W., Dhatariya, K., Dungan, K., Hershman, J.M., Hofland, J., Kalra, S., et al., Eds.; MDText.com, Inc.: South Dartmouth, MA, USA, 2000.
3. Wardle, J.; Carnell, S.; Haworth, C.M.; Plomin, R. Evidence for a strong genetic influence on childhood adiposity despite the force of the obesogenic environment. *Am. J. Clin. Nutr.* **2008**, *87*, 398–404. [CrossRef] [PubMed]
4. Singh, R.K.; Kumar, P.; Mahalingam, K. Molecular genetics of human obesity: A comprehensive review. *Comptes Rendus Biol.* **2017**, *340*, 87–108. [CrossRef] [PubMed]
5. Duis, J.; Butler, M.G. Syndromic and Nonsyndromic Obesity: Underlying Genetic Causes in Humans. *Adv. Biol.* **2022**, e2101154. [CrossRef] [PubMed]
6. Butler, M.G. Single Gene and Syndromic Causes of Obesity: Illustrative Examples. *Prog. Mol. Biol. Transl. Sci.* **2016**, *140*, 1–45.
7. Farooqi, I.S. Genetic and hereditary aspects of childhood obesity. *Best Pract. Res. Clin. Endocrinol. Metab.* **2005**, *19*, 359–374. [CrossRef]
8. Xia, Q.; Grant, S.F. The genetics of human obesity. *Ann. N. Y. Acad. Sci.* **2013**, *1281*, 178–190. [CrossRef]
9. Choquet, H.; Meyre, D. Genetics of Obesity: What have we Learned? *Curr. Genom.* **2011**, *12*, 169–179. [CrossRef]
10. Lyon, H.N.; Hirschhorn, J.N. Genetics of common forms of obesity: A brief overview. *Am. J. Clin. Nutr.* **2005**, *82* (Suppl. S1), 215S–217S. [CrossRef]
11. Dietrich, J.; Lovell, S.; Veatch, O.J.; Butler, M.G. PHIP gene variants with protein modeling, interactions, and clinical phenotypes. *Am. J. Med. Genet. Part A* **2022**, *188*, 579–589. [CrossRef]
12. Friedman, J.M.; Halaas, J.L. Leptin and the regulation of body weight in mammals. *Nature* **1998**, *395*, 763–770. [CrossRef] [PubMed]
13. Vohra, M.S.; Benchoula, K.; Serpell, C.J.; Hwa, W.E. AgRP/NPY and POMC neurons in the arcuate nucleus and their potential role in treatment of obesity. *Eur. J. Pharmacol.* **2022**, *915*, 174611. [CrossRef] [PubMed]
14. Franks, P.W.; Brage, S.; Luan, J.; Ekelund, U.; Rahman, M.; Farooqi, I.S.; Halsall, I.; O'Rahilly, S.; Wareham, N.J. Leptin predicts a worsening of the features of the metabolic syndrome independently of obesity. *Obes. Res.* **2005**, *13*, 1476–1484. [CrossRef] [PubMed]
15. Krude, H.; Gruters, A. Implications of proopiomelanocortin (POMC) mutations in humans: The POMC deficiency syndrome. *Trends Endocrinol. Metab.* **2000**, *11*, 15–22. [CrossRef]
16. Hilado, M.A.; Randhawa, R.S. A novel mutation in the proopiomelanocortin (POMC) gene of a Hispanic child: Metformin treatment shows a beneficial impact on the body mass index. *J. Pediatr. Endocrinol. Metab.* **2018**, *31*, 815–819. [CrossRef]
17. Gregoric, N.; Groselj, U.; Bratina, N.; Debeljak, M.; Zerjav Tansek, M.; Suput Omladic, J.; Kovac, J.; Battelino, T.; Kotnik, P.; Avbelj Stefanija, M. Two Cases With an Early Presented Proopiomelanocortin Deficiency-A Long-Term Follow-Up and Systematic Literature Review. *Front. Endocrinol.* **2021**, *12*, 689387. [CrossRef]
18. Yeo, G.S.; Farooqi, I.S.; Aminian, S.; Halsall, D.J.; Stanhope, R.G.; O'Rahilly, S. A frameshift mutation in MC4R associated with dominantly inherited human obesity. *Nat. Genet.* **1998**, *20*, 111–112. [CrossRef]
19. Tao, Y.X. The melanocortin-4 receptor: Physiology, pharmacology, and pathophysiology. *Endocr. Rev.* **2010**, *31*, 506–543. [CrossRef]
20. Frayling, T.M.; Timpson, N.J.; Weedon, M.N.; Zeggini, E.; Freathy, R.M.; Lindgren, C.M.; Perry, J.R.; Elliott, K.S.; Lango, H.; Rayner, N.W.; et al. A common variant in the FTO gene is associated with body mass index and predisposes to childhood and adult obesity. *Science* **2007**, *316*, 889–894. [CrossRef]
21. Scuteri, A.; Sanna, S.; Chen, W.M.; Uda, M.; Albai, G.; Strait, J.; Najjar, S.; Nagaraja, R.; Orru, M.; Usala, G.; et al. Genome-wide association scan shows genetic variants in the FTO gene are associated with obesity-related traits. *PLoS Genet.* **2007**, *3*, e115. [CrossRef]
22. Dina, C.; Meyre, D.; Gallina, S.; Durand, E.; Korner, A.; Jacobson, P.; Carlsson, L.M.; Kiess, W.; Vatin, V.; Lecoeur, C.; et al. Variation in FTO contributes to childhood obesity and severe adult obesity. *Nat. Genet.* **2007**, *39*, 724–726. [CrossRef] [PubMed]
23. Cho, Y.S.; Go, M.J.; Kim, Y.J.; Heo, J.Y.; Oh, J.H.; Ban, H.J.; Yoon, D.; Lee, M.H.; Kim, D.J.; Park, M.; et al. A large-scale genome-wide association study of Asian populations uncovers genetic factors influencing eight quantitative traits. *Nat. Genet.* **2009**, *41*, 527–534. [CrossRef] [PubMed]
24. Wen, W.; Cho, Y.S.; Zheng, W.; Dorajoo, R.; Kato, N.; Qi, L.; Chen, C.H.; Delahanty, R.J.; Okada, Y.; Tabara, Y.; et al. Meta-analysis identifies common variants associated with body mass index in east Asians. *Nat. Genet.* **2012**, *44*, 307–311. [CrossRef] [PubMed]
25. Okada, Y.; Kubo, M.; Ohmiya, H.; Takahashi, A.; Kumasaka, N.; Hosono, N.; Maeda, S.; Wen, W.; Dorajoo, R.; Go, M.J.; et al. Common variants at CDKAL1 and KLF9 are associated with body mass index in east Asian populations. *Nat. Genet.* **2012**, *44*, 302–306. [CrossRef] [PubMed]

26. Kalantari, N.; Keshavarz Mohammadi, N.; Izadi, P.; Gholamalizadeh, M.; Doaei, S.; Eini-Zinab, H.; Salonurmi, T.; Rafieifar, S.; Janipoor, R.; Azizi Tabesh, G. A complete linkage disequilibrium in a haplotype of three SNPs in Fat Mass and Obesity associated (FTO) gene was strongly associated with anthropometric indices after controlling for calorie intake and physical activity. *BMC Med. Genet.* **2018**, *19*, 146. [CrossRef]
27. Loos, R.J.F.; Yeo, G.S.H. The genetics of obesity: From discovery to biology. *Nat. Rev. Genet.* **2022**, *23*, 120–133. [CrossRef]
28. Castro, G.V.; Latorre, A.F.S.; Korndorfer, F.P.; de Carlos Back, L.K.; Lofgren, S.E. The Impact of Variants in Four Genes: MC4R, FTO, PPARG and PPARGC1A in Overweight and Obesity in a Large Sample of the Brazilian Population. *Biochem. Genet.* **2021**, *59*, 1666–1679. [CrossRef]
29. Dastgheib, S.A.; Bahrami, R.; Setayesh, S.; Salari, S.; Mirjalili, S.R.; Noorishadkam, M.; Sadeghizadeh-Yazdi, J.; Akbarian, E.; Neamatzadeh, H. Evidence from a meta-analysis for association of MC4R rs17782313 and FTO rs9939609 polymorphisms with susceptibility to obesity in children. *Diabetes Metab. Syndr.* **2021**, *15*, 102234. [CrossRef]
30. Resende, C.M.M.; Silva, H.; Campello, C.P.; Ferraz, L.A.A.; de Lima, E.L.S.; Beserra, M.A.; Muniz, M.T.C.; da Silva, L.M.P. Polymorphisms on rs9939609 FTO and rs17782313 MC4R genes in children and adolescent obesity: A systematic review. *Nutrition* **2021**, *91–92*, 111474. [CrossRef]
31. Dumesic, D.A.; Oberfield, S.E.; Stener-Victorin, E.; Marshall, J.C.; Laven, J.S.; Legro, R.S. Scientific Statement on the Diagnostic Criteria, Epidemiology, Pathophysiology, and Molecular Genetics of Polycystic Ovary Syndrome. *Endocr. Rev.* **2015**, *36*, 487–525. [CrossRef]
32. Glueck, C.J.; Goldenberg, N. Characteristics of obesity in polycystic ovary syndrome: Etiology, treatment, and genetics. *Metab. Clin. Exp.* **2019**, *92*, 108–120. [CrossRef] [PubMed]
33. Ewens, K.G.; Jones, M.R.; Ankener, W.; Stewart, D.R.; Urbanek, M.; Dunaif, A.; Legro, R.S.; Chua, A.; Azziz, R.; Spielman, R.S.; et al. FTO and MC4R gene variants are associated with obesity in polycystic ovary syndrome. *PLoS ONE* **2011**, *6*, e16390. [CrossRef]
34. Tu, X.; Yu, C.; Gao, M.; Zhang, Y.; Zhang, Z.; He, Y.; Yao, L.; Du, J.; Sun, Y.; Sun, Z. LEPR gene polymorphism and plasma soluble leptin receptor levels are associated with polycystic ovary syndrome in Han Chinese women. *Pers. Med.* **2017**, *14*, 299–307. [CrossRef] [PubMed]
35. Dasouki, M.J.; Youngs, E.L.; Hovanes, K. Structural Chromosome Abnormalities Associated with Obesity: Report of Four New subjects and Review of Literature. *Curr. Genom.* **2011**, *12*, 190–203. [CrossRef] [PubMed]
36. Cheon, C.K. Genetics of Prader-Willi syndrome and Prader-Will-Like syndrome. *Ann. Pediatr. Endocrinol. Metab.* **2016**, *21*, 126–135. [CrossRef] [PubMed]
37. Bellad, A.; Bandari, A.K.; Pandey, A.; Girimaji, S.C.; Muthusamy, B. A Novel Missense Variant in PHF6 Gene Causing Borjeson-Forssman-Lehman Syndrome. *J. Mol. Neurosci.* **2020**, *70*, 1403–1409. [CrossRef]
38. Hidestrand, P.; Vasconez, H.; Cottrill, C. Carpenter syndrome. *J. Craniofac. Surg.* **2009**, *20*, 254–256. [CrossRef]
39. Gupta, D.; Goyal, S. Cornelia de-Lange syndrome. *J. Indian Soc. Pedod. Prev. Dent.* **2005**, *23*, 38–41. [CrossRef]
40. Raible, S.E.; Mehta, D.; Bettale, C.; Fiordaliso, S.; Kaur, M.; Medne, L.; Rio, M.; Haan, E.; White, S.M.; Cusmano-Ozog, K.; et al. Clinical and molecular spectrum of CHOPS syndrome. *Am. J. Med. Genet. Part A* **2019**, *179*, 1126–1138. [CrossRef]
41. Abidi, F.E.; Cardoso, C.; Lossi, A.M.; Lowry, R.B.; Depetris, D.; Mattei, M.G.; Lubs, H.A.; Stevenson, R.E.; Fontes, M.; Chudley, A.E.; et al. Mutation in the 5′ alternatively spliced region of the XNP/ATR-X gene causes Chudley-Lowry syndrome. *Eur. J. Hum. Genet.* **2005**, *13*, 176–183. [CrossRef]
42. Rogers, R.C.; Abidi, F.E. Coffin-Lowry Syndrome. In *GeneReviews((R))*; Adam, M.P., Mirzaa, G.M., Pagon, R.A., Wallace, S.E., Bean, L.J.H., Gripp, K.W., Amemiya, A., Eds.; University of Washington: Seattle, WA, USA, 1993.
43. Kleefstra, T.; de Leeuw, N. Kleefstra, T.; de Leeuw, N. Kleefstra Syndrome. In *GeneReviews((R))*; Adam, M.P., Mirzaa, G.M., Pagon, R.A., Wallace, S.E., Bean, L.J.H., Gripp, K.W., Amemiya, A., Eds.; University of Washington: Seattle, WA, USA, 1993.
44. Milani, D.; Manzoni, F.M.; Pezzani, L.; Ajmone, P.; Gervasini, C.; Menni, F.; Esposito, S. Rubinstein-Taybi syndrome: Clinical features, genetic basis, diagnosis, and management. *Ital. J. Pediatr.* **2015**, *41*, 4. [CrossRef] [PubMed]
45. Kagami, M.; Nagasaki, K.; Kosaki, R.; Horikawa, R.; Naiki, Y.; Saitoh, S.; Tajima, T.; Yorifuji, T.; Numakura, C.; Mizuno, S.; et al. Temple syndrome: Comprehensive molecular and clinical findings in 32 Japanese patients. *Genet. Med.* **2017**, *19*, 1356–1366. [CrossRef] [PubMed]
46. Yearwood, E.L.; McCulloch, M.R.; Tucker, M.L.; Riley, J.B. Care of the patient with Prader-Willi syndrome. *Medsurg. Nurs.* **2011**, *20*, 113–122. [PubMed]
47. Cassidy, S.B.; Driscoll, D.J. Prader-Willi syndrome. *Eur. J. Hum. Genet. EJHG* **2009**, *17*, 3–13. [CrossRef] [PubMed]
48. Bittel, D.C.; Butler, M.G. Prader-Willi syndrome: Clinical genetics, cytogenetics and molecular biology. *Expert Rev. Mol. Med.* **2005**, *7*, 1–20. [CrossRef]
49. Gardner, R.M.; Sutherland, G.R.; Shaffer, L.G. *Chromosome Abnormalities and Genetic Counseling*, 4th ed.; Oxford University Press: New York, NY, USA, 2012.
50. Bachere, N.; Diene, G.; Delagnes, V.; Molinas, C.; Moulin, P.; Tauber, M. Early diagnosis and multidisciplinary care reduce the hospitalization time and duration of tube feeding and prevent early obesity in PWS infants. *Horm. Res.* **2008**, *69*, 45–52. [CrossRef]
51. Butler, J.V.; Whittington, J.E.; Holland, A.J.; McAllister, C.J.; Goldstone, A.P. The transition between the phenotypes of Prader-Willi syndrome during infancy and early childhood. *Dev. Med. Child Neurol.* **2010**, *52*, e88–e93. [CrossRef]

52. Oldzej, J.; Manazir, J.; Gold, J.A.; Mahmoud, R.; Osann, K.; Flodman, P.; Cassidy, S.B.; Kimonis, V.E. Molecular subtype and growth hormone effects on dysmorphology in Prader-Willi syndrome. *Am. J. Med. Genet. Part A* **2020**, *182*, 169–175. [CrossRef]
53. Mahmoud, R.; Leonenko, A.; Butler, M.G.; Flodman, P.; Gold, J.A.; Miller, J.L.; Roof, E.; Dykens, E.; Driscoll, D.J.; Kimonis, V. Influence of molecular classes and growth hormone treatment on growth and dysmorphology in Prader-Willi syndrome: A multicenter study. *Clin. Genet.* **2021**, *100*, 29–39. [CrossRef]
54. Miller, J.L.; Lynn, C.H.; Driscoll, D.C.; Goldstone, A.P.; Gold, J.A.; Kimonis, V.; Dykens, E.; Butler, M.G.; Shuster, J.J.; Driscoll, D.J. Nutritional phases in Prader-Willi syndrome. *Am. J. Med. Genet. Part A* **2011**, *155*, 1040–1049. [CrossRef]
55. Bereket, A.; Atay, Z. Current status of childhood obesity and its associated morbidities in Turkey. *J. Clin. Res. Pediatr. Endocrinol.* **2012**, *4*, 1–7. [CrossRef] [PubMed]
56. Brambilla, P.; Crino, A.; Bedogni, G.; Bosio, L.; Cappa, M.; Corrias, A.; Delvecchio, M.; Di Candia, S.; Gargantini, L.; Grechi, E.; et al. Metabolic syndrome in children with Prader-Willi syndrome: The effect of obesity. *Nutr. Metab. Cardiovasc. Dis. NMCD* **2011**, *21*, 269–276. [CrossRef] [PubMed]
57. Miller, J.L.; Goldstone, A.P.; Couch, J.A.; Shuster, J.; He, G.; Driscoll, D.J.; Liu, Y.; Schmalfuss, I.M. Pituitary abnormalities in Prader-Willi syndrome and early onset morbid obesity. *Am. J. Med. Genet. Part A* **2008**, *146*, 570–577. [CrossRef] [PubMed]
58. Butler, J.V.; Whittington, J.E.; Holland, A.J.; Boer, H.; Clarke, D.; Webb, T. Prevalence of, and risk factors for, physical ill-health in people with Prader-Willi syndrome: A population-based study. *Dev. Med. Child Neurol.* **2002**, *44*, 248–255. [CrossRef] [PubMed]
59. Li, G.; Vega, R.; Nelms, K.; Gekakis, N.; Goodnow, C.; McNamara, P.; Wu, H.; Hong, N.A.; Glynne, R. A role for Alstrom syndrome protein, alms1, in kidney ciliogenesis and cellular quiescence. *PLoS Genet.* **2007**, *3*, e8. [CrossRef]
60. Choudhury, A.R.; Munonye, I.; Sanu, K.P.; Islam, N.; Gadaga, C. A review of Alstrom syndrome: A rare monogenic ciliopathy. *Intractable Rare Dis. Res.* **2021**, *10*, 257–262. [CrossRef]
61. Hunter, J.E.; Berry-Kravis, E.; Hipp, H.; Todd, P.K. FMR1 Disorders. In *GeneReviews((R))*; Adam, M.P., Mirzaa, G.M., Pagon, R.A., Wallace, S.E., Bean, L.J.H., Gripp, K.W., Amemiya, A., Eds.; University of Washington: Seattle, WA, USA, 1993.
62. Gantois, I.; Popic, J.; Khoutorsky, A.; Sonenberg, N. Metformin for Treatment of Fragile X Syndrome and Other Neurological Disorders. *Annu. Rev. Med.* **2019**, *70*, 167–181. [CrossRef]
63. Nowicki, S.T.; Tassone, F.; Ono, M.Y.; Ferranti, J.; Croquette, M.F.; Goodlin-Jones, B.; Hagerman, R.J. The Prader-Willi phenotype of fragile X syndrome. *J. Dev. Behav. Pediatr. JDBP* **2007**, *28*, 133–138. [CrossRef]
64. Raspa, M.; Bailey, D.B.; Bishop, E.; Holiday, D.; Olmsted, M. Obesity, food selectivity, and physical activity in individuals with fragile X syndrome. *Am. J. Intellect. Dev. Disabil.* **2010**, *115*, 482–495. [CrossRef]
65. Kidd, S.A.; Lachiewicz, A.; Barbouth, D.; Blitz, R.K.; Delahunty, C.; McBrien, D.; Visootsak, J.; Berry-Kravis, E. Fragile X syndrome: A review of associated medical problems. *Pediatrics* **2014**, *134*, 995–1005. [CrossRef]
66. Choo, T.H.; Xu, Q.; Budimirovic, D.; Lozano, R.; Esler, A.N.; Frye, R.E.; Andrews, H.; Velinov, M. Height and BMI in fragile X syndrome: A longitudinal assessment. *Obesity* **2022**, *30*, 743–750. [CrossRef] [PubMed]
67. Presson, A.P.; Partyka, G.; Jensen, K.M.; Devine, O.J.; Rasmussen, S.A.; McCabe, L.L.; McCabe, E.R. Current estimate of Down Syndrome population prevalence in the United States. *J. Pediatr.* **2013**, *163*, 1163–1168. [CrossRef] [PubMed]
68. Asim, A.; Kumar, A.; Muthuswamy, S.; Jain, S.; Agarwal, S. Down syndrome: An insight of the disease. *J. Biomed. Sci.* **2015**, *22*, 41. [CrossRef] [PubMed]
69. Hendrix, C.G.; Prins, M.R.; Dekkers, H. Developmental coordination disorder and overweight and obesity in children: A systematic review. *Obes. Rev.* **2014**, *15*, 408–423. [CrossRef]
70. Liou, T.H.; Pi-Sunyer, F.X.; Laferrere, B. Physical disability and obesity. *Nutr. Rev.* **2005**, *63*, 321–331. [CrossRef]
71. Maiano, C.; Normand, C.L.; Aime, A.; Begarie, J. Lifestyle interventions targeting changes in body weight and composition among youth with an intellectual disability: A systematic review. *Res. Dev. Disabil.* **2014**, *35*, 1914–1926. [CrossRef]
72. Magge, S.N.; O'Neill, K.L.; Shults, J.; Stallings, V.A.; Stettler, N. Leptin levels among prepubertal children with Down syndrome compared with their siblings. *J. Pediatr.* **2008**, *152*, 321–326. [CrossRef]
73. Hill, D.L.; Parks, E.P.; Zemel, B.S.; Shults, J.; Stallings, V.A.; Stettler, N. Resting energy expenditure and adiposity accretion among children with Down syndrome: A 3-year prospective study. *Eur. J. Clin. Nutr.* **2013**, *67*, 1087–1091. [CrossRef]
74. Nordstrom, M.; Retterstol, K.; Hope, S.; Kolset, S.O. Nutritional challenges in children and adolescents with Down syndrome. *Lancet Child Adolesc. Health* **2020**, *4*, 455–464. [CrossRef]
75. Fructuoso, M.; Rachdi, L.; Philippe, E.; Denis, R.G.; Magnan, C.; Le Stunff, H.; Janel, N.; Dierssen, M. Increased levels of inflammatory plasma markers and obesity risk in a mouse model of Down syndrome. *Free Radic. Biol. Med.* **2018**, *114*, 122–130. [CrossRef]
76. Florea, L.; Caba, L.; Gorduza, E.V. Bardet-Biedl Syndrome-Multiple Kaleidoscope Images: Insight into Mechanisms of Genotype-Phenotype Correlations. *Genes* **2021**, *12*, 1353. [CrossRef]
77. Mantovani, G.; Elli, F.M. Inactivating PTH/PTHrP Signaling Disorders. *Front. Horm. Res.* **2019**, *51*, 147–159. [PubMed]
78. Thiele, S.; de Sanctis, L.; Werner, R.; Grotzinger, J.; Aydin, C.; Juppner, H.; Bastepe, M.; Hiort, O. Functional characterization of GNAS mutations found in patients with pseudohypoparathyroidism type Ic defines a new subgroup of pseudohypoparathyroidism affecting selectively Gsalpha-receptor interaction. *Hum. Mutat.* **2011**, *32*, 653–660. [CrossRef] [PubMed]
79. Butler, M.G. Imprinting disorders in humans: A review. *Curr. Opin. Pediatr.* **2020**, *32*, 719–729. [CrossRef] [PubMed]
80. Ong, K.K.; Amin, R.; Dunger, D.B. Pseudohypoparathyroidism—another monogenic obesity syndrome. *Clin. Endocrinol.* **2000**, *52*, 389–391. [CrossRef] [PubMed]

81. Delaval, K.; Wagschal, A.; Feil, R. Epigenetic deregulation of imprinting in congenital diseases of aberrant growth. *BioEssays* **2006**, *28*, 453–459. [CrossRef]
82. Fischbach, B.V.; Trout, K.L.; Lewis, J.; Luis, C.A.; Sika, M. WAGR syndrome: A clinical review of 54 cases. *Pediatrics* **2005**, *116*, 984–988. [CrossRef]
83. Breslow, N.E.; Norris, R.; Norkool, P.A.; Kang, T.; Beckwith, J.B.; Perlman, E.J.; Ritchey, M.L.; Green, D.M.; Nichols, K.E.; National Wilms Tumor Study Group. Characteristics and outcomes of children with the Wilms tumor-Aniridia syndrome: A report from the National Wilms Tumor Study Group. *J. Clin. Oncol.* **2003**, *21*, 4579–4585. [CrossRef]
84. Gul, D.; Ogur, G.; Tunca, Y.; Ozcan, O. Third case of WAGR syndrome with severe obesity and constitutional deletion of chromosome (11)(p12p14). *Am. J. Med. Genet.* **2002**, *107*, 70–71. [CrossRef]
85. Marlin, S.; Couet, D.; Lacombe, D.; Cessans, C.; Bonneau, D. Obesity: A new feature of WAGR (del 11p) syndrome. *Clin. Dysmorphol.* **1994**, *3*, 255–257. [CrossRef]
86. Tiberio, G.; Digilio, M.C.; Giannotti, A. Obesity and WAGR syndrome. *Clin. Dysmorphol.* **2000**, *9*, 63–64. [CrossRef] [PubMed]
87. Han, J.C.; Liu, Q.R.; Jones, M.; Levinn, R.L.; Menzie, C.M.; Jefferson-George, K.S.; Adler-Wailes, D.C.; Sanford, E.L.; Lacbawan, F.L.; Uhl, G.R.; et al. Brain-derived neurotrophic factor and obesity in the WAGR syndrome. *N. Engl. J. Med.* **2008**, *359*, 918–927. [CrossRef] [PubMed]
88. Rodrigues, J.M.; Fernandes, H.D.; Caruthers, C.; Braddock, S.R.; Knutsen, A.P. Cohen Syndrome: Review of the Literature. *Cureus* **2018**, *10*, e3330. [CrossRef]
89. Wang, H.; Falk, M.J.; Wensel, C.; Traboulsi, E.I. Cohen Syndrome. In *GeneReviews((R))*; Adam, M.P., Mirzaa, G.M., Pagon, R.A., Wallace, S.E., Bean, L.J.H., Gripp, K.W., Amemiya, A., Eds.; University of Washington: Seattle, WA, USA, 1993.
90. Limoge, F.; Faivre, L.; Gautier, T.; Petit, J.M.; Gautier, E.; Masson, D.; Jego, G.; El Chehadeh-Djebbar, S.; Marle, N.; Carmignac, V.; et al. Insulin response dysregulation explains abnormal fat storage and increased risk of diabetes mellitus type 2 in Cohen Syndrome. *Hum. Mol. Genet.* **2015**, *24*, 6603–6613. [CrossRef] [PubMed]
91. Smith, A.C.M.; Boyd, K.E.; Brennan, C.; Charles, J.; Elsea, S.H.; Finucane, B.M.; Foster, R.; Gropman, A.; Girirajan, S.; Haas-Givler, B. Smith-Magenis Syndrome. In *GeneReviews((R))*; Adam, M.P., Mirzaa, G.M., Pagon, R.A., Wallace, S.E., Bean, L.J.H., Gripp, K.W., Amemiya, A., Eds.; University of Washington: Seattle, WA, USA, 1993.
92. Stamou, M.I.; Georgopoulos, N.A. Kallmann syndrome: Phenotype and genotype of hypogonadotropic hypogonadism. *Metabolism* **2018**, *86*, 124–134. [CrossRef]
93. Markham, A. Setmelanotide: First Approval. *Drugs* **2021**, *81*, 397–403. [CrossRef] [PubMed]
94. Farooqi, I.S.; Matarese, G.; Lord, G.M.; Keogh, J.M.; Lawrence, E.; Agwu, C.; Sanna, V.; Jebb, S.A.; Perna, F.; Fontana, S.; et al. Beneficial effects of leptin on obesity, T cell hyporesponsiveness, and neuroendocrine/metabolic dysfunction of human congenital leptin deficiency. *J. Clin. Investig.* **2002**, *110*, 1093–1103. [CrossRef]
95. Lindgren, A.C.; Hagenas, L.; Muller, J.; Blichfeldt, S.; Rosenborg, M.; Brismar, T.; Ritzen, E.M. Effects of growth hormone treatment on growth and body composition in Prader-Willi syndrome: A preliminary report. The Swedish National Growth Hormone Advisory Group. *Acta Paediatr.* **1997**, *423*, 60–62. [CrossRef]
96. Lindgren, A.C.; Hagenas, L.; Muller, J.; Blichfeldt, S.; Rosenborg, M.; Brismar, T.; Ritzen, E.M. Growth hormone treatment of children with Prader-Willi syndrome affects linear growth and body composition favourably. *Acta Paediatr.* **1998**, *87*, 28–31. [CrossRef]
97. Eiholzer, U.; Gisin, R.; Weinmann, C.; Kriemler, S.; Steinert, H.; Torresani, T.; Zachmann, M.; Prader, A. Treatment with human growth hormone in patients with Prader-Labhart-Willi syndrome reduces body fat and increases muscle mass and physical performance. *Eur. J. Pediatr.* **1998**, *157*, 368–377. [CrossRef]
98. Whitman, B.Y.; Myers, S.; Carrel, A.; Allen, D. The behavioral impact of growth hormone treatment for children and adolescents with Prader-Willi syndrome: A 2-year, controlled study. *Pediatrics* **2002**, *109*, E35. [CrossRef] [PubMed]
99. Goldstone, A.P.; Holland, A.J.; Hauffa, B.P.; Hokken-Koelega, A.C.; Tauber, M.; Speakers Contributors at the Second Expert Meeting of the Comprehensive Care of Patients with PWS. Recommendations for the diagnosis and management of Prader-Willi syndrome. *J. Clin. Endocrinol. Metab.* **2008**, *93*, 4183–4197. [CrossRef] [PubMed]
100. Festen, D.A.; de Lind van Wijngaarden, R.; van Eekelen, M.; Otten, B.J.; Wit, J.M.; Duivenvoorden, H.J.; Hokken-Koelega, A.C. Randomized controlled GH trial: Effects on anthropometry, body composition and body proportions in a large group of children with Prader-Willi syndrome. *Clin. Endocrinol.* **2008**, *69*, 443–451. [CrossRef] [PubMed]
101. Medscape. FDA Approves First Drug to Treat Children with Prader-Willi Syndrome Medscape Medical News [Online], 2000. Available online: http://www.medscape.com/viewarticle/411964 (accessed on 14 May 2010).
102. Butler, M.G.; Smith, B.K.; Lee, J.; Gibson, C.; Schmoll, C.; Moore, W.V.; Donnelly, J.E. Effects of growth hormone treatment in adults with Prader-Willi syndrome. *Growth Horm. IGF Res.* **2013**, *23*, 81–87. [CrossRef] [PubMed]

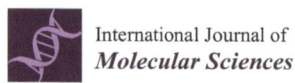
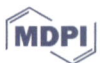

Case Report

Connective Tissue Disorders and Fragile X Molecular Status in Females: A Case Series and Review

Merlin G. Butler [1,*], Waheeda A. Hossain [1], Jacob Steinle [1], Harry Gao [2], Eleina Cox [2], Yuxin Niu [2], May Quach [2] and Olivia J. Veatch [1]

1. Department of Psychiatry & Behavioral Sciences, University of Kansas Medical Center, 3901 Rainbow Blvd. MS 4015, Kansas City, KS 66160, USA
2. Fulgent Genetics, 4978 Santa Anita Ave., Temple City, CA 91780, USA
* Correspondence: mbutler4@kumc.edu; Tel.: +1-(913)-588-1800; Fax: +1-(913)-588-1305

Abstract: Fragile X syndrome (FXS) is the most common inherited cause of intellectual disabilities and the second most common cause after Down syndrome. FXS is an X-linked disorder due to a full mutation of the CGG triplet repeat of the *FMR1* gene which codes for a protein that is crucial in synaptogenesis and maintaining functions of extracellular matrix-related proteins, key for the development of normal neuronal and connective tissue including collagen. In addition to neuropsychiatric and behavioral problems, individuals with FXS show physical features suggestive of a connective tissue disorder including loose skin and joint laxity, flat feet, hernias and mitral valve prolapse. Disturbed collagen leads to hypermobility, hyperextensible skin and tissue fragility with musculoskeletal, cardiovascular, immune and other organ involvement as seen in hereditary disorders of connective tissue including Ehlers–Danlos syndrome. Recently, *FMR1* premutation repeat expansion or carrier status has been reported in individuals with connective tissue disorder-related symptoms. We examined a cohort of females with features of a connective tissue disorder presenting for genetic services using next-generation sequencing (NGS) of a connective tissue disorder gene panel consisting of approximately 75 genes. In those females with normal NGS testing for connective tissue disorders, the *FMR1* gene was then analyzed using CGG repeat expansion studies. Three of thirty-nine females were found to have gray zone or intermediate alleles at a 1:13 ratio which was significantly higher ($p < 0.05$) when compared with newborn females representing the general population at a 1:66 ratio. This association of connective tissue involvement in females with intermediate or gray zone alleles reported for the first time will require more studies on how the size variation may impact *FMR1* gene function and protein directly or in relationship with other susceptibility genes involved in connective tissue disorders.

Keywords: *FMR1* gene; fragile X syndrome; *FMR1* gray zone or intermediate alleles; connective tissue-related disorders

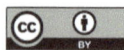

Citation: Butler, M.G.; Hossain, W.A.; Steinle, J.; Gao, H.; Cox, E.; Niu, Y.; Quach, M.; Veatch, O.J. Connective Tissue Disorders and Fragile X Molecular Status in Females: A Case Series and Review. *Int. J. Mol. Sci.* 2022, 23, 9090. https://doi.org/10.3390/ijms23169090

Academic Editor: Motohiro Okada

Received: 29 June 2022
Accepted: 9 August 2022
Published: 13 August 2022

Publisher's Note: MDPI stays neutral with regard to jurisdictional claims in published maps and institutional affiliations.

Copyright: © 2022 by the authors. Licensee MDPI, Basel, Switzerland. This article is an open access article distributed under the terms and conditions of the Creative Commons Attribution (CC BY) license (https://creativecommons.org/licenses/by/4.0/).

1. Introduction

Fragile X syndrome (FXS) is the most common inherited cause of intellectual disabilities and autism spectrum disorder. FXS is the second most common cause of intellectual disability after Down syndrome [1,2]. FXS is an X-linked disorder due to a full mutation of the CGG triplet repeat in the 5′-untranslated region of the fragile X messenger ribonucleoprotein 1 (*FMR1*) gene, formerly named fragile X mental retardation 1, located at Xq27.3, and the most prevalent cause of intellectual disability in males. It affects 1 in 5000 to 7000 men, and 1 in 4000 to 6000 women [1,3,4]. The findings include neuro-behavioral disturbances, communication and social deficits with intellectual disability and facial dysmorphism. Other physical features are suggestive of a connective tissue disorder involving ligaments, muscles, the skeleton and the genitourinary, cardiovascular and immune systems [5,6].

Reported physical findings in FXS include a long, narrow face which is seen in 83% of affected individuals and more commonly in adults. Macrocephaly is seen in 50% to 81% of individuals; prominent ears in 75%; a prominent jaw in 80% seen mostly in adults; flat feet in 29% to 69%; joint hypermobility in 57% and less commonly in adults; palmar and plantar creases, hernias and mitral valve prolapse in >20% of cases; and macro-orchidism in 95% with onset in adolescence or during adulthood (e.g., [1,7–11]). The *FMR1* protein (FMRP) is encoded by the X-linked *FMR1* gene. This protein is crucial in maintaining functions of extracellular matrix-related proteins and key for the development and function of neuronal and connective tissue including collagen. Similarly, disturbed collagen leads to clinical outcomes seen in hereditary disorders of connective tissue (e.g., Ehlers–Danlos syndrome (EDS), Marfan syndrome, osteogenesis imperfecta) (e.g., [12]). These heterogeneous groups of genetic disorders are due to numerous distinct mutations or variants. They are characterized by variable expressivity of joint hypermobility, hyperextensible skin and tissue fragility with musculoskeletal, cardiovascular, immune and other organ system involvement as similarly recognized in those affected with FXS (e.g., [1]).

The normal number of triplet repeats in the *FMR1* gene is less than 45. As this trinucleotide repeat expands beyond this range, the gene is potentially disturbed and may impact the function of the encoded protein. The intermediate or gray zone range consists of 45 to 54 repeats. The premutation or carrier status represents those with 55 to 200 repeats. The premutation can lead to a reduction in FMRP which is crucial in maintaining functions of extracellular matrix-related proteins including matrix metallopeptidase 9 and elastin supporting involvement in the clinical presentation of those females with connective tissue disorders. In addition, elevated *FMR1* mRNA can also cause protein sequestration and result in RNA toxicity which may affect several gene families and proteins involving multiple organ systems along with immune mediation and inflammation seen in those with connective tissue disorders [13–15]. Due to expansion to full mutation with over 200 CGG repeats, the *FMR1* gene becomes epigenetically hypermethylated and shuts down, leading to a deficit of its encoded protein (FMRP). An abnormal *FMR1* gene repeat expansion seen in premutation alters protein levels impacting neuronal and connective tissue structure and function (e.g., [6]), leading to hypermobility and other features of a connective tissue disorder (CTD) [5].

To evaluate the potential connection between the triplet repeat expansion in the *FMR1* gene and presentation of connective tissue disorder-related symptoms, we performed CLIA/CAP polymerase chain reaction (PCR) testing of *FMR1* CGG repeats and AGG interruptions—which may induce stability of the CGG expansion region by decreasing further expansion in females with premutation (e.g., [16,17])—in a cohort of females with features of a CTD. These individuals had undergone prior clinical genetic evaluation and testing of a CTD gene-specific panel using next-generation sequencing (NGS), but no potentially damaging variants were identified in genes included on this panel. Herein, we present *FMR1* gene testing results in females with features of a CTD and previous normal DNA testing for connective tissue disorders in the clinical setting and compared to the general population.

2. Results

We report our experience utilizing a patient cohort consisting of 100 consecutive unrelated patients presenting for genetic evaluation for a CTD using NGS of a customized CTD gene panel ordered and undertaken at Fulgent Genetics (Temple City, CA) and describe three females with a gray zone *FMR1* gene allele. The most common reason for referral was a suspected connective tissue disorder (n = 71), followed by EDS (n = 18), joint hyperflexibility (n = 7), Marfan syndrome (n = 3) and Chiari malformation (n = 1). Eighty of the one hundred patients were females, and forty-eight were found to not have any pathogenic, likely pathogenic or predicted potentially pathogenic variants using a customized connective tissue disorder gene panel [18]. DNA was then available to test for *FMR1* gene CGG repeat expansions in 39 of the 48 females as features of connective tissue disorders have been reported in those affected with fragile X syndrome (e.g., [5]). The average age (SD) of the females tested for the *FMR1* repeat expansion was 33y (13), with an average (SD) Beighton score of 5.9 (1.5). Sixteen of the females had no variants identified using NGS of hereditary disorders of connective tissue-related genes, while twenty-three females were found with variants of unknown clinical significance but not meeting pathogenicity criteria and interpreted as non-disease-causing.

Three of the thirty-nine females tested for the *FMR1* repeat expansion in our patient cohort were found with a 1:13 ratio of having an intermediate repeat expansion (45–54 repeats) (see Table 1). A chi-square test with Yates's correction was calculated comparing this intermediate or gray zone frequency to that reported by Tassone et al. [19] in a representative sample involving several ethnic groups in the United States having a 1:66 ratio or 105 of 6889 newborn females studied. The chi-square test value was 6.02 with one degree of freedom, and the one-tailed p-value was 0.007; the two-tailed p-value was 0.014, with both being significant based on the threshold of $p < 0.05$. The report by Tassone et al. [19] in a large cohort of newborn females was selected as relevant for estimating the frequency of *FMR1* gene findings in the general population.

Table 1. Molecular and clinical findings in three adult females with FMR1 gray zone repeats in a cohort of females presenting for genetic services.

Participants	Age (Years)	CGG Repeats	AGG Interruptions (Number; Allele Size)	Immune-Mediated Disorder or Inflammation	Beighton Hyperflexibility Score
Case #1	26	20, 51 *	(1; 20 or 51 *) (1; 51 *)	Polyarthralgia, hypothyroidism, migraines	7 out of 9
Case #2	45	33, 48 *	(1; 33 or 48 *) (1; 48 *)	Positive anti-nuclear antibody (ANA), migraines	3 out of 8
Case #3	44	24, 50 *	(0; 24) (2; 50 *)	Fibromyalgia, polymyositis, lupus, migraines, family history of Churg–Strauss vasculitis	4 out of 6

* Designates the intermediate or gray zone repeats.

3. Discussion

Several clinical findings and physical features seen in FXS can overlap with those diagnosed with a hereditary connective tissue disorder such as hypermobile EDS. The findings in EDS do include a long, narrow face, ear and jaw problems, flat feet with joint hypermobility, loose skin, hernias and mitral valve prolapse as similarly seen in FXS (e.g., [1,2,7–10]). EDS has been classified into 13 subtypes and related to 19 separate genes (e.g., [12]) showing all three inheritance patterns (autosomal recessive, autosomal dominant or X-linked). Overall, EDS is considered an uncommon inherited disease with an estimated prevalence ranging from 1 in 2500 to 5000 individuals including the classic form. Other forms of connective tissue disorders are less common (e.g., Marfan syndrome), with a prevalence of 1 in 5000 to 10,000 individuals. Some types of EDS are exceedingly rare such as EDS type VIIC, dermatosparaxis type (OMIM:255410), with fewer than 20 patients reported (e.g., [20]).

Females in our study presented with features of a connective tissue disorder, and potentially related findings including immune/autoimmune problems such as fibromyalgia showed the frequency of an intermediate *FMR1* repeat expansion to be significantly higher than in the general population ascertained through surveying newborn females [19]. For example, 45% of *FMR1* premutation carrier females were found in other studies to have an immune-mediated disorder (IMD) with autoimmune thyroiditis (24%) followed by fibromyalgia (10%) in a survey of 344 carrier females (age 19 to 81y) [15]. Autoimmune thyroid disorder and fibromyalgia have also been reported to be associated with women having a premutation and fragile X-associated tremor/ataxia syndrome (FXTAS) (e.g., [21]).

Additionally, about one fifth of those females with premutations had fragile X premature ovarian insufficiency (FXPOI), and one fourth had chronic muscle pain. The pathogenesis of premutation disorders is apparently related to a gain-of-function effect from 1.5- to 8-fold elevated levels due to an expanded CGG repeat *FMR1* mRNA, leading to RNA toxicity [22]. Toxicity is thought to be due to sequestration of RNA-binding proteins, including DROSHA and DGCR8 which are critical for maturing miRNAs including a role in processing *FMR1* [23]. The role of miRNA in regulating autoimmunity in T-cell lymphocytes with potential consequences of miRNA dysregulation in developing IMDs may be due to abnormal control of T-cell function and upregulation of the innate immune response through increased or prolonged inflammatory cytokine production [24]. In addition, *FMR1* premutations lead to dysregulation of the hypothalamic–pituitary axis and enhanced release of the stress hormone cortisol, impacting the immune system and resulting in inflammation including of the central nervous system [25]. Mis-splicing of a variety of messages could lead to several forms of autoimmunity including MS, SLE and RA [26]. Furthermore, miRNA dysregulation was found to be associated with infertility and corpus luteum failure as a possible role in FXPOI secondary to RNA toxicity [15,27].

Previously, Tassanakijpanich et al. [6] also noted an association between CGG repeat expansions in the *FMR1* gene and connective tissue problems in five females with a hypermobile EDS phenotype and having a premutation carrier status (allele sizes in these five females ranged from 66 to 150 CGG repeats) and RNA toxicity compounding problems for connective tissue through mitochondrial dysfunction and inflammation. Hence, our study of females with features of a connective tissue disorder with negative NGS testing of known connective tissue disorder genes and *FMR1* gene studies found a 1:13 ratio for an intermediate allele status.

No premutation cases were found in our study, but an intermediate expansion was seen in a subset of females with connective tissue problems. Fragile X AGG analysis has provided risk predictions for 45–69-repeat alleles having intermediate and small premutation alleles based on fragile X repeat instability upon transmission [28]. The number of AGG interruptions and the length of uninterrupted CGG repeats at the 3′ end have been correlated with repeat instability upon transmission. Maternal alleles with no AGGs conferred the greatest risk for unstable transmission. The magnitude of repeat expansion was larger for alleles lacking AGG interruptions. The number of AGG interruptions in our three females with gray zone alleles each showed two interruptions which is an expected number or range as reported in female premutation cohorts studied (e.g., 57 females with premutations had a mean $\pm$ standard deviation = 0.7 $\pm$ 0.7, with a range from 0 to 2) [17].

Many genes and their encoded proteins are important for the development of features seen in connective tissue disorders and will require further characterization, with secondary gene effects potentially playing a role. Gene–gene interactions and collagen-related protein or biological pathways that may or may not be disturbed should be studied in those with features of CTD with or without recognized CTD gene involvement. Potential sex effects were raised by Tassanakijpanich et al. [6] due to the observation that most patients presenting with connective tissue disorders are females, showing sex skewness as many more females inherit fragile X premutations compared with men [19]. The role of X chromosome inactivation should also be considered with level of disease involvement for X-linked genes in females. Sex steroid differences do occur between the sexes, with variable effects of sex steroids on muscle tone and tendon/ligament strength being notably different in males and females, further suggesting a significant role in the expression of CTD findings, with more females affected. Furthermore, pain perception and modulation differ between sexes, which may impact musculoskeletal pain which is observed as a feature most often in females affected with a CTD [29].

The status of the gray zone or intermediate repeat expansion and clinical involvement is not clearly established, but evidence suggests an expanding role for gray zone allele involvement with a similar phenotype and manifestations, as discussed and seen in females with the premutation status [30]. For example, the clinical phenotype of adult fragile

X gray zone allele carriers in our study is similar to that observed with the *FMR1* gene premutation status including neurological, molecular and cognitive aspects [31]. Gray zone alleles have been reported to expand over two generations to a full mutation, but this typically takes over two generations [32]. Additionally, signs of parkinsonism and earlier death have been reported in adult males having the gray zone allele [33], while studies show that those with premutation alleles are associated with fragile X-associated primary ovarian insufficiency in females, motor ataxia or movement disorders and, more recently, connective tissue-related disorders (e.g., [5,6,34]). We now report a possible association of connective tissue involvement in females with the intermediate or gray zone allele, but additional studies are needed.

The authors would welcome investigations to further understand the role of the *FMR1* gene and altered FMRP with disturbed relationships involving connective tissue development and function. Notably, 60% of the females presenting for genetic services and NGS testing of a CTD-specific gene panel in our report did not have any potentially damaging variants identified in CTD recognized genes. By using leftover DNA available following these initial screens, we were able to readily examine the *FMR1* status using the PCR methodology and follow-up with AGG interruption studies from a commercially based laboratory conducting genetic testing (Fulgent Genetics). Gray zone alleles and FMRP should be studied to determine if altered or reduced protein levels are present which could also impact potential therapeutic interventions. Hence, special emphasis should be placed on the disturbance of the *FMR1* mRNA and encoded protein in those with the intermediate or gray zone allele, if present, and how this size variation may affect *FMR1* gene function directly or its relationship with other inter-related or susceptibility genes including for connective tissue disorders.

4. Materials and Methods

4.1. Subjects

Over a 3.5-year interval between 2016 and 2020, 100 unrelated consecutive patients were referred for genetic evaluation with features of a connective tissue disorder and seen at the University of Kansas Medical Center (KUMC) Genetics Clinic directed by one of the coauthors (MGB), an ABMG board-certified clinical geneticist. There were 80 females and 20 males, with an average age ($\pm$SD) of 33 ± 14 years and an age range of 7 to 68 years [18]. The average Beighton hyperflexibility score was 5.9 ± 1.9 in this cohort, with a number greater than or equal to 5 considered to be abnormal in young adults. Age, gender and medical and family histories were obtained along with recorded physical and phenotypic features. Those identified with associated features of hereditary connective tissue disorders included a positive Beighton hyperflexibilty score (i.e., 5 out of 9 measures) followed by easy bruising, stretchable thin skin with poor scarring, scoliosis and joint dislocations, instability or pain.

4.2. Molecular Genetics and Case Reports

4.2.1. Molecular Genetics

Approximately 75 genes are recognized to cause hereditary connective tissue disorders, as examined using a comprehensive connective tissue disorder gene panel with NGS performed at Fulgent Genetics. This is a Clinical Laboratory Improvement Amendments (CLIA) approved and accredited commercial laboratory using established guidelines required for certification following informed consent obtained from all participants prior to collection of buccal samples for DNA extraction. The NGS data included gene name, inheritance, variant type (missense, nonsense, frameshift, indel), coding position, amino acid substitution, zygosity and pathogenicity status (pathogenic, likely pathogenic, unknown clinical significance) based on the American College of Medical Genetics (ACMG) recommendations (http://www.acmg.net/ (8 February 2022)). For each gene variant, the likelihood of being protein-damaging and influencing the expression of a disorder-related phenotype (potentially pathogenic) was determined and calculated using approximately ten in silico prediction programs, amino acid evolutionary conservation reported in primate and mammal genome databases, variant and allele frequencies found in human genomic databases (e.g., Broad Institute GnomAD) and Grantham distance scores greater than 100 for missense variants following standard protocols (e.g., [18]). Variants not meeting internal quality control standards were confirmed by Sanger sequencing.

FMR1 gene CGG triplet repeat sizes were determined using a CLIA/CAP-approved PCR methodology on the same DNA sample performed by Fulgent Genetics previously with NGS of CTD gene-specific panels. Those with FMR1 gene repeat expansion had AGG interruptions analyzed using the FMR1 Asuragen kit (Austin, TX). There were 48 females out of 80 tested, and no ACMG-classified pathogenic, likely pathogenic or predicted potentially pathogenic variants were identified in genes from the comprehensive connective tissue disorder panel. Of these 48 females, 39 had sufficient DNA remaining for FMR1 gene repeat expansion testing. The full FMR1 repeat expansion is seen in 99% of patients with FXS [35]. Of the 39 females, 3 showed a gray zone FMR1 gene variant status, while the other 36 showed a normal FMR1 gene pattern. A description of the clinical, medical, genetic and family history information of the three females can be found below, and the laboratory flow chart for the genetic testing results is illustrated in Figure 1.

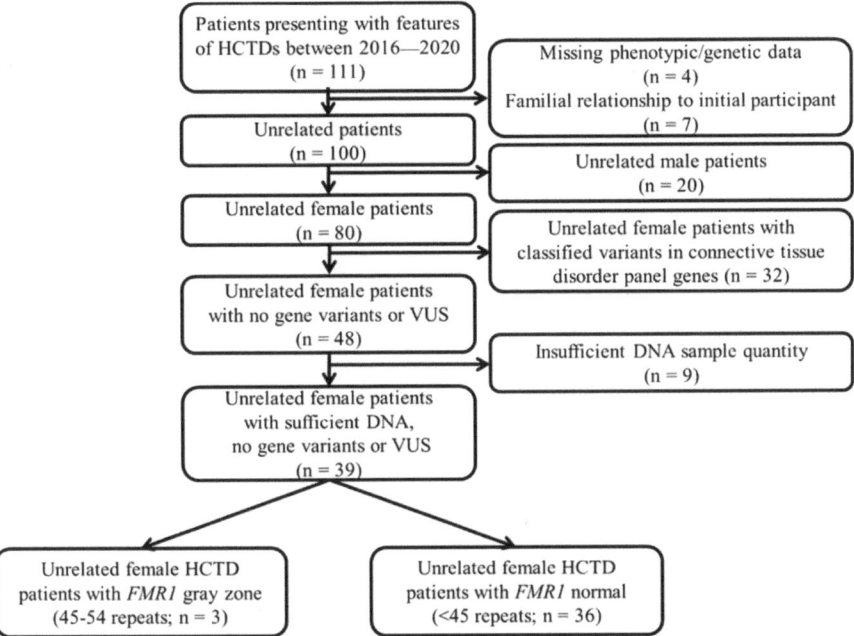

Figure 1. FMR1 gene repeat testing in female patients presenting for heritable connective tissue disorders (HCTDs). Flow chart with details for patients who presented to the genetics clinic over a 3.5-year period. Next-generation sequencing results for genes included on commercially available connective tissue disorder testing panels were evaluated for 80 unrelated female patients. Unrelated female patients with no variants or variants of unknown significance (VUS) reported as ACMG-classified pathogenic, likely pathogenic or determined potentially pathogenic based on allele frequency, biological conservation, Grantham distance and damaging in silico predictions were followed up with FMR1 triplet repeat testing using an approved polymerase chain reaction (PCR), given a sufficient DNA sample was available.

4.2.2. Case Reports

Case #1

A 26-year-old female was seen in the Genetics Clinic at KUMC for evaluation of a connective tissue disorder. She presented with hypermobility, polyarthralgia, easy bruisability and joint laxity of both major and minor joints. She complained about joint pain, a tingling sensation and hand and lower back pain with extensive hyperflexibility, particularly of her wrists, shoulders, elbows and knees. She had right shoulder subluxation which required repair on two separate occasions along with repair of labral tears of both hips. She had loose ligaments/capsules repaired on her left shoulder. She has persistent tachycardia and was diagnosed with hypothyroidism. She had a heart murmur in the past, but cardiac evaluation found no structural defects or anomalies. She has a history of weekly migraine headaches.

A three-generation pedigree was obtained. Her parents are both alive but adopted with no available family histories. She has an older brother with psychiatric and behavioral problems. No consanguinity was noted.

On physical examination, she was well developed and nourished with a normal blood pressure and heart rate. Her weight was 55.3 kg (40th percentile) and height was 160 cm (25th percentile), with a body mass index of 21.6 kg/m^2. Her head circumference was 54 cm (40th percentile), total hand length was 17.7 cm (50th percentile) and middle finger length was 7.2 cm (40th percentile). Her Beighton hyperflexibility score was 7 out of 9, indicating a possible connective tissue disorder with a score greater than 5. She exhibited positive signs for hyperextensible bilateral knees, bilateral fifth digits and bilateral hyperextensible thumbs to wrists and placed both palms on the floor upon standing and bending forward. The rest of the physical examination was normal including abdomen, HEENT (head, eyes, ears, nose and throat), neurological, pulmonary, cardiac, cutaneous and psychiatric.

Clinical genetic testing was ordered using next-generation sequencing (NGS) for CTDs based on her physical examination and medical history (as described above). These test results as a component of their medical care showed no pathogenic, likely pathogenic or potentially pathogenic variants and were interpreted as normal. This test was then followed by an *FMR1* gene triplet repeat expansion study using an approved PCR of available DNA, and a normal allele (20) and an intermediate (51) repeat expansion size allele were found. AAG interruptions were also studied, and one AGG interruption was found prior to 20 repeats which could belong to either allele. A second AGG interruption occurred after 20 repeats, which would belong to the 51-repeat allele.

Case #2

A 45-year-old female was seen in the Genetics Clinic at KUMC for evaluation of a connective tissue disorder. She presented with migraine headaches, carpel tunnel syndrome and dislocated thumbs requiring previous surgical intervention during adulthood, decreased muscle mass, non-trauma-related ankle and heel sprains, spontaneous nose bleeds and easy bruising, thin loose skin with poor scarring, myopia and astigmatism. She also presented with bipolar disorder, depression, insomnia, gastro-esophageal reflux disease (GERD), asthma and vitamin D deficiency.

She was born without any congenital anomalies but exhibited hypermobility since childhood. She has a history of heart palpitations and syncope. She has a history of hidradenitis involving several subcutaneous sweat glands that were removed from the axillary regions.

A three-generation pedigree was obtained and showed that she has two sons (17 and 12 years of age), with her older son having bipolar disorder and joint laxity. She has a 36-year-old brother with a history of depression. Her mother died at 70 years of age due to leukemia. Her mother also had a history of nose bleeds, joint laxity, high blood pressure and severe depression. Her maternal grandmother died at the age of 50 years due to heart issues, and her maternal grandfather died at the age of 70 years due to a stroke. Her father is 74 years of age and has high blood pressure, a pacemaker and dementia. Her paternal grandmother died from a stroke and dementia. Her paternal grandfather died from an unexplained heart disease. No consanguinity was noted.

On physical examination, her blood pressure and heart rate were within normal range. Her weight was 84.1 kg (80th percentile) and height was 174 cm (90th percentile), with a body mass index of 27.8 kg/m^2. In addition, her head circumference was 57 cm (60th percentile), ear length was 6.1 cm (55th percentile), total hand length was 18.8 cm (75th percentile) and middle finger length was 7.7 cm (75th percentile). Her Beighton heteroflexibility score was 3 out of 8 (had left thumb surgery and could not score for mobility). Her right shoulder was lower than her left shoulder upon standing. The rest of her physical examination was within normal range other than the features noted historically above. The *FMR1* gene triplet repeat expansion study using PCR of available DNA showed a normal allele (33) and an intermediate (48) repeat expansion size allele. AAG interruptions were also studied, and one AGG interruption was found prior to 33 repeats, which could belong to either allele. A second AGG interruption occurred after 33 repeats and would belong to the 48-repeat allele.

Case #3

A 44-year-old female was seen in the Genetics Clinic at KUMC. She presented with concerns about fibromyalgia, tachycardia, migraines, tinnitus and hypertension with subluxation of her major and minor joints caused by a connective tissue disorder such as EDS.

A three-generation pedigree was obtained and showed that both of her sons (13 and 16 years of age) had features of a connective tissue disorder including postural orthostatic tachycardia (POTs). Her 16-year-old nephew has scoliosis and elbow dislocations. Her 72-year-old mother has a history of Churg–Strauss vasculitis, and her 73-year-old father has a history of six separate abdominal hernias. Her maternal grandmother died in her 80 s from an unknown cause. Her maternal grandfather passed away at a young age with a history of a heart attack and high cholesterol. Her paternal grandmother and paternal grandfather both died at the age of 70 years with a history of breast cancer and mesothelioma, respectively.

On physical examination, her blood pressure was 114/72 and heart rate was 99. Her weight was 91.4 kg (95th percentile) and height was 166 cm (70th percentile), with a body mass index of 33.1 kg/m^2. Her Beighton hyperflexibility score was 4 out of 6. She has a history of loose, thin and stretchable skin and numerous vertical striae on her abdomen. The rest of her physical examination was within normal range including HEENT, pulmonary/cardiac, neurological and psychiatric. The *FMR1* gene triplet repeat expansion study using PCR of available DNA showed a normal allele (24) and an intermediate (50) repeat expansion size allele. AAG interruptions were also studied, and two AGG interruptions were found, with both occurring after 24 repeats and therefore belonging to the 50-repeat allele.

4.3. Statistical Analyses

A chi-square test with Yates's correction was used for statistical analysis of the *FMR1* triplet repeat status in this study to determine differences in the frequency of females in our cohort with no significant connective tissue gene variants identified and their *FMR1* status. We then performed comparisons with the reported *FMR1* gene repeat status in the general population of females. The threshold for statistical significance was set at $p < 0.05$.

Author Contributions: M.G.B. planned the investigation, examined the patients and ordered the tests; W.A.H. and J.S. compiled and analyzed the data; W.A.H., M.G.B., J.S. and O.J.V. contributed to the writing of the manuscript; H.G., Y.N. and M.Q. participated in the laboratory and curation activities with generation of laboratory results and interpretations; E.C. maintained communication and logistics of samples and results between Fulgent Genetics and the other coauthors. All authors have read and agreed to the published version of the manuscript.

Funding: This research received no external funding.

Institutional Review Board Statement: This article is a scholarly report of a clinical cohort of patients with connective tissue disorders who were tested as part of their medical care. IRB approval was not required because it was not part of a research project. The results presented in this paper have been deidentified and will not affect the patients' clinical care, nor will they have the potential to cause the patients any harm.

Informed Consent Statement: All pertinent private and protected health information about each patient was eliminated prior to collation and analysis of data.

Data Availability Statement: Data sharing is not applicable to this article as the original data presented in this study are included, further inquiries can be directed to the corresponding authors.

Conflicts of Interest: There are no conflicts of interest to report. Harry Gao, Eleina Cox, Yuxin Niu and May Quach are employees of Fulgent Genetics, a for-profit firm offering genetic testing as a fee-for-service.

References

1. McLennan, Y.; Polussa, J.; Tassone, F.; Hagerman, R. Fragile X Syndrome. *Eur. J. Hum. Genet.* **2011**, *12*, 216–224. [CrossRef]
2. Hagerman, R.J.; Berry-Kravis, E.; Hazlett, H.C.; Bailey, D.B.; Moine, H.; Kooy, R.F.; Tassone, F.; Gantois, I.; Sonenberg, N.; Mandel, J.L.; et al. Fragile X Syndrome. *Nat. Rev. Dis. Primers* **2017**, *3*, 17065. [CrossRef] [PubMed]
3. Hunter, J.; Rivero-Arias, O.; Angelov, A.; Kim, E.; Fotheringham, I.; Leal, J. Epidemiology of Fragile X Syndrome: A Systematic Review and Meta-Analysis. *Am. J. Med. Genet. A* **2014**, *164A*, 1648–1658. [CrossRef] [PubMed]
4. Ciaccio, C.; Fontana, L.; Milani, D.; Tabano, S.; Miozzo, M.; Esposito, S. Fragile X Syndrome: A Review of Clinical and Molecular Diagnoses. *Ital. J. Pediatr.* **2017**, *43*, 39. [CrossRef] [PubMed]
5. Ramírez-Cheyne, J.A.; Duque, G.A.; Ayala-Zapata, S.; Saldarriaga-Gil, W.; Hagerman, P.; Hagerman, R.; Payán-Gómez, C. Fragile X Syndrome and Connective Tissue Dysregulation. *Clin. Genet.* **2019**, *95*, 262–267. [CrossRef] [PubMed]
6. Tassanakijpanich, N.; McKenzie, F.J.; McLennan, Y.A.; Makhoul, E.; Tassone, F.; Jasoliya, M.J.; Romney, C.; Petrasic, I.C.; Napalinga, K.; Buchanan, C.B.; et al. Hypermobile Ehlers-Danlos Syndrome (HEDS) Phenotype in Fragile X Premutation Carriers: Case Series. *J. Med. Genet.* **2022**, *59*, 687–690. [CrossRef]
7. Butler, M.G.; Allen, G.A.; Haynes, J.L.; Singh, D.N.; Watson, M.S.; Breg, W.R. Anthropometric Comparison of Mentally Retarded Males with and without the Fragile X Syndrome. *Am. J. Med. Genet.* **1991**, *38*, 260–268. [CrossRef]
8. Butler, M.G.; Pratesi, R.; Watson, M.S.; Breg, W.R.; Singh, D.N. Anthropometric and Craniofacial Patterns in Mentally Retarded Males with Emphasis on the Fragile X Syndrome. *Clin. Genet.* **1993**, *44*, 129–138. [CrossRef]
9. Hagerman, R.; Hoem, G.; Hagerman, P. Fragile X and Autism: Intertwined at the Molecular Level Leading to Targeted Treatments. *Mol. Autism* **2010**, *1*, 12. [CrossRef]
10. Rajaratnam, A.; Shergill, J.; Salcedo-Arellano, M.; Saldarriaga, W.; Duan, X.; Hagerman, R. Fragile X Syndrome and Fragile X-Associated Disorders. *F1000Research* **2017**, *6*, 2112. [CrossRef]
11. Baeza-Velasco, C.; Cohen, D.; Hamonet, C.; Vlamynck, E.; Diaz, L.; Cravero, C.; Cappe, E.; Guinchat, V. Autism, Joint Hypermobility-Related Disorders and Pain. *Front. Psychiatry* **2018**, *9*, 656. [CrossRef] [PubMed]
12. Malfait, F.; Francomano, C.; Byers, P.; Belmont, J.; Berglund, B.; Black, J.; Bloom, L.; Bowen, J.M.; Brady, A.F.; Burrows, N.P.; et al. The 2017 International Classification of the Ehlers-Danlos Syndromes. *Am. J. Med. Genet. C Semin. Med. Genet.* **2017**, *175*, 8–26. [CrossRef] [PubMed]
13. Coffey, S.M.; Cook, K.; Tartaglia, N.; Tassone, F.; Nguyen, D.V.; Pan, R.; Bronsky, H.E.; Yuhas, J.; Borodyanskaya, M.; Grigsby, J.; et al. Expanded Clinical Phenotype of Women with the *FMR1* Premutation. *Am. J. Med. Genet. A* **2008**, *146A*, 1009–1016. [CrossRef]
14. Rodriguez-Revenga, L.; Madrigal, I.; Pagonabarraga, J.; Xunclà, M.; Badenas, C.; Kulisevsky, J.; Gomez, B.; Milà, M. Penetrance of *FMR1* Premutation Associated Pathologies in Fragile X Syndrome Families. *Eur. J. Hum. Genet.* **2009**, *17*, 1359–1362. [CrossRef]
15. Winarni, T.I.; Chonchaiya, W.; Sumekar, T.A.; Ashwood, P.; Morales, G.M.; Tassone, F.; Nguyen, D.V.; Faradz, S.M.H.; Van de Water, J.; Cook, K.; et al. Immune-Mediated Disorders among Women Carriers of Fragile X Premutation Alleles. *Am. J. Med. Genet. A* **2012**, *158A*, 2473–2481. [CrossRef]
16. Nolin, S.L.; Glicksman, A.; Ersalesi, N.; Dobkin, C.; Brown, W.T.; Cao, R.; Blatt, E.; Sah, S.; Latham, G.J.; Hadd, A.G. Fragile X Full Mutation Expansions Are Inhibited by One or More AGG Interruptions in Premutation Carriers. *Genet. Med.* **2015**, *17*, 358–364. [CrossRef]
17. Friedman-Gohas, M.; Kirshenbaum, M.; Michaeli, A.; Domniz, N.; Elizur, S.; Raanani, H.; Orvieto, R.; Cohen, Y. Does the Presence of AGG Interruptions within the CGG Repeat Tract Have a Protective Effect on the Fertility Phenotype of Female FMR_1 Premutation Carriers? *J. Assist. Reprod. Genet.* **2020**, *37*, 849–854. [CrossRef] [PubMed]
18. Steinle, J.; Hossain, W.A.; Veatch, O.J.; Strom, S.P.; Butler, M.G. Next-generation Sequencing and Analysis of Consecutive Patients Referred for Connective Tissue Disorders. *Am. J. Med. Genet. Part A*, 2022; ajmg.a.62905, ahead of print. [CrossRef]

19. Tassone, F.; Iong, K.P.; Tong, T.-H.; Lo, J.; Gane, L.W.; Berry-Kravis, E.; Nguyen, D.; Mu, L.Y.; Laffin, J.; Bailey, D.B.; et al. FMR1 CGG Allele Size and Prevalence Ascertained through Newborn Screening in the United States. *Genome Med.* **2012**, *4*, 100. [CrossRef] [PubMed]
20. Desai, A.; Connolly, J.J.; March, M.; Hou, C.; Chiavacci, R.; Kim, C.; Lyon, G.; Hadley, D.; Hakonarson, H. Systematic Data-Querying of Large Pediatric Biorepository Identifies Novel Ehlers-Danlos Syndrome Variant. *BMC Musculoskelet. Disord.* **2016**, *17*, 80. [CrossRef]
21. Jacquemont, S.; Hagerman, R.J.; Leehey, M.A.; Hall, D.A.; Levine, R.A.; Brunberg, J.A.; Zhang, L.; Jardini, T.; Gane, L.W.; Harris, S.W.; et al. Penetrance of the Fragile X-Associated Tremor/Ataxia Syndrome in a Premutation Carrier Population. *JAMA* **2004**, *291*, 460–469. [CrossRef]
22. Tassone, F.; Hagerman, R.J.; Taylor, A.K.; Gane, L.W.; Godfrey, T.E.; Hagerman, P.J. Elevated Levels of *FMR1* MRNA in Carrier Males: A New Mechanism of Involvement in the Fragile-X Syndrome. *Am. J. Hum. Genet.* **2000**, *66*, 6–15. [CrossRef] [PubMed]
23. Garcia-Arocena, D.; Hagerman, P.J. Advances in Understanding the Molecular Basis of FXTAS. *Hum. Mol. Genet.* **2010**, *19*, R83–R89. [CrossRef] [PubMed]
24. Dai, R.; Ahmed, S.A. MicroRNA, a New Paradigm for Understanding Immunoregulation, Inflammation, and Autoimmune Diseases. *Transl. Res.* **2011**, *157*, 163–179. [CrossRef] [PubMed]
25. Chang, L.; Sundaresh, S.; Elliott, J.; Anton, P.A.; Baldi, P.; Licudine, A.; Mayer, M.; Vuong, T.; Hirano, M.; Naliboff, B.D.; et al. Dysregulation of the Hypothalamic-Pituitary-Adrenal (HPA) Axis in Irritable Bowel Syndrome. *Neurogastroenterol. Motil.* **2009**, *21*, 149–159. [CrossRef]
26. Evsyukova, I.; Somarelli, J.A.; Gregory, S.G.; Garcia-Blanco, M.A. Alternative Splicing in Multiple Sclerosis and Other Autoimmune Diseases. *RNA Biol.* **2010**, *7*, 462–473. [CrossRef]
27. Otsuka, M.; Zheng, M.; Hayashi, M.; Lee, J.-D.; Yoshino, O.; Lin, S.; Han, J. Impaired MicroRNA Processing Causes Corpus Luteum Insufficiency and Infertility in Mice. *J. Clin. Investig.* **2008**, *118*, 1944–1954. [CrossRef]
28. Nolin, S.L.; Sah, S.; Glicksman, A.; Sherman, S.L.; Allen, E.; Berry-Kravis, E.; Tassone, F.; Yrigollen, C.; Cronister, A.; Jodah, M.; et al. Fragile X AGG Analysis Provides New Risk Predictions for 45-69 Repeat Alleles. *Am. J. Med. Genet. A* **2013**, *161A*, 771–778. [CrossRef]
29. Wijnhoven, H.A.H.; de Vet, H.C.W.; Picavet, H.S.J. Explaining Sex Differences in Chronic Musculoskeletal Pain in a General Population. *Pain* **2006**, *124*, 158–166. [CrossRef]
30. Hall, D.A. In the Gray Zone in the Fragile X Gene: What Are the Key Unanswered Clinical and Biological Questions? *Tremor Other Hyperkinetic Mov.* **2014**, *4*, 208. [CrossRef]
31. Debrey, S.M.; Leehey, M.A.; Klepitskaya, O.; Filley, C.M.; Shah, R.C.; Kluger, B.; Berry-Kravis, E.; Spector, E.; Tassone, F.; Hall, D.A. Clinical Phenotype of Adult Fragile X Gray Zone Allele Carriers: A Case Series. *Cerebellum* **2016**, *15*, 623–631. [CrossRef]
32. Fernandez-Carvajal, I.; Walichiewicz, P.; Xiaosen, X.; Pan, R.; Hagerman, P.J.; Tassone, F. Screening for Expanded Alleles of the *FMR1* Gene in Blood Spots from Newborn Males in a Spanish Population. *J. Mol. Diagn.* **2009**, *11*, 324–329. [CrossRef] [PubMed]
33. Hall, D.A.; Nag, S.; Ouyang, B.; Bennett, D.A.; Liu, Y.; Ali, A.; Zhou, L.; Berry-Kravis, E. Fragile X Gray Zone Alleles Are Associated with Signs of Parkinsonism and Earlier Death. *Mov. Disord.* **2020**, *35*, 1448–1456. [CrossRef] [PubMed]
34. Loesch, D.; Hagerman, R. Unstable Mutations in the *FMR1* Gene and the Phenotypes. *Adv. Exp. Med. Biol.* **2012**, *769*, 78–114. [CrossRef] [PubMed]
35. Sitzmann, A.F.; Hagelstrom, R.T.; Tassone, F.; Hagerman, R.J.; Butler, M.G. Rare *FMR1* Gene Mutations Causing Fragile X Syndrome: A Review. *Am. J. Med. Genet. A* **2018**, *176*, 11–18. [CrossRef] [PubMed]

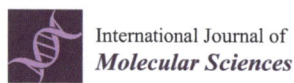
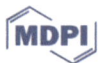

Article

Defining the 3′ Epigenetic Boundary of the *FMR1* Promoter and Its Loss in Individuals with Fragile X Syndrome

David E. Godler [1,2,*], Yoshimi Inaba [1], Minh Q. Bui [3], David Francis [4], Cindy Skinner [5], Charles E. Schwartz [5] and David J. Amor [2,6]

1. Diagnosis and Development, Murdoch Children's Research Institute, Royal Children's Hospital, Melbourne, VIC 3052, Australia; inachoku@hotmail.com
2. Department of Paediatrics, Faculty of Medicine, Dentistry and Health Sciences, University of Melbourne, Parkville, VIC 3052, Australia; david.amor@mcri.edu.au
3. Centre for Epidemiology and Biostatistics, Melbourne School of Population and Global Health, University of Melbourne, Melbourne, VIC 3052, Australia; mbui@unimelb.edu.au
4. Victorian Clinical Genetics Services and Murdoch Children's Research Institute, The Royal Children's Hospital, Melbourne, VIC 3052, Australia; david.francis@vcgs.org.au
5. Center for Molecular Studies, J.C. Self Research Institute of Human Genetics, Greenwood Genetic Center, Greenwood, SC 29646, USA; cskinner@ggc.org (C.S.); charles.schwartz224@gmail.com (C.E.S.)
6. Neurodisability and Rehabilitation, Murdoch Children's Research Institute, Royal Children's Hospital, Melbourne, VIC 3052, Australia
* Correspondence: david.godler@mcri.edu.au

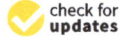

Citation: Godler, D.E.; Inaba, Y.; Bui, M.Q.; Francis, D.; Skinner, C.; Schwartz, C.E.; Amor, D.J. Defining the 3′Epigenetic Boundary of the *FMR1* Promoter and Its Loss in Individuals with Fragile X Syndrome. *Int. J. Mol. Sci.* **2023**, *24*, 10712. https://doi.org/10.3390/ijms241310712

Academic Editor: Lidia Larizza

Received: 1 May 2023
Revised: 20 June 2023
Accepted: 21 June 2023
Published: 27 June 2023

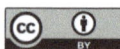

Copyright: © 2023 by the authors. Licensee MDPI, Basel, Switzerland. This article is an open access article distributed under the terms and conditions of the Creative Commons Attribution (CC BY) license (https://creativecommons.org/licenses/by/4.0/).

Abstract: This study characterizes the DNA methylation patterns specific to fragile X syndrome (FXS) with a full mutation (FM > 200 CGGs), premutation (PM 55–199 CGGs), and X inactivation in blood and brain tissues at the 3′ boundary of the *FMR1* promoter. Blood was analyzed from 95 controls and 462 individuals (32% males) with FM and PM alleles. Brain tissues (62% males) were analyzed from 12 controls and 4 with FXS. There was a significant increase in intron 1 methylation, extending to a newly defined 3′ epigenetic boundary in the FM compared with that in the control and PM groups ($p < 0.0001$), and this was consistent between the blood and brain tissues. A distinct intron 2 site showed a significant decrease in methylation for the FXS groups compared with the controls in both sexes ($p < 0.01$). In all female groups, most intron 1 (but not intron 2 sites) were sensitive to X inactivation. In all PM groups, methylation at the 3′ epigenetic boundary and the proximal sites was significantly decreased compared with that in the control and FM groups ($p < 0.0001$). In conclusion, abnormal *FMR1* intron 1 and 2 methylation that was sensitive to X inactivation in the blood and brain tissues provided a novel avenue for the detection of PM and FM alleles through DNA methylation analysis.

Keywords: fragile X syndrome; FMR1; epigenetic boundary; premutation; methylation intellectual disability

1. Introduction

Fragile X syndrome (FXS) is the most common heritable form of intellectual disability and is the second-most common cause of comorbid autism (1 in 3600 males and 1 in 6000 females) [1]. FXS usually results from expansions of a trinucleotide CGG repeat in the 5′ untranslated region (UTR) of the *FMR1* gene to ≥200 repeats, called full mutation (FM), with the normal range being <45 repeats [2]. The FM is associated with a decrease in the expression of *FMR1* due to promoter methylation, with subsequent loss of its protein product (FMRP), which is important for normal neurodevelopment [3,4]. FM males with mosaicism for CGG size and methylation have been reported to have better intellectual function than those without mosaicism [5]. In addition, approximately 5% of males with an FM have been reported to have a completely unmethylated promoter (UFM), associated with the expression of *FMR1* mRNA and FMRP, and an IQ within the normal range [6–8].

Smaller CGG expansions, defined as premutation (PM, 55–199 repeats), do not cause FXS but have been associated with elevated levels of *FMR1* mRNA linked to RNA toxicity [9]. These PM alleles are more common, with frequencies reported between 1 in 400 and 1 in 800 in males and between 1 in 300 and 1 in 400 in females [10]. The RNA toxicity associated with PM alleles has been linked to late onset disorders, fragile X-associated tremor/ataxia syndrome (FXTAS), and fragile X-associated primary ovarian insufficiency (FXPOI) [10–12]. However, the CGG size and *FMR1* mRNA levels have been shown to have limited utility as predictors of which individuals with PM alleles become symptomatic [11]. It has also been shown that CGG size-dependent toxicity may be related to elevated mRNA levels of the gene *ASFMR1*, which spans the CGG expansion in the antisense direction. *ASFMR1* has several transcriptional start sites located at 5′ of the CpG island and in intron 2 of *FMR1* [12]. While the role of CpG island methylation 5′ of the expansion in *FMR1* silencing has been characterized, there is minimal understanding of the role of the epi-genotype beyond the CpG island in PM- and FM-related disorders.

Our previous findings suggest that the *FMR1* promoter is much larger than originally thought [3,13–16], expanding on the 5′ side to an epigenetic boundary located ~800 bp upstream of the CGG expansion [3], which is consistent with the findings of Naumann et al. [17] reporting the location of this boundary to be 65–70 CpG pairs upstream of the CGG repeat expansion. This boundary is located within a region that we named Fragile X-Related Epigenetic Element 1 (FREE1) [3,18], which also contains one of the *ASFMR1* transcription start sites [12,19]. By examining methylation within the *FMR1* 'minimal' promoter [20] and the adjacent regions in transformed lymphoblast cell lines from FXS individuals, 'high-functioning' individuals with UFM alleles, and controls, we identified new regions differentially methylated in individuals with *FMR1*-related disorders [3,16], with Fragile X-Related Element 2 (FREE2) located largely within *FMR1* intron 1 and Fragile X-Related Element 3 (FREE3) located within *FMR1* intron 2. This study characterized the normal and pathological methylation of these regions in venous blood and brain tissues to: (1) determine the associations between differential methylation within these regions and the presence of FM and PM alleles and X-inactivation and (2) provide novel avenues for the detection of expanded *FMR1* alleles through DNA methylation analyses.

2. Results

2.1. The FMR1 Methylation Map

In this study, we define the amplicon of the previously described FREE2 region as FREE2(A) [3], with methylation presented in units as described in our earlier publications [15–19]. The amplicons extending 3′ from FREE2(A) were named FREE2(B), FREE2(C), FREE2(D), FREE2(E), and FREE3 (Figure 1). A more detailed genomic organization of the targeted regions, including the number of differentially methylated CpG sites examined, is described in the additional files (Note S1, Figures S1 and S2, and Tables S1 and S2).

2.2. Inter-Group Methylation Comparisons in the Venous Blood of Males

Inter-group comparisons of methylation were performed between 73 males with FXS and FM alleles, 27 males with mosaicism for FM and PM alleles, and 21 males with mosaicism for FM alleles and smaller expansions. Of the CGG size mosaics, 23 were mosaic for the PM and FM alleles, 4 were unusual mosaic cases for either normal-sized FM alleles (29/1300 CGG and 30/175 CGG) or intermediate-sized FM alleles (41/800 CGG and 50/763 CGG). There was a significant increase in intron 1 methylation extending ~1.5 kb 3′ from the CGG expansion to a novel epigenetic boundary in these FM groups, compared with that in 27 control males with normal-sized alleles, 39 males with PM, and 5 with unmethylated FM (UFM) alleles ($p < 0.0001$) (Figures 2 and S3). At the 3′ boundary, three CpG units of FREE2(E) showed a progressive increase in methylation in the control, PM, and UFM groups. However, in all FM groups other than UFM, the difference in methylation between these three CpG units of FREE2(E) was not as large when compared with the control and PM groups. This suggests that there is a transfer of methylation from the adjacent 3′ regions that may be caused by the presence of FM expansions, contributing to loss of the 3′ epigenetic boundary in intron 1 in males with FXS.

This postulate was consistent with the 'high-functioning' males with UFM alleles expressing normal or elevated levels of *FMR1* being completely unmethylated within the CpG island [6–8] and within intron 1 upstream of the 3′ boundary. Two out of five UFM males showed methylation of intron 1 units (B)CpG2 and (C)CpG4 marginally above the male control range. It is of note that one of the males with a UFM of 323–517 CGGs was the first 'high-functioning' male with an FM allele reported to develop FXTAS [8]. He also showed the highest methylation for (B)CpG2 and (C)CpG4 of all individuals with a UFM allele (Figure 2E).

2.3. Inter-Group Methylation Comparisons in the Venous Blood of Females

There was a significant increase in intron 1 methylation, extending ~1.5 kb 3′ from the CGG repeat to a novel epigenetic boundary for 132 females with an FM compared with 75 female controls and 157 females with a PM ($p < 0.0001$) (Figures 3 and S4). In contrast to the males with FM alleles, for the females with FM alleles, methylation of this region for most CpG units was not significantly increased in the CGG size mosaic group compared with the female controls and females with a PM (Figure S4). The female control baseline levels of methylation within this intron 1 region were also different from the males, with the female control methylation output ratio (MOR) being between ~0.1 and ~0.5. This is in line with the previously reported levels of methylation resulting from X inactivation [21], also suggesting that X inactivation-sensitive CpG sites extend downstream from the expansion up to the 3′ epigenetic boundary. While methylation also increased above the control range at the 3′ epigenetic boundary for most of females with an FM (Figure 3C), for the females with a PM, methylation at €CpG4, (E)CpG5, a€(E)CpG6, methylation was significantly decreased compared with the controls ($p < 0.0001$). This suggests that methylation in this region is sensitive to X inactivation and presence of PM and FM alleles in females (Figure S4).

2.4. Abnormally Decreased Methylation of the Intron 1 3′ Boundary and Intron 2 Sites in Males with a PM Allele

The males with a PM had significantly decreased methylation at the 3′ epigenetic boundary compared with the males with an FM and the male controls ($p < 0.0001$) (Figure 4). This PM-specific decrease was observed for the comparisons of the male controls to (1) all 39 males with a PM collapsed into one group (Figure 4) and (2) the male PM group split into two independent cohorts based on the site of participant recruitment (US cohort $n = 21$; Australian cohort $n = 18$) (Figure 5). Moreover, the (E)CpG4 unit 3′ of this epigenetic boundary showed the greatest overlap in methylation values between the controls and PM ranges in males, with intergroup comparison showing a decrease in methylation of marginal significance in the PM group compared with the male controls ($p = 0.047$).

The intron 2 (F3)CpG1 unit within FREE3 showed an inverse methylation pattern to that observed for most intron 1 sites within FREE2 and to the methylation status of the *FMR1* minimal promoter within the CpG island 5′ of the CGG expansion. This inverse pattern involved a significant decrease in methylation in FM only and the groups mosaic for the PM and FM alleles ($p < 0.0001$). The MOR for these ranged between 0.6 and 0.95, compared with the MOR range between 0.9 and 1 for the control, PM, and UFM male groups (Figure 4E). Interestingly, for intron 2 (F3)CpG2, the PM group showed a significant decrease in methylation compared with the male controls ($p < 0.0001$) and males with a UFM ($p = 0.04$). However, there was no significant change in methylation for intron 2 (F3)CpG2 for the PM group compared with the FM group (Figure 4F). Furthermore, (F3)CpG2 methylation was also significantly decreased in the males with a PM and FM mosaic groups compared with the male controls ($p < 0.0001$).

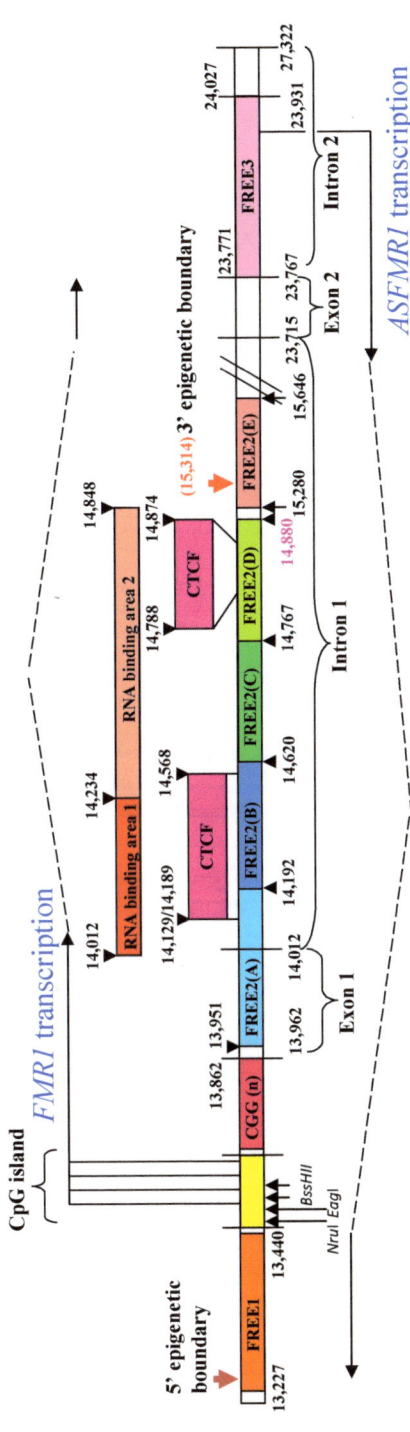

Figure 1. Genetic and epigenetic organization of the 5′ portion of the *FMR1* locus (sequence numbering from GenBank L29074) and locations of target amplicons. The intron and exon regions 5′ and 3′ of the *FMR1* CGG expansion are presented in relation to *FMR1* and *ASFMR1* transcription start sites (the broken lines indicate spliced out regions). Fragile X-Related Epigenetic Elements 1 and 2 (FREE1 and FREE2), the *FMR1* CpG island, and methylation-sensitive restriction sites (*NruI*, *EagI*, and *BssHII*) analyzed using routine fragile X Southern blot testing. A CGG repeat is located within 5′ (UTR) of the *FMR1* gene. *ASFMR1* spans the CGG expansion in the antisense direction and is also regulated by another promoter located in intron 2 of *FMR1*. FREE2 is located downstream of the CGG expansion. The FREE3 region is located within intron 2 of *FMR1* downstream of the second *ASFMR1* promoter. Primers utilized for MALDI-TOF methylation analysis targeted six regions at the Xq27.3 locus, designated as FREE1, FREE2(A) (described as amplicon 5 in Godler et al. [3]), FREE2(B), FREE2(C), FREE2(D), FREE2(E), and FREE3 (color-coded). Red boxes indicate regions pulled down by ChIRP to show RNA binding to intron 1 DNA in the control and FXS human embryonic stem cells (hESCs) at day 45 of differentiation, with RNA area 1 showing the greatest binding intensity (Figure S1). The FREE2 sequences amplified by forward and reverse primers used in the chromatin isolation by the RNA purification (ChiRP) technique are indicated in Figure S1.

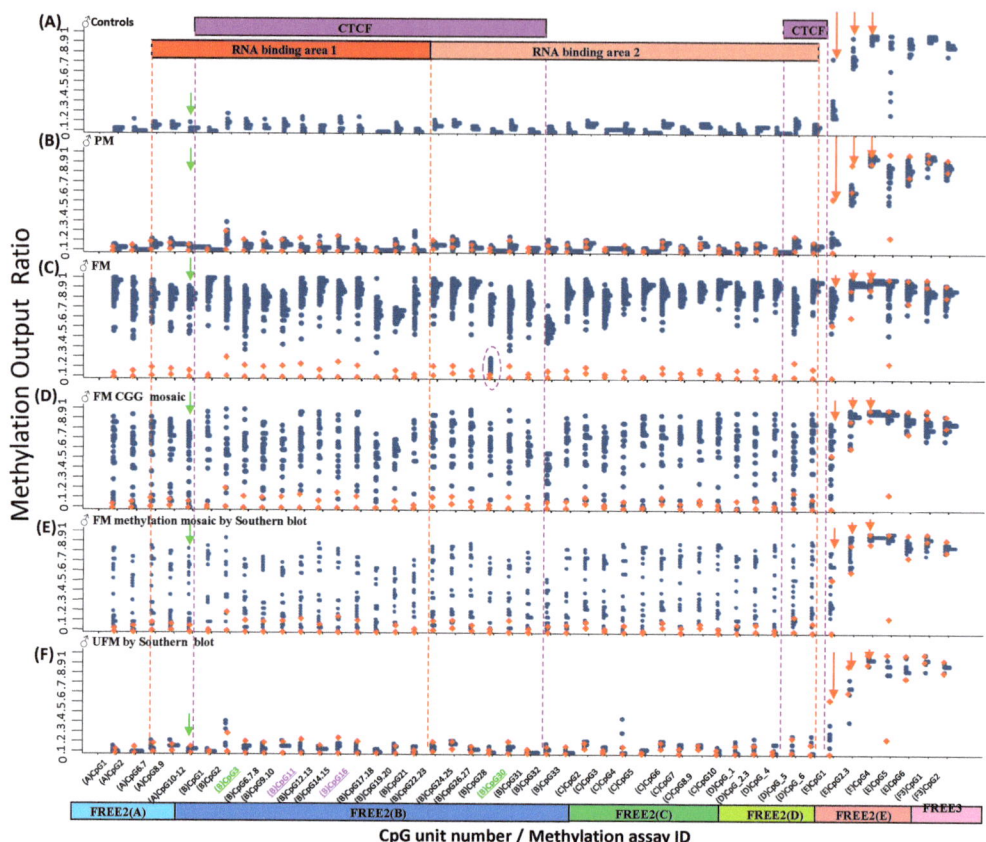

Figure 2. *FMR1* methylation in venous blood 3′ of the CGG expansion in males. (**A**) Male controls with CGG < 40 (*n* = 20). (**B**) Males with a PM (*n* = 39). (**C**) Males with an FM and FXS (100% methylated by Southern blot) (*n* = 73). (**D**) Males with an FM and CGG size mosaicism (*n* = 27). (**E**) Males with an FM and incomplete methylation through Southern blot (*n* = 21). (**F**) 'High-functioning' males (*n* = 5) with a UFM identified by Southern blot. Red dots overlayed onto plots (**B**–**F**) represent the upper and lower normal methylation range (two standard deviations from the mean methylation of male controls with normal CGG size alleles). On the x axis, the (B)CpG3 and (B)CpG30 units (in green) had fragments of the same mass. (B)CpG11 and (B)CpG16 (in purple) also had fragments of the same mass. The EpiTYPER mass spectrometry approach could only provide the mean methylation for these fragments of the same mass. The green arrow indicates methylation of CpG units 10–12, previously described to be significantly associated with the type and severity of cognitive impairment in a female carrier of expanded *FMR1* alleles. The purple oval indicates methylation of a CpG unit which separates the male FM group into two distinct groups. The red arrows indicate methylation CpG units at the novel 3′ epigenetic boundary. The purple boxes represent the CTCF binding sites. The red boxes indicate regions pulled down by ChIRP to show RNA binding to DNA in the control and FXS hESCs in earlier studies (Figure S1).

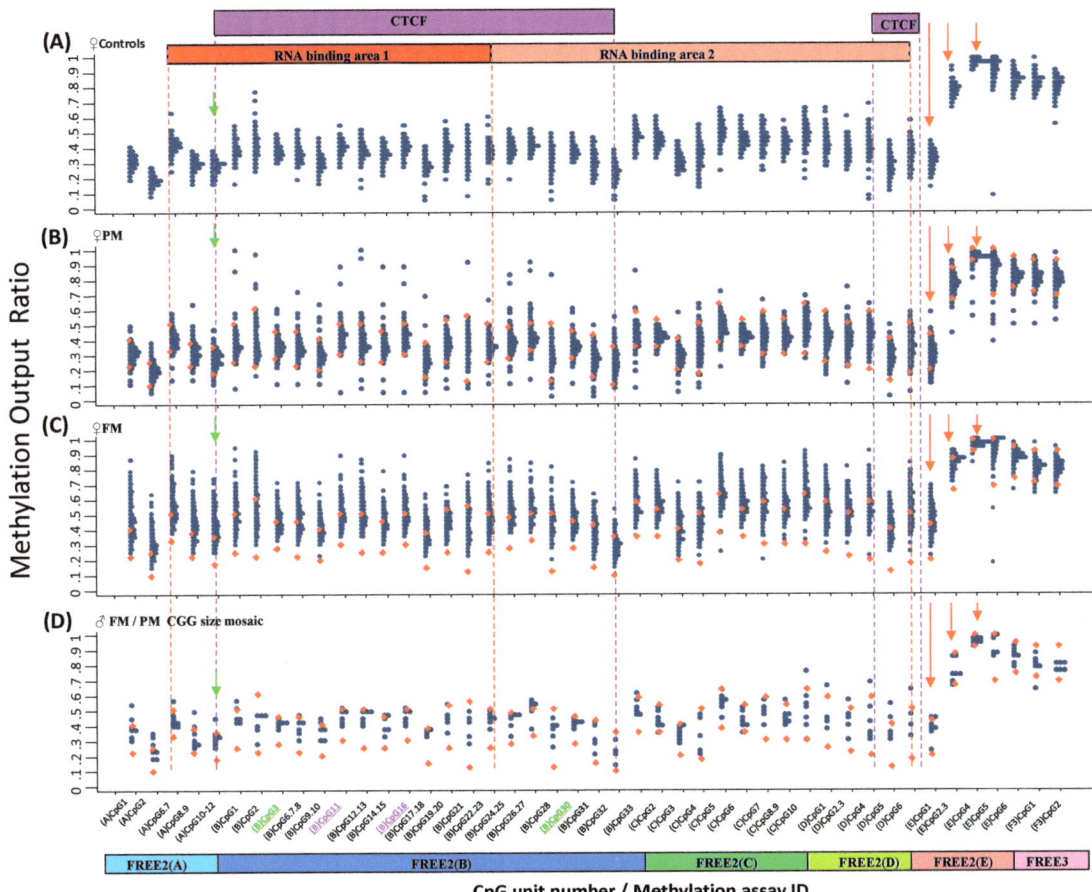

Figure 3. *FMR1* methylation in venous blood at 3′ of the CGG expansion in females. (**A**) Female controls with CGG < 40 (*n* = 75). (**B**) Females with a PM (*n* = 157). (**C**) Females with an FM (*n* = 132). (**D**) Female mosaic for PM and FM alleles (*n* = 8). The red dots overlayed onto plots (**B**–**D**) represent the upper and lower normal methylation range (two standard deviations from the mean methylation of the female control group with normal size CGG alleles). On the x axis, the (B)CpG3 and (B)CpG30 units (in green) had fragments of the same mass. (B)CpG11 and (B)CpG16 (in purple) also had fragments of the same mass. The EpiTYPER mass spectrometry approach could only provide mean methylation for these fragments of the same mass. The green arrow indicates methylation of CpG units 10–12, which we previously described to be significantly associated with the type and severity of cognitive impairment in a female carrier of expanded *FMR1* alleles. The purple oval indicates methylation of a CpG unit, which separates the female with an FM into two distinct subgroups. The red arrows point to methylation of CpG units at the novel 3′ epigenetic boundary. The purple boxes represent CTCF binding sites. The red boxes indicate regions pulled down by ChIRP to show RNA binding to DNA in the control and FXS hESCs in earlier studies (Figure S1).

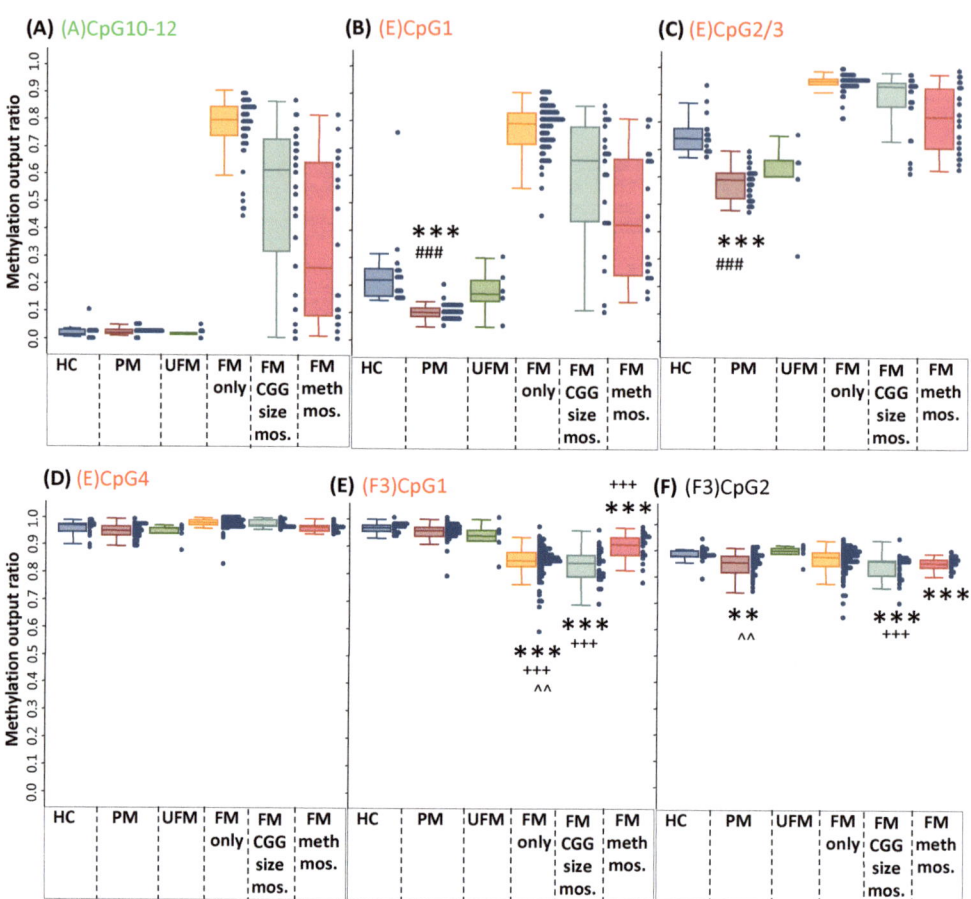

Figure 4. *FMR1* methylation at the exon1/intron 1 boundary, the intron 1 3′ epigenetic boundary, and the intron 2 region overlapping with the *ASFMR1* promoter in venous blood of males. Nonparametric tests for intergroup comparisons were performed in males for methylation of 6 CpG units for 21 control males with CGG size < 40 (HC), 39 males with a PM, 5 'high-functioning' males with a UFM, 73 males with an FM affected by FXS (FM only; 100% methylated by Southern blot), 27 males with an FM CGG size mosaicism (including PM/FM, GZ/FM, and normal size/FM), and 21 males with an FM partially methylated from Southern blot assessments (FM meth. mos.) (n = 21). (**A**) FREE2 CpG10–12. (**B**–**D**) FREE2 3′ epigenetic boundary CpG 1–4 sites. (**E**,**F**) FREE3 CpG1 and 2. Note: Selected comparisons of significant decrease in methylation $p < 0.0001$ are indicated by *** compared with HC, ### compared with FM, and +++ compared with PM. For ^^, $p < 0.05$ compared with UFM, and ** is $p < 0.05$ compared with HC. The exact p values for these intergroup comparisons are presented in Table S4 and Figure S3.

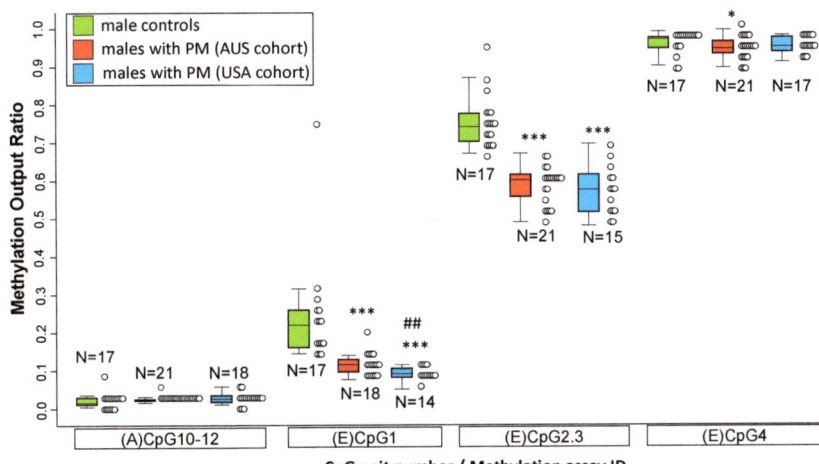

Figure 5. PM-specific hypomethylation of the 3′ epigenetic boundary within *FMR1* intron 1 in venous blood of males. Comparison of methylation at FREE2 (A)CpG10–12 for the exon1/intron 1 border and the 3′ epigenetic boundary within intron 1 between control males (HC) and males with a PM from the USA cohort (CGG55–130) and the Australian cohort (CGG57–170). Note: *** $p < 0.0001$; * $p < 0.05$ compared with HC; ## $p < 0.05$ compared with the USA PM cohort. The exact p values for these intergroup comparisons are presented in Table S3 and Figure S3.

2.5. Inter-Group Methylation Comparisons in Brain Tissues and Blood

To determine if the presence of FM alleles is associated with abnormal methylation of the intron 1 and 2 regions in the prefrontal cortex (PFC), we compared the methylation in the brain tissues of males with FXS and male controls with normal-sized alleles. In the PFC, the 3′ epigenetic boundary was lost in the males with FXS, with the methylation output ratio elevated (MOR approaching one) compared with the male controls (MOR < 0.1) (Figure 6A,B). All CpG sites within the FREE2 region within *FMR1* intron 1 5′ of the 3′ boundary were hypermethylated in the PFCs of the males with FXS compared with the controls. The male with FXS with the lowest level of methylation in the PFC across all of the intron 1 sites of all males with only FM alleles was the only mosaic for PM and FM alleles in this group.

To determine if X inactivation is associated with increased methylation within these loci between different areas of the brain and the peripheral tissues, we compared the methylation in this region between male and female control groups in the venous blood, PFC, and cerebellum (Figures 6C,D and 7). The mean methylation output ratio in the venous blood and all brain tissues of the female controls was significantly elevated for 40 CpG sites, snapping across a 1.5 kB region within *FMR1* intron 1 in the female controls compared with the male controls. In contrast, the methylation of two CpG sites—(E)CpG4 and 5 5′of the 3′epigenetic boundary in intron 1 and the (F3)CpG1 site at the 5′ end of *FMR1* intron 2 (FREE3: *ASFMR1* promoter)—was significantly decreased in the PFCs and cerebella of the female controls compared with the corresponding brain tissues in the male controls. This difference, however, was not preserved in the venous blood comparisons (Figure 6C,D).

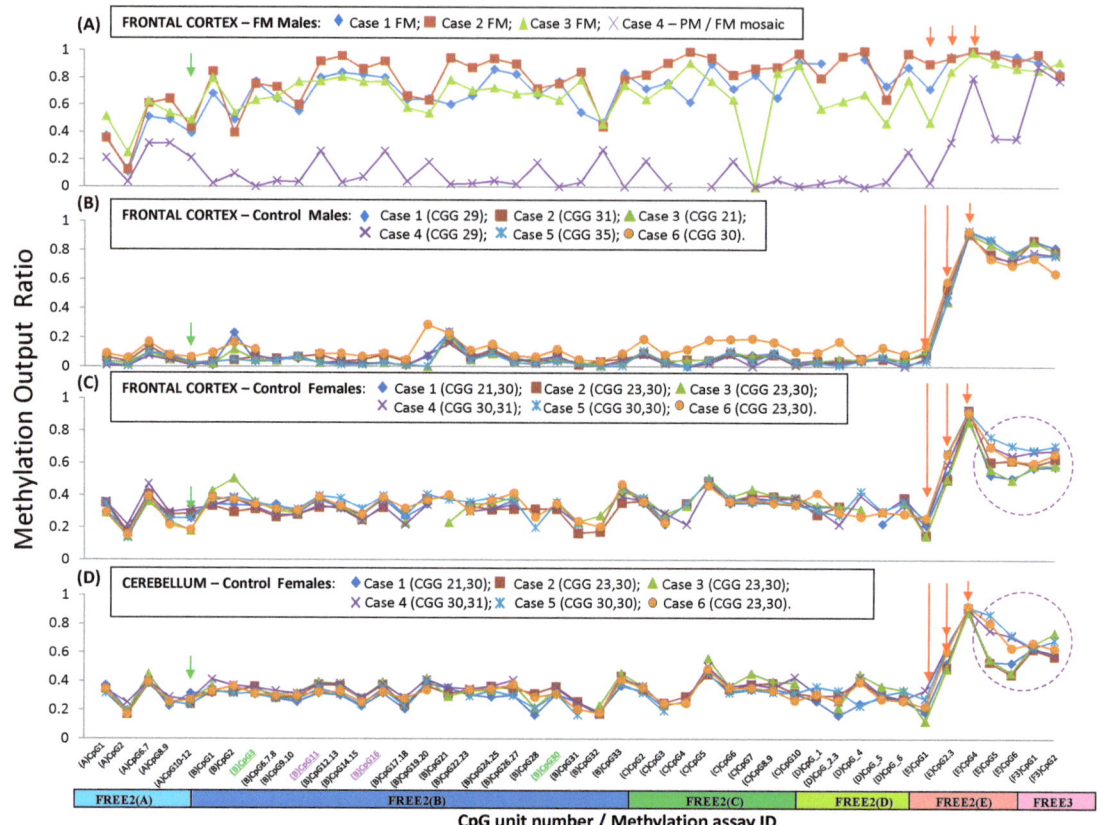

Figure 6. *FMR1* methylation in brain tissues 3′ of the CGG expansion in males and females. (**A**) Prefrontal cortexes of males with an FM (*n* = 4). (**B**) Prefrontal cortexes of male controls (CGG < 40) (*n* = 6). (**C**) Prefrontal cortexes of female controls (CGG < 40) (*n* = 6). (**D**) Cerebella of female controls (CGG < 40) (*n* = 6). On the x axis, the (B)CpG3 and (B)CpG30 units (in green) had fragments of the same mass. (B)CpG11 and (B)CpG16 (in purple) also had fragments of the same mass. The EpiTYPER mass spectrometry approach could only provide the mean methylation for these fragments of the same mass. The green arrow indicates methylation of CpG units 10–12, which we previously described to be significantly associated with the type and severity of cognitive impairment in a female carrier of expanded *FMR1* alleles. The red arrows point to methylation of CpG units at the novel 3′ epigenetic boundary.

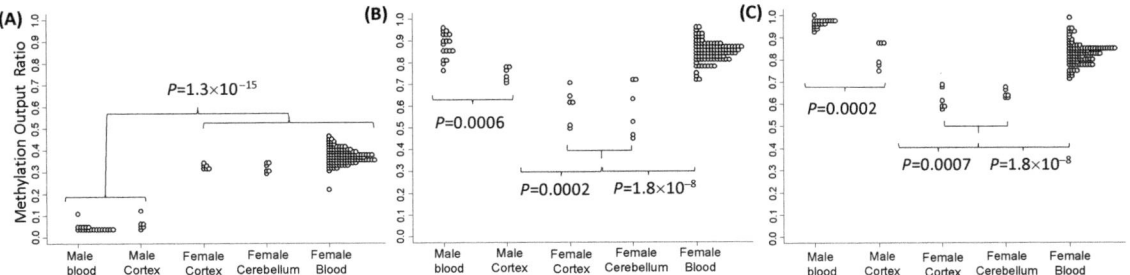

Figure 7. *FMR1* intron 1 and 2 methylation pattern variation in postmortem brain tissue and blood in individuals with *FMR1* CGG allele sizes in the normal range. Mean methylation output ratio in prefrontal cortex (PFC) from six male controls, PFCs and cerebellum were from six female controls and venous blood of 75 female and 20 male controls across (**A**) 40 CpG sites snapping across a 1.5 kB region within *FMR1* intron 1, (**B**) 2 CpG sites (E)CpG4 and 5 5′ of the intron 1 epigenetic boundary, and (**C**) (F3)CpG1 at the 5′ end of *FMR1* intron 2 (*ASFMR1* promoter).Interestingly, methylation of two CpG sites (E)CpG4 and five at 5′ of the 3′ epigenetic boundary in intron 1, as well as the (F3)CpG1 site at the 5′ end of *FMR1* intron 2 (*ASFMR1* promoter), was significantly decreased in the PFCs of the male controls compared with the venous blood of the male controls (Figure 6C,D). This suggested presence of PFC-specific methylation for these CpG sites.

3. Discussion

This study used the EpiTYPER system on the DNA from venous blood and brain tissues to characterize, at the single CpG level, the methylation of *FMR1* introns 1 and 2. The methylation patterns within these intragenic regions were compared between males and females to define the regions sensitive to X inactivation and between individuals with PM and FM alleles and controls to provide novel avenues for the detection of expanded *FMR1* alleles through DNA methylation analysis. These regions are different from the *FMR1* CpG island and the 'minimal' *FMR1* promoter described by Kumari and Usdin [20]. Most recently, we have shown that the methylation of CpG sites 6 or 7 and 10–12 at the 5′ end of the *FMR1* intron 1 were most informative in predicting the likelihood of adult females with a PM exhibiting dysexecutive and psychiatric symptoms [11]. This study defined additional regions differentially methylated within *FMR1* introns 1 and 2 due to the presence of expanded *FMR1* alleles in the blood and brain tissues to provide: (1) better understanding of the differentially methylated regions, which may be involved in the regulation of *FMR1* and *ASFMR1* expression, and (2) new targets for the development of biomarkers for DNA methylation-based screening for expanded *FMR1* alleles, which may also have prognostic utility for *FMR1*-associated disorders.

3.1. Evidence Suggesting the FMR1 Promoter Is Larger Than the FMR1 CpG Island including FMR1 Intronic Sequences

The *FMR1* promoter, which is sensitive to methylation changes, has been previously suggested to be primarily located within the CpG island upstream of the CGG expansion, as reviewed in [22]. This was based on limited studies showing that *FMR1* regulatory regions which are functionally influenced by methylation changes are located within this region [20,23]. Kumari and Usdin [20] defined the 5′ end of the 'minimal' *FMR1* promoter to be 355 bp upstream of the CGG expansion and its 3′ end to be 60 bp downstream of the CGG expansion. This 'minimal' promoter was suggested to encompass the *FMR1* CpG island consisting of the 52 CpG sites 5′ of the CGG expansion and 4 *FMR1* transcription start sites [23]. Moreover, Kumari and Usdin [20] suggested that this promoter encompasses the CGG expansion and a portion of *FMR1* exon 1. There was no evidence presented by this group for differential methylation of the *FMR1* intron 1 or 2 sequences in individuals with expanded *FMR1* alleles nor any suggestion of it being included as part of the *FMR1* promoter.

We demonstrated that increased methylation of the *FMR1* intron 1 sites, specifically CpG10–12, located within FREE2(A) was associated with an increased CGG size within the FM range in males, with its analytical superiority to methylation-sensitive Southern blot (used in current FXS diagnostics) and FMRP immunostaining in the blood as a predictor of cognitive impairment in females with an FM [3,14,21] and the dysexecutive-psychiatric phenotype in adult females with PM alleles. Interestingly, a 5′ 380–400 base pair CTCF binding region within intron 1 (*ChIP-seq K562 Sg1* and 2 from ENCODE/University of Washington; 2012) is located in ~100 base pairs 3′ of the intron 1/exon 1 boundary and overlaps with the CpG10–12 at the 5′ end of FREE2 that was clinically most informative in our earlier FM and PM studies (Figure 1). Furthermore, it has been recently shown that as few as one abnormally methylated CpG site strategically positioned at an exon/intron boundary can impact the methylation of the upstream promoter region, gene expression, and the severity of the phenotype at other disease-related loci [24]. Methylation of the FREE2 CpG sites proximal to the intron 1/exon 1 boundary in FM females could interfere with splicing of *FMR1* intron 1 and result in intron retention.

Of potential functional relevance to our observations are also previous reports of abnormal methylation of exonic CpG sites at other loci inhibiting the binding of CTCF, with exon exclusion resulting from aberrant splicing [25]. Evidence showing the formation of RNA:DNA duplexes within this region and that disruption of these duplexes can reactivate the *FMR1* gene in FXS cell lines also suggests that *FMR1* intron 1 upstream of the 3′ boundary should be considered as part of the *FMR1* promoter [26]. Together with our previous findings and those from this study, this evidence indicates that the boundaries of the *FMR1* promoter and the model of epigenetic regulation of *FMR1* should be redefined to include *FMR1* intron 1 CpG sites expanding up to the 3′ epigenetic boundary targeted by the FREE2(E) assay (Figures 2 and 3).

3.2. Hypomethylation of FMR1 Intron 2: Novel FXS Biomarkers

Earlier, we found that the CpG sites proximal to the *ASFMR1* transcription start site within *FMR1* intron 2, which we named FREE3 [16], were hypomethylated in FXS lymphoblast cell lines lacking FMRP, with reduced *ASFMR1* expression compared with the controls and UFM cell lines [16]. Here, we showed that in the primary cells from the blood, the same CpG sites also had significantly decreased methylation in the FM, PM/FM CGG size and methylation mosaic males and females compared with the control, PM, and UFM groups. In addition, consistent with our previous and current observations of FXS-specific hypomethylation in intron 2, Alisch et al. [27] described the results for one CpG site within intron 2 that showed FXS-specific hypomethylation, which partially overlapped with the range of methylation values for the controls. In this study, we found that (F3)CpG1 showed the most significant decrease in methylation in the FM FXS groups in both males and females compared with the controls and compared with the 'high-functioning' males with UFM alleles (Figure S3). This suggests that decreased methylation of intron 2, specifically for the sites proximal to the *ASFMR1* promoter, are novel epigenetic biomarkers hypomethylated in individuals with FM alleles.

3.3. Hypomethylation of the 3′ Epigenetic Boundary in Individuals with a PM

This is the first study to identify several epigenetic biomarkers at the novel 3′ epigenetic boundary that are differentially methylated in all males with a PM. We found that in males with a PM, methylation of the 3′ boundary was decreased compared with the control group, regardless of whether all 39 PM males were considered as one group or split into two independent cohorts based on the site of recruitment. Females with a PM also showed significantly decreased methylation at the 3′ boundary and several CpG sites downstream of the boundary compared with the controls ((E)CpG4, 5, and 6) (Figure S4). These markers therefore have the potential to be used to screen for the presence of PM alleles using DNA methylation testing.

3.4. Differentially Methylated Regions Associated with Expanded FMR1 Alleles and X Chromosome Inactivation Conserved between Tissues

This study has demonstrated the following: (1) The 3′ epigenetic boundary identified by the FREE2(E) assay is lost in the brain tissues (as in the venous blood) in males with FXS but not in the controls with normal-sized alleles. All CpG sites within the FREE2 region 5′ of the 3′ epigenetic boundary were hypermethylated in the examined brain tissues of males with FXS compared with the controls, as in the venous blood. (2) The mean methylation for 40 CpG sites spanning across a 1.5 kB region within *FMR1* intron 1 at the 3′ epigenetic boundary in the venous blood and all brain tissues of the female controls with alleles in the normal range was significantly elevated compared with those tissues from the male controls. This strongly suggests that X inactivation causes an increase in DNA methylation across tissues, spanning from FREE2(A) to the 3′ epigenetic boundary identified by the FREE2(E) assay. (3) Differential methylation sensitive to X inactivation within *FMR1* intron 1 up to the 3′ epigenetic boundary was conserved between different regions of the brain in the female controls (prefrontal cortex and cerebellum). This observation highlights the functional importance of the 3′ epigenetic boundary identified in this study.

Interestingly, the CpG sites downstream of the 3′ epigenetic boundary within *FMR1* introns 1 and 2 showed hypomethylation in the females compared to the male controls. This, however, was not preserved in the blood, suggesting that this X inactivation-specific hypomethylation was restricted to the brain tissues. In the male controls, these CpG sites also showed significantly decreased methylation in the brain tissues compared with the venous blood of the male controls. Together, these fundings suggest that the 3′ epigenetic boundary defined in this study is of functional significance, playing a role as an 'insulator' to prevent a 'methylation spillover' from the gene bogy of *FMR1* to the *FMR1* promoter conserved across different tissues. This postulate is in line with the location of a CTCF binding site immediately at 5′ of this boundary (Figure 1), which has been described to act as such an insulator in other settings [17].

3.5. Limitations

While this study has several strengths, an important limitation is that no data were available on the level of *FMR1* or *ASFMR1* mRNA, FMRP, or the clinical status (other than for males with a UFM), especially in relation to the presence and severity of *FMR1*-associated disorders in the individuals with PM and FM alleles included in this study. Moreover, functional studies were not performed to examine how loss of the 3′ epigenetic boundary impacts the binding of CTCF and expression of *FMR1*, *ASFMR1*, and FMRP. Future studies should explore (1) the clinical significance of this PM-specific 3′ boundary hypomethylation and how it may be related to the levels of *FMR1* and *ASFMR1* RNA toxicity, as well as the levels of FMRP in different tissues, and (2) the functional significance of its loss and gain in different cell types.

Another limitation is the relatively small number of brain tissues included in this study. Because FXS is a rare disorder, the numbers (4 FXS for PFC and 12 controls for PFC and cerebella) are reasonable to support the main conclusions, with large-sized effects regarding: (1) conservation of the 3′ epigenetic boundary between tissues in the controls examined, (2) its complete loss due to the presence of an FM, and (3) its relationship with X-inactivation. The relatively small sample size for brain tissues included in this study should be also viewed in light of previous studies [28,29] examining molecular changes in brain tissues from individuals with FXS and the controls, which had a comparable number of brain samples used. Future studies should re-examine our observations in larger cohorts and in different brain regions than those examined in this study.

3.6. Conclusions

In summary, this study has characterized 45 novel epigenetic biomarker sites where differential methylation is associated with the presence of expanded *FMR1* alleles (but not in high-functioning males with UFM alleles) and X inactivation. These patterns of methylation were also conserved between blood and brain tissues based on comparisons between individuals with FM alleles affected by FXS and neurotypical controls, as well as between the controls of different sexes. Importantly, almost all males with a PM were found to have methylation levels of the 3′ epigenetic boundary in their venous blood below the control range. Significantly decreased methylation of the CpG sites proximal to this boundary was also observed in females with a PM. Therefore, the methylation status of the 3′ boundary and proximal sites may provide a novel way to screen for PM alleles using DNA methylation testing and may have potential diagnostic and prognostic relevance to *FMR1*-associated disorders, which should be examined in future studies.

While FXTAS, FXPOI, and other comorbidities have been linked to PM alleles [30–33], these are of incomplete penetrance, with no avenues currently available to predict reliably who is most at risk. Unfortunately, this study did not have formal assessment or clinical status information available for individuals with PM alleles that would have allowed examination of the relationships between the phenotype(s) and the levels of hypomethylation of the 3′ epigenetic boundary. Future studies should explore the clinical significance of this PM-specific 3′ boundary hypomethylation and how or if it may be used as a prognostic biomarker to predict who is most at risk of developing PM-associated disorders.

4. Materials and Methods

4.1. Cohort Description

This study examined methylation in DNA samples from a total of 557 participants, which were collected as parts of previous studies [8,14,21,34]. The cohort consisted of 185 males (aged from birth to 82 years) and 372 females (aged from birth to 80 years). For the males, there were 20 controls (CGG < 40), 39 PM males, 5 UFM males (identified through cascade testing and determined to be unmethylated under Southern blot analysis), 73 FXS-affected FM males (identified through investigation of developmental delay or ASD and 100% methylated through Southern blot analysis), 21 FM methylation mosaics, and 27 PM/FM size mosaics under Southern blot analysis. Formal cognitive assessments were performed for three of the UFM males using the Wechsler Intelligence Test, which is appropriate for chronological age, with a Full-Scale IQ (FSIQ) between 71 and 81, as described previously [8,14,35]. For the females, there were 75 controls (CGG < 40), 157 PM females, 132 FM females (identified through investigation of developmental delay and cascade testing), and 8 were mosaics for PM and FM alleles under Southern blot analysis. For 527 individuals with expanded FMR1 alleles and controls, blood DNA was collected as part of FXS cascade testing and routine molecular microarray testing through VCGS and the Greenwood Genetic Center as described previously [21]. These samples were de-identified before use in this study and as such did not have information on formal assessments or clinical history to allow for accurate assessment of heterogeneity in the clinical picture of the presented groups. An additional 30 females with an FM were recruited through the VCGS. All control brain tissues were provided by the Victorian Brain Bank Network with brain tissues from 4 males affected by FXS from earlier studies [28,29] provided by Flora Tassone from the Department of Biochemistry and Molecular Medicine at the University of California's Davis School of Medicine in Sacramento, California, USA. Details on the postmortem brain tissue processing, age, and the clinical phenotype are given in Table S6. This study received ethical approval by The Royal Children's Hospital Human Research Ethics Committee (single site reference numbers HREC 34227 and HREC 33066 and multi-site HREC reference number HREC/13/RCHM/24, approved on 24 May 2013).

4.2. Molecular Analyses

Processing of the venous blood DNA samples and the CGG repeat sizing using PCR was conducted as previously described [36]. For samples with greater than 55 repeats, methylation-sensitive Southern blotting was performed as previously described [3]. Briefly, 7–9 μg of DNA was digested with EcoRI and NruI (located within FMR1 CpG island), and the StB12.3 probe was used to estimate the range of FMR1 allele CGG sizes and CpG island methylation. For the males, Southern blot methylation was used to classify the expanded alleles as either unmethylated, partially methylated, or fully methylated. For the alleles that were estimated to have greater than 150 CGGs and methylated by Southern blotting, the classification of FM was given. The PM allele classification was given to alleles estimated to be between 55 and 200 repeats that were unmethylated by Southern blotting. FMR1 intron 1 and intron 2 methylation was assessed in the same samples using the EpiTYPER system as previously described [3]. The primer sequences and the PCR conditions are listed in Table S5.

4.3. Data Analyses

Testing for normality distribution of MOR was conducted using the Shapiro–Wilk test at a significance level $p = 0.05$. For intergroup comparisons, depending on the results of this test, we used either a two-sample t test for the means if the data were normal or a nonparametric Mann–Whitney test for the median if the data were not normal. All analyses were conducted using the publicly available R statistical computing package [37].

Supplementary Materials: The following supporting information can be downloaded at: https://www.mdpi.com/article/10.3390/ijms241310712/s1.

Author Contributions: D.E.G., Y.I. and D.J.A. made substantial contributions to the conception and design, data acquisition, analysis and interpretation, and compiling the first draft of the manuscript. M.Q.B. made significant contributions to the statistical analysis and data interpretation. C.E.S., D.F., D.J.A. and C.S. provided access to clinical samples and CGG sizing from diagnostic testing. All authors were involved in drafting the article or revising it critically for important intellectual content. All authors have read and agreed to the published version of the manuscript.

Funding: This work was supported by the Victorian government's Operational Infrastructure Support Program, Murdoch Children's Research Institute, Royal Children's Hospital Foundation, National Health and Medical Research Council, an Australia development grant (No. 1017263 to D.E.G.), the E.W. Al Thrasher Award of the USA (to D.E.G.), Martin & E.H. Flack Trust of Australia (to DEG), Pierce Armstrong Trust (to D.E.G.), National Health and Medical Research Council, Australia project grants (Nos. 104299 and 1103389 to D.E.G.), Next Generation Clinical Researchers Program—Career Development Fellowship funded by the Medical Research Future Fund (MRFF1141334 to D.E.G.), and in part by a grant from the South Carolina Department of Disabilities and Special Needs (SCDDSN) to C.E.S.

Institutional Review Board Statement: The study was conducted in accordance with the Declaration of Helsinki, and received ethical approval by The Royal Children's Hospital Human Re-search Ethics Committee (single site reference numbers HREC 34227 and HREC 33066 and multi-site HREC reference number HREC/13/RCHM/24, approved on 24 May 2013).

Informed Consent Statement: Informed consent was obtained from all subjects or if subjects were under 18, it was obtained from a parent and/or legal guardian when their samples were submitted for clinical testing, as part of FXS cascade testing and routine molecular microarray testing through VCGS and the Greenwood Genetic Center as described previously [21]. All samples from these individuals were de-identified before use in this study.

Data Availability Statement: The data that support the findings of this study are available on request from the corresponding author. The data are not publicly available due to privacy or ethical restrictions.

Acknowledgments: The authors would like to thank all study participants and their families for their involvement in this study. We thank Benjamin Ong from the EpiTYPER Platform Facility (MCRI) and Xin Li and Elva Z Shi for performing some of the laboratory work for this study, including methylation analysis and fragile X CGG sizing. We would like to thank the Victorian Brain Bank Network and acknowledge the generosity shown by the donors and donor families in donating tissue for the research presented in this study. We would also like to thank Flora Tassone from the Department of Biochemistry and Molecular Medicine at the University of California's Davis School of Medicine in Sacramento, California, USA for providing brain tissue from four individuals affected by fragile X syndrome from earlier studies [28,29]. This study is dedicated to the memory of Ethan Francis Schwartz (1996–1998).

Conflicts of Interest: D.E.G. and Y.I. are inventors for patents related to the technologies described in this study. D.E.G. is the executive director of E.D.G. Innovations & Consulting, which receives funds from the intellectual property related to these patents. He has also acted as a paid consultant for Bellberry, Ltd. and Actinogen Medical, Pty, Ltd. No other authors have conflicts or competing interests to declare.

Abbreviations

FXS	Fragile X syndrome
FM	Full mutations
PM	Permutation
UFM	FM found to be unmethylated by Southern blot analysis
FMRP	*FMR1* protein
UTR	Untranslated region
FXTAS	Fragile X-associated tremor/ataxia syndrome
FXPOI	fragile X-associated primary ovarian insufficiency
FREE1	Fragile X-Related Epigenetic Element 1
FREE2	Fragile X-Related Epigenetic Element 2
FREE3	Fragile X-Related Epigenetic Element 3
MOR	Methylation output ratio
FMR1-IT1	FMR1 intronic transcript 1
VCGS	Victorian Clinical Genetics Services

References

1. Hagerman, R.J.; Berry-Kravis, E.; Kaufmann, W.E.; Ono, M.Y.; Tartaglia, N.; Lachiewicz, A.; Kronk, R.; Delahunty, C.; Hessl, D.; Visootsak, J.; et al. Advances in the treatment of fragile X syndrome. *Pediatrics* **2009**, *123*, 378–390. [CrossRef] [PubMed]
2. Verkerk, A.J.; Pieretti, M.; Sutcliffe, J.S.; Fu, Y.H.; Kuhl, D.P.; Pizzuti, A.; Reiner, O.; Richards, S.; Victoria, M.F.; Zhang, F.P.; et al. Identification of a gene (FMR-1) containing a CGG repeat coincident with a breakpoint cluster region exhibiting length variation in fragile X syndrome. *Cell* **1991**, *65*, 905–914. [CrossRef] [PubMed]
3. Godler, D.E.; Tassone, F.; Loesch, D.Z.; Taylor, A.K.; Gehling, F.; Hagerman, R.J.; Burgess, T.; Ganesamoorthy, D.; Hennerich, D.; Gordon, L.; et al. Methylation of novel markers of fragile X alleles is inversely correlated with FMRP expression and FMR1 activation ratio. *Hum. Mol. Genet.* **2010**, *19*, 1618–1632. [CrossRef] [PubMed]
4. Loesch, D.Z.; Huggins, R.M.; Hagerman, R.J. Phenotypic variation and FMRP levels in fragile X. *Ment. Retard. Dev. Disabil. Res. Rev.* **2004**, *10*, 31–41. [CrossRef]
5. Nolin, S.L.; Glicksman, A.; Houck, G.E., Jr.; Brown, W.T.; Dobkin, C.S. Mosaicism in fragile X affected males. *Am. J. Med. Genet.* **1994**, *51*, 509–512. [CrossRef]
6. Hagerman, R.J.; Hull, C.E.; Safanda, J.F.; Carpenter, I.; Staley, L.W.; O'Connor, R.A.; Seydel, C.; Mazzocco, M.M.; Snow, K.; Thibodeau, S.N.; et al. High functioning fragile X males: Demonstration of an unmethylated fully expanded FMR-1 mutation associated with protein expression. *Am. J. Med. Genet.* **1994**, *51*, 298–308. [CrossRef]
7. Jarmolowicz, A.I.; Baker, E.K.; Bartlett, E.; Francis, D.; Ling, L.; Gamage, D.; Delatycki, M.B.; Godler, D.E. Fragile X syndrome full mutation in cognitively normal male identified as part of an Australian reproductive carrier screening program. *Am. J. Med. Genet. A* **2021**, *185*, 1498–1503. [CrossRef]
8. Loesch, D.Z.; Sherwell, S.; Kinsella, G.; Tassone, F.; Taylor, A.; Amor, D.; Sung, S.; Evans, A. Fragile X-associated tremor/ataxia phenotype in a male carrier of unmethylated full mutation in the FMR1 gene. *Clin. Genet.* **2012**, *82*, 88–92. [CrossRef]
9. Maenner, M.J.; Baker, M.W.; Broman, K.W.; Tian, J.; Barnes, J.K.; Atkins, A.; McPherson, E.; Hong, J.; Brilliant, M.H.; Mailick, M.R. FMR1 CGG expansions: Prevalence and sex ratios. *Am. J. Med. Genet. Part B Neuropsychiatr. Genet. Off. Publ. Int. Soc. Psychiatr. Genet.* **2013**, *162B*, 466–473. [CrossRef]
10. Kraan, C.M.; Bui, Q.M.; Field, M.; Archibald, A.D.; Metcalfe, S.A.; Christie, L.M.; Bennetts, B.H.; Oertel, R.; Smith, M.J.; du Sart, D.; et al. FMR1 allele size distribution in 35,000 males and females: A comparison of developmental delay and general population cohorts. *Genet. Med.* **2018**, *20*, 1627–1634. [CrossRef]

11. Cornish, K.M.; Kraan, C.M.; Bui, Q.M.; Bellgrove, M.A.; Metcalfe, S.A.; Trollor, J.N.; Hocking, D.R.; Slater, H.R.; Inaba, Y.; Li, X.; et al. Novel methylation markers of the dysexecutive-psychiatric phenotype in FMR1 premutation women. *Neurology* **2015**, *84*, 1631–1638. [CrossRef]
12. Ladd, P.D.; Smith, L.E.; Rabaia, N.A.; Moore, J.M.; Georges, S.A.; Hansen, R.S.; Hagerman, R.J.; Tassone, F.; Tapscott, S.J.; Filippova, G.N. An antisense transcript spanning the CGG repeat region of FMR1 is upregulated in premutation carriers but silenced in full mutation individuals. *Hum. Mol. Genet.* **2007**, *16*, 3174–3187. [CrossRef]
13. Godler, D.E.; Slater, H.R.; Bui, Q.M.; Ono, M.; Gehling, F.; Francis, D.; Amor, D.J.; Hopper, J.L.; Hagerman, R.; Loesch, D.Z. FMR1 intron 1 methylation predicts FMRP expression in blood of female carriers of expanded FMR1 alleles. *J. Mol. Diagn. JMD* **2011**, *13*, 528–536. [CrossRef] [PubMed]
14. Godler, D.E.; Slater, H.R.; Bui, Q.M.; Storey, E.; Ono, M.Y.; Gehling, F.; Inaba, Y.; Francis, D.; Hopper, J.L.; Kinsella, G.; et al. Fragile X mental retardation 1 (FMR1) intron 1 methylation in blood predicts verbal cognitive impairment in female carriers of expanded FMR1 alleles: Evidence from a pilot study. *Clin. Chem.* **2012**, *58*, 590–598. [CrossRef]
15. Godler, D.E. Assay for Determining Epigenetic Profiles of Markers of Fragile x Alleles. Google Patents AU2009900668A, 17 February 2010.
16. Godler, D.E. Treatment and Diagnosis of Epigenetic Disorders and Conditions. Google Patents WO2012019235A1, 16 February 2012.
17. Naumann, A.; Hochstein, N.; Weber, S.; Fanning, E.; Doerfler, W. A distinct DNA-methylation boundary in the 5′-upstream sequence of the FMR1 promoter binds nuclear proteins and is lost in fragile X syndrome. *Am. J. Hum. Genet.* **2009**, *85*, 606–616. [CrossRef] [PubMed]
18. Godler, D. Novel epigenetic markers of the Fragile X alleles. Google Patents PCT/AU2010/000169, 17 February 2010.
19. Khalil, A.M.; Faghihi, M.A.; Modarresi, F.; Brothers, S.P.; Wahlestedt, C. A novel RNA transcript with antiapoptotic function is silenced in fragile X syndrome. *PLoS ONE* **2008**, *3*, e1486. [CrossRef]
20. Kumari, D.; Usdin, K. Interaction of the transcription factors USF1, USF2, and alpha -Pal/Nrf-1 with the FMR1 promoter. Implications for Fragile X mental retardation syndrome. *J. Biol. Chem.* **2001**, *276*, 4357–4364.
21. Godler, D.E.; Inaba, Y.; Shi, E.Z.; Skinner, C.; Bui, Q.M.; Francis, D.; Amor, D.J.; Hopper, J.L.; Loesch, D.Z.; Hagerman, R.J.; et al. Relationships between age and epi-genotype of the FMR1 exon 1/intron 1 boundary are consistent with non-random X-chromosome inactivation in FM individuals, with the selection for the unmethylated state being most significant between birth and puberty. *Hum. Mol. Genet.* **2013**, *22*, 1516–1524. [CrossRef]
22. Bagni, C.; Tassone, F.; Neri, G.; Hagerman, R. Fragile X syndrome: Causes, diagnosis, mechanisms, and therapeutics. *J. Clin. Investig.* **2012**, *122*, 4314–4322. [CrossRef]
23. Pietrobono, R.; Pomponi, M.G.; Tabolacci, E.; Oostra, B.; Chiurazzi, P.; Neri, G. Quantitative analysis of DNA demethylation and transcriptional reactivation of the FMR1 gene in fragile X cells treated with 5-azadeoxycytidine. *Nucleic Acids Res.* **2002**, *30*, 3278–3285. [CrossRef] [PubMed]
24. Kuehnen, P.; Mischke, M.; Wiegand, S.; Sers, C.; Horsthemke, B.; Lau, S.; Keil, T.; Lee, Y.A.; Grueters, A.; Krude, H. An Alu element-associated hypermethylation variant of the POMC gene is associated with childhood obesity. *PLoS Genet.* **2012**, *8*, e1002543. [CrossRef] [PubMed]
25. Shukla, S.; Kavak, E.; Gregory, M.; Imashimizu, M.; Shutinoski, B.; Kashlev, M.; Oberdoerffer, P.; Sandberg, R.; Oberdoerffer, S. CTCF-promoted RNA polymerase II pausing links DNA methylation to splicing. *Nature* **2011**, *479*, 74–79. [CrossRef]
26. Colak, D.; Zaninovic, N.; Cohen, M.S.; Rosenwaks, Z.; Yang, W.Y.; Gerhardt, J.; Disney, M.D.; Jaffrey, S.R. Promoter-bound trinucleotide repeat mRNA drives epigenetic silencing in fragile X syndrome. *Science* **2014**, *343*, 1002–1005. [CrossRef]
27. Alisch, R.S.; Wang, T.; Chopra, P.; Visootsak, J.; Conneely, K.N.; Warren, S.T. Genome-wide analysis validates aberrant methylation in fragile X syndrome is specific to the FMR1 locus. *BMC Med. Genet.* **2013**, *14*, 18. [CrossRef] [PubMed]
28. Hunsaker, M.R.; Greco, C.M.; Tassone, F.; Berman, R.F.; Willemsen, R.; Hagerman, R.J.; Hagerman, P.J. Rare intranuclear inclusions in the brains of 3 older adult males with fragile x syndrome: Implications for the spectrum of fragile x-associated disorders. *J. Neuropathol. Exp. Neurol.* **2011**, *70*, 462–469. [CrossRef]
29. Schwartz, P.H.; Tassone, F.; Greco, C.M.; Nethercott, H.E.; Ziaeian, B.; Hagerman, R.J.; Hagerman, P.J. Neural progenitor cells from an adult patient with fragile X syndrome. *BMC Med. Genet.* **2005**, *6*, 2. [CrossRef]
30. Greco, C.M.; Hagerman, R.J.; Tassone, F.; Chudley, A.E.; Del Bigio, M.R.; Jacquemont, S.; Leehey, M.; Hagerman, P.J. Neuronal intranuclear inclusions in a new cerebellar tremor/ataxia syndrome among fragile X carriers. *Brain* **2002**, *125 Pt 8*, 1760–1771. [CrossRef]
31. Hagerman, R.J.; Leehey, M.; Heinrichs, W.; Tassone, F.; Wilson, R.; Hills, J.; Grigsby, J.; Gage, B.; Hagerman, P.J. Intention tremor, parkinsonism, and generalized brain atrophy in male carriers of fragile X. *Neurology* **2001**, *57*, 127–130. [CrossRef]
32. Jacquemont, S.; Hagerman, R.J.; Leehey, M.A.; Hall, D.A.; Levine, R.A.; Brunberg, J.A.; Zhang, L.; Jardini, T.; Gane, L.W.; Harris, S.W.; et al. Penetrance of the fragile X-associated tremor/ataxia syndrome in a premutation carrier population. *JAMA* **2004**, *291*, 460–469. [CrossRef] [PubMed]
33. Farzin, F.; Perry, H.; Hessl, D.; Loesch, D.; Cohen, J.; Bacalman, S.; Gane, L.; Tassone, F.; Hagerman, P.; Hagerman, R. Autism spectrum disorders and attention-deficit/hyperactivity disorder in boys with the fragile X premutation. *J. Dev. Behav. Pediatr.* **2006**, *27* (Suppl. S2), S137–S144. [CrossRef] [PubMed]

34. Aliaga, S.M.; Slater, H.R.; Francis, D.; Du Sart, D.; Li, X.; Amor, D.J.; Alliende, A.M.; Santa Maria, L.; Faundes, V.; Morales, P.; et al. Identification of Males with Cryptic Fragile X Alleles by Methylation-Specific Quantitative Melt Analysis. *Clin. Chem.* **2016**, *62*, 343–352. [CrossRef] [PubMed]
35. Tassone, F.; Hagerman, R.J.; Loesch, D.Z.; Lachiewicz, A.; Taylor, A.K.; Hagerman, P.J. Fragile X males with unmethylated, full mutation trinucleotide repeat expansions have elevated levels of FMR1 messenger RNA. *Am. J. Med. Genet.* **2000**, *94*, 232–236. [CrossRef] [PubMed]
36. Khaniani, M.S.; Kalitsis, P.; Burgess, T.; Slater, H.R. An improved Diagnostic PCR Assay for identification of Cryptic Heterozygosity for CGG Triplet Repeat Alleles in the Fragile X Gene (FMR1). *Mol. Cytogenet.* **2008**, *1*, 5. [CrossRef]
37. RDevelopmentCoreTeam. *A Language and Environment for Statistical Computing*; R Foundation for statistical computing; The R Foundation: Indianapolis, IN, USA, 2009.

Disclaimer/Publisher's Note: The statements, opinions and data contained in all publications are solely those of the individual author(s) and contributor(s) and not of MDPI and/or the editor(s). MDPI and/or the editor(s) disclaim responsibility for any injury to people or property resulting from any ideas, methods, instructions or products referred to in the content.

Review

DNA Methylation Episignatures in Neurodevelopmental Disorders Associated with Large Structural Copy Number Variants: Clinical Implications

Kathleen Rooney [1,2] and Bekim Sadikovic [1,2,*]

1. Department of Pathology and Laboratory Medicine, Western University, London, ON N6A 3K7, Canada; kathleen.rooney@lhsc.on.ca
2. Verspeeten Clinical Genome Centre, London Health Sciences Centre, London, ON N6A 5W9, Canada
* Correspondence: bekim.sadikovic@lhsc.on.ca; Tel.: +1-519-685-8500 (ext. 53074)

Abstract: Large structural chromosomal deletions and duplications, referred to as copy number variants (CNVs), play a role in the pathogenesis of neurodevelopmental disorders (NDDs) through effects on gene dosage. This review focuses on our current understanding of genomic disorders that arise from large structural chromosome rearrangements in patients with NDDs, as well as difficulties in overlap of clinical presentation and molecular diagnosis. We discuss the implications of epigenetics, specifically DNA methylation (DNAm), in NDDs and genomic disorders, and consider the implications and clinical impact of copy number and genomic DNAm testing in patients with suspected genetic NDDs. We summarize evidence of global methylation episignatures in CNV-associated disorders that can be used in the diagnostic pathway and may provide insights into the molecular pathogenesis of genomic disorders. Finally, we discuss the potential for combining CNV and DNAm assessment into a single diagnostic assay.

Keywords: DNA methylation; episignature; epigenetics; copy number variant; neurodevelopmental disorder; genomic disorder

1. Introduction

Neurodevelopmental disorders (NDDs) are a class of neurological and neuropsychiatric conditions that manifest in childhood during the developmental phase and persist throughout life [1]. They affect development of the central nervous system and can lead to brain dysfunction, resulting in limitations or impairment in cognition, motor performance, vision, hearing, speech and behavior [2]. NDDs include, but are not limited to, autistic spectrum disorder (ASD), intellectual disability (ID), attention deficit hyperactivity disorder (ADHD) and epilepsy, all of which show high rates of comorbidity and phenotypic overlap [3]. They are estimated to affect approximately 3% of children worldwide [4,5] and therefore, collectively represent a significant impact to families and health care systems.

NDDs present with a broad range of genetic and phenotypic heterogeneity, and clinical presentations are often non-specific. Genetics plays an important role in the etiology of hereditary NDDs. Genetic mutations associated with NDDs vary in size from single nucleotide variants (SNVs) to whole chromosome aneuploidies [6]. Due to the phenotypic overlap exhibited, in addition to targeted gene sequencing approaches, genetic testing often involves global genomic screening including chromosomal microarray analysis (CMA), exome or whole genome sequencing (WES, WGS), or classically G-banded chromosome karyotyping (karyotyping). CMA, considered the first-tier diagnostic test for patients with NDDs, has been used clinically for nearly two decades [7,8] to detect structural imbalances involving deletion or duplication of genetic material, collectively termed copy number variants (CNVs). Whilst some of the first CMAs included bacterial artificial chromosome

(BAC) clones in an array-based comparative genomic hybridization (aCGH) with genome-wide coverage at approximately 1 Mb intervals [9,10], more recent platforms involving oligonucleotide or high-resolution single nucleotide polymorphism (SNP) arrays may reach a resolution of a few hundred base pairs [11,12]. Therefore, genomic imbalances beyond the resolution of karyotyping (minimum detection sizes 3–7 Mb) [13,14] are now routinely detected. SNP arrays offer the highest resolution of commercially available microarrays and are designed to determine genotype, structural imbalances, genomic aneuploidy, and loss of heterozygosity [15].

Microarray platforms can be customized to increase coverage and resolution in clinically relevant regions and regions associated with well-defined genomic syndromes. In addition to probe-coverage enriched regions, clinical use microarray platforms have probes equally spaced across the rest of the genome, termed "backbone" coverage. The combination of high probe densities and optimized targeted design is aimed at reducing the rate of ambiguous findings termed variants of uncertain significance (VUSs), since, at this time, there is a limited understanding of the impact of CNVs outside of protein coding regions.

2. The Role of CNVs in Genomic Disorders

Structural variants, defined as "alterations that involve segments of DNA larger than 1 kb" [13], include CNVs linked to phenotypic variation and disease susceptibility [16]. CNVs can contain millions of nucleotides, multiple genes and regulatory elements. Tuzun et al. suggested that individuals carry on average 250 CNVs [17]. As such, compared with SNVs, CNVs are reported to be responsible for more than ten times the total heritable sequence differences observed in the general population [18]. CNVs are also described as polymorphisms in association with several non-pathological conditions, e.g., those involved in variation in olfactory perception [19]. The presence of CNVs in non-pathological conditions can present challenges in the interpretation and classification of variants, especially in the absence of functional studies.

Genomic disorders are a group of genetic conditions caused by CNVs affecting dosage sensitive genes or genes critical for normal development or maintenance and/or their regulatory elements [20]. Recurrent disorders, those with common start and stop breakpoints, include CNVs that are similar in size and gene content, and typically present with similar phenotypes, e.g., deletions and duplications of 17p11.2 (Smith–Magenis and Potocki–Lupski syndrome), 7q11.23 (Williams syndrome), 15q11.2 (Prader–Willi/Angelman syndrome) and 17q21.31 (Koolen–de Vries syndrome) [6,21,22]. In contrast, non-recurrent disorders show variability in size and gene content (typically there is a common region of overlap). Phenotypes in these patients vary substantially, e.g., deletions of 22q13.3 in Phelan–McDermid syndrome (PHMDS) or deletions of 9q34.3 in Kleefstra syndrome [6].

Segmental duplications (also known as low copy repeats; LCRs) are blocks of DNA ranging from 1–400 kb that occur throughout the genome and typically share a high level (>90%) of sequence identity [23,24]. Many structural rearrangements, including CNVs, are mediated by LCRs through non-allelic homologous recombination (NAHR) [25]. These LCRs are highly prone to rearrangements which can result in genomic imbalances, including those associated with the common CNV-related disorders.

A recent study assessed the prevalence and inheritance of CNVs associated with NDDs and estimated recurrent CNVs present in approximately 1 in 200 live births [26]. These results indicate that while individual CNVs may be rare, collectively they contribute significantly to NDDs. The most common CNVs observed in NDDs are those associated with genomic disorders [6], and a recent study estimated deletions of the 16p11.2 proximal region, 17q12, and 1q21.1 regions, and duplications of 15q11.2, 22q11.2, and the 16p11.2 distal region as the most common [26]. These findings vary from previous studies where duplications of 2q13 and deletions of 22q11.2, 15q11.2 and 1p36 were among the most common [21]. These differences likely reflect increased resolution of microarray platforms, as well as a decrease in ascertainment bias.

Considerable research to date has focused on genes within the CNV regions of genomic disorders and how dosage sensitivity may be responsible for the observed phenotypes. While this research has identified some causative or candidate genes for specific Mendelian disorders and phenotypes, the genetic contribution for the majority of the observed clinical phenotypes in CNV disorders are not well defined [21]. One example of a disorder where a contributory gene has been identified is the 5q35 deletion. 5q35 deletion is predominantly mediated by NAHR and is associated with Sotos syndrome 1, where haploinsufficiency of the nuclear receptor-binding set domain protein (*NSD1*) gene contained within this region is shown, on its own, to be causative for Sotos [27]. This is similar to findings in Smith–Magenis syndrome, where deletions of 17p11.2 are responsible for 90% of causative variants, while approximately 5% are the result of point mutations in the retinoic acid-induced 1 (*RAI1*) gene contained within this region [22–28]. This is in contrast to disorders such as 16p11.2 and 22q11.2 deletion and duplication syndromes where no single candidate gene has been identified.

Overall, CNVs may contribute to the clinical features observed in genomic disorders through dosage sensitivity, via haploinsufficiency (as described for Sotos and Smith–Magenis), triplosensitivity (e.g., 22q11.2 duplication syndrome) or imprinting effects (Prader-Willi and Angelman syndromes), or through disruption of gene expression via positional effects, including disruption of transcriptional regulatory elements and changes in the chromatin structure.

3. Clinical Identification of CNVs in Patients with NDDs

CMA screening for CNVs in patients with NDDs has an estimated diagnostic yield of approximately 15–20% [21–29], which is a significant increase from karyotyping (3%) [7]. Newer molecular techniques such as WES or WGS in patients with developmental delay (DD) or ID have a reported diagnostic yield of approximately 25–36% [30–33]. Although these technological advancements have improved diagnostic capabilities in these disorders, half to two thirds of patients with suspected genetic conditions remain without a diagnosis [32–34].

This 'diagnostic odyssey', the time from initial consultation to diagnosis, often involves multiple clinical evaluations and laboratory tests spanning years [35,36], resulting in significant social and economic burden on both families and health care systems. In addition to CMA as the first-tier screen [7], in males with DD it is often accompanied by assessment for Fragile-X syndrome (FRX). FRX is an X-linked dominant condition and the most common inherited cause of ID. FRX results from abnormal expansion of the CGG trinucleotide repeat (>200 repeats) located in the promoter of the fragile X messenger ribonucleoprotein 1 (*FMR1*) gene, resulting in promotor DNA hypermethylation and gene silencing [37]. FRX can also be the result of deletions of Xq27.3 containing the *FMR1* gene [38]. Reflexive genetic testing, whereby the results of previous tests are used to guide further investigations, include DNA methylation (DNAm) analysis in individuals with CNVs at common imprinting loci, e.g., 15q11.1 and 11p15.5 regions. The average time to diagnosis in patients referred for genetic testing is estimated at 1–8 years [7,35–39], and the cost to healthcare is often difficult to estimate or missing from research. Recent studies describe the substantial positive medical and psychosocial outcome of receiving a genetic diagnosis [40,41]. Therefore, development of novel diagnostic technologies or testing strategies to shorten the diagnostic odyssey or increase the diagnostic yield represent an ongoing priority in NDD research [42].

Many recent studies have demonstrated disruption of genomic DNAm as a functional consequence of genetic defects in patients with NDDs [43–46]. There is emerging evidence of similar DNAm disruptions as epigenetic biomarkers for CNV disorders and their associated clinical phenotypes.

4. The Role of Epigenetics in NDDs and Subsequent Episignature Mapping

Epigenetics refers to mitotically heritable gene regulatory mechanisms without changes in the DNA sequence [47,48]. Epigenetic regulation of gene expression occurs at the level of chromatin and typically involves processes that modify chromatin or histones, the proteins around which DNA is wrapped, or covalent modifications in the associated DNA molecule [49]. DNAm is the most extensively studied epigenetic modification and refers to the mechanism of addition or removal of a methyl group to cytosine nucleotides [50]. Most cytosines subject to DNAm are adjacent to guanine residues and referred to as CpG dinucleotides (CpGs) [50]. High density clusters of CpGs, often associated with gene promoters, are referred to as CpG islands [50]. Unmethylated (hypomethylated) CpGs and CpG islands are generally associated with open, transcriptionally accessible chromatin, while DNA hypermethylation correlates with compact, transcriptionally repressive chromatin [51]. The majority of CpGs in the human genome are methylated except for those contained within CpG islands [52]. Therefore, in addition to affecting chromatin states and stability, disruptions in DNAm patterns can alter gene expression [51].

An increasing number of chromatin and epigenetic regulatory genes are becoming implicated in a variety of NDDs. Mutations in these genes result in DNAm episignatures, whole genome methylation changes, which are routinely detectable in the peripheral blood of patients affected by these disorders [43]. An episignature is defined as a recurring epigenetic pattern associated with a common genetic or environmental etiology in a disorder-specific patient population. Episignatures are highly sensitive and specific biomarkers that can be used to help resolve ambiguous clinical and genetic findings, and for screening patients with suspected genetic conditions [45]. Episignatures have the potential to provide insight into functional effects of certain mutations and genomic alterations on widespread DNAm and their contribution to the pathophysiology of genetic disorders [46].

Histone modifications refer to the chemical modification of histone tails by processes including methylation, acetylation, phosphorylation and ubiquitination. Histone tails are loosely structured protein segments that can mediate interaction between nucleosomes, and their modifications can result in either condensed or more relaxed chromatin, ultimately exhibiting an effect on gene transcription, as well as accessibility of DNA to other chromatin remodeling factors, including those involved in DNA methylation. Our group and others have identified unique episignatures in multiple NDDs that are the consequence of mutations in genes associated with histone modification [44], including, e.g., Kabuki syndrome caused by mutations in the lysine-specific methyltransferase 2D gene (*KMT2D*) [53]. We have mapped episignatures in several other histone modifying genes including lysine-specific methyltransferase 2B (*KMT2B*), set domain-containing protein 2 (*SETD2*), creb-binding protein (*CREBBP*), lysine acetyltransferase 6A (*KAT6A*) and lysine demethylase 4B (*KDM4B*) [43]. In addition, unique episignatures have also been reported in genes associated with the removal of histone methylation marks, the so-called "eraser" genes, such as the histone lysine demethylase 5C gene (*KDM5C*) in Claes–Jensen syndrome [54]. Histone modifications work in concert with DNAm to affect chromatin remodeling and gene expression.

The DNAm reaction is catalyzed by enzymes known as DNA methyltransferases (DNMT), which are responsible for mediating the transfer of the methyl group from S-adenosylmethionine (SAM) to cytosine residues. Robust episignatures have been reported in NDDs caused by mutations in the DNA methyltransferase genes *DNMT1*, *DNMT3A* and *DNMT3B* [44,55]. These genes are involved in the establishment and maintenance of DNAm during DNA replication and are termed "writers" since they are responsible for the addition of the methyl group to cytosines. Unique episignatures in two disorders are associated with mutations in *DNMT1*, hereditary sensory neuropathy with dementia and hearing loss (HSNDHL), and autosomal dominant cerebellar ataxia, deafness and narcolepsy (ADCADN) ([56,57]), while loss of function mutations in *DNMT3A* result in an episignature in Tatton–Brown–Rahman syndrome (TBRS) [44,58]. Mutations in *DNMT3B*, which cause immunodeficiency, centromere instability and facial anomalies (ICF) syndrome, also result in genomic defects in DNAm [59]. We recently demonstrated a genome-wide DNA hypermethylation episignature in a DNA demethylation gene Tet methylcytosine dioxygenase 3 (*TET3*), an "eraser" gene that opposes the writer function of *DNMT1* [60]. Mutations in the highly conserved catalytic domain of TET3 cause Beck–Fahrner syndrome (BEFAHRS). Inheritance patterns of BEFAHRS vary and include autosomal dominant or recessive forms [61]. Through episignature mapping, we were able to differentiate between affected individuals with mono- and bi-allelic mutations [60].

To date, chromatin remodeling genes comprise the largest group of epigenetic modifier genes with mapped episignatures, e.g., truncating mutations in the SNF2-related CBP activator protein gene (*SRCAP*) result in an episignature specific for Floating-Harbor syndrome [62]. Schenkel et al. reported a unique methylation profile associated with mutations in the ATRX chromatin remodeler gene *ATRX* in alpha-thalassemia X-linked intellectual disability syndrome [63]. In addition, our group previously described a shared DNAm episignature in Coffrin–Siris and Nicolaides–Baraitser syndromes (NCBRS) [64], which are two phenotypically similar NDDs associated with mutations in subunits of the BAF chromatin remodeling complex (commonly referred to as BAFopathies). This study described a shared BAFopathies episignature and supported the findings from previous studies suggesting that these conditions represent a disease spectrum rather than two distinct disorders [65]. Furthermore, this study indicates that methylation analysis may uncover or provide further support for the "relatedness" of genes and their disorders. In a subsequent study by our group, we described a new syndrome involving the BAF complex and the SWI/SNF-related matrix-associated, actin-dependent regulator of the chromatin gene (*SMARCA2*)—a gene reported in multiple individuals with NCBRS. This new syndrome was identified based on unique methylation patterns observed in individuals with intragenic variants located in the helicase domain of the *SMARCA2* gene compared to individuals with pathogenic variants located outside the helicase domain [66]. In support of these findings, clinical features of patients with *SMARCA2* helicase domain mutations exhibited a common phenotype distinct from NCBRS. Similarly, functional studies in yeast supported a different molecular mechanism underlying these two disorders [66]. Therefore, by analyzing variants from multiple regions within a gene, we were able to identify two unique episignatures and uncover functional data to explain the phenotypic differences seen between patients harboring variants in the same gene, resulting in the discovery of a new syndrome.

Interestingly, two distinct domain-specific episignatures have also been described in Helsmoortel-van der Aa syndrome associated with dominant negative truncating mutations in the activity-dependent neuroprotector homeobox gene (*ADNP*), which has chromatin regulatory functions [67]. These signatures were partially opposing, with mutations in the N- and C-terminus resulting in a predominantly hypomethylated signature; in contrast, mutations centered on the nuclear localization sequence resulted in a predominant hypermethylation signature. A subsequent study confirmed phenotypic differences between patients that correlated with the two episignatures [68].

Genes whose primary function is not associated with epigenetic and chromatin regulatory mechanisms, such as ubiquitin-conjugating enzyme E2 A (*UBE2A*) and spermine synthase (*SMS*) in X-linked syndromic forms of mental retardation—Nascimento and Snyder–Robinson types, respectively [44]—have also shown evidence of unique episignatures. The *UBE2A* gene at Xq24 encodes the RAD6 ubiquitin-conjugating enzyme and has been recently shown to be involved in histone modifications that control gene expression [69,70]. The *SMS* gene at Xp22.11 encodes for an enzyme involved in polyamine synthesis and recycling and is directly related to decarboxylated SAM. Previous studies have suggested that alterations in this polyamine synthesis could result in an excess of SAM and may lead to aberrant DNAm status [71].

Taken together, these studies show that DNAm episignatures can be detected in genes with various functions and provide strong evidence for the clinical utility of episignatures as diagnostic biomarkers in NDDs [43,44,72], while also enabling broader understanding of the clinical associations and biological roles of DNAm in genetic disorders.

5. Current Episignature Detection in NDDs

We recently described an approach to episignature mapping and development of a clinical EpiSign classifier in 65 genetic syndromes [43] involving bisulfite converted peripheral blood samples analyzed using methylation microarrays. Blood presents itself as the ideal tissue type for episignature development as it is a common clinical sample type and is easily accessible. Since episignatures represent a fundamental defect in NDDs caused by genetic variation in the germline, DNAm changes will be present in all subsequent tissues. This microarray technology enables a genome-wide, cost-effective, standardized, scalable and high throughput assessment of DNAm patterns, amenable to clinical validation in a diagnostic laboratory setting. This technology enables simultaneous assessment of up to 850,000 CpGs across the genome. By applying a custom bioinformatic pipeline to the methylation data obtained from these arrays, we are able to identify sensitive and disorder-specific episignatures. Using unsupervised machine learning models (MLMs), the sensitivity of an episignature can be assessed. Construction of multiclass supervised MLMs to compare a patient's DNAm data against controls and samples from other clinically validated episignatures at the same time, through the use of an expansive tissue-specific database, should be applied to confirm the specificity of a signature [44]. These methods rely on the ability to perform concurrent assessment of multiple disorders and controls, and highlights the importance of development of large-scale reference databases. To use episignatures in different tissues, a reference database would be required to establish the unique DNAm changes in the particular tissue that arise in development during differentiation and determine how this may impact the specific episignature. Our group has focused on episignatures in blood and has not assessed peripheral blood episignatures in other tissue types. Use of these supervised and unsupervised MLMs is also important when we consider the scalability of testing, as the list of episignatures continues to expand, requiring these algorithms to be capable of handling large amounts of data and computations in a cost-effective and timely fashion.

The ability to detect episignatures is highly contingent upon the intensity (effect size) and extent (number of differentially methylated CpGs) of the observed DNAm changes [44]. Some disorders, such as Sotos or TBRS, are associated with robust changes to the extent of involvement of tens of thousands of CpGs. In contrast, disorders such as the BAFopathies only exhibit a few hundred differentially methylated CpGs [64]. In light of this, sample size can play a role in the ability to detect episignatures in disorders associated with mild or moderate DNAm changes.

When analyzing methylation effects, it is important to consider confounding biological factors such as age, sex and blood cell composition, which are known to be associated with changes in methylation patterns in healthy individuals [73,74]. Methods should be in place to account for such factors when trying to decipher which observed methylation changes contribute to the underlying NDD.

To identify regions containing methylation changes, referred to as differentially methylated regions (DMRs), a 'bump hunting' approach [75] can be used, which typically considers regions containing 3–5 CpGs with greater than 10% methylation change between case samples and controls, and gaps of no more than 500 bp between neighboring CpGs [53]. DMRs can be useful in determining significant downstream effects of gene disruption and pathogenesis of disorders such as up- and down-regulated gene expression.

The complex bioinformatic pipeline required to identify episignatures, and to overcome previously mentioned confounding variables, relies heavily on a large-scale tissue-specific reference DNAm database, as well as bioinformatic and clinical genetic expertise [45]. Broadening utility of episignature assessment in the clinical setting involve screening of patients with suspected NDDs, as well as a functional assay for reclassification of VUSs.

6. The Use of Episignatures in the Diagnosis of NDDs

EpiSign is a clinical genome-wide DNAm test that has been available since 2019 that can detect over 60 disorders in more than 80 genes associated with Mendelian disorders through assessment of peripheral blood DNA [43]. A list of the current disorders detectable by EpiSign version 3 are listed in Table 1.

Table 1. EpiSign v3 assay gene content.

Syndrome	Episignature Abbreviation	Underlying Gene(s) or Region	OMIM
Alpha-thalassemia mental retardation syndrome	ATRX	ATRX	301040
Angelman syndrome	Angelman	UBE3A	105830
Arboleda–Tham syndrome	ARTHS	KAT6A	616268
Autism, susceptibility to, 18	AUTS18	CHD8	615032
Beck–Fahrner syndrome	BEFAHRS	TET3	618798
Beckwith–Wiedemann syndrome	BWS	Chr11p15 (ICR1, KCNQ1OT1, CDKN1C)	130650
Blepharophimosis intellectual disability SMARCA2 syndrome	BIS	SMARCA2	619293
Börjeson–Forssman–Lehmann syndrome	BFLS	PHF6	301900
Cerebellar ataxia, deafness, and narcolepsy, autosomal dominant	ADCADN	DNMT1	604121
CHARGE syndrome	CHARGE	CHD7	214800
Chr16p11.2 deletion syndrome	Chr16p11.2del	Chr16p11.2 deletion	611913
Coffin–Siris syndrome-1, 2 (CSS1,2)	CSS_c.6200	ARID1A; ARID1B	135900; 614607
Coffin–Siris 1–4 (CSS1–4) and Nicolaides–Baraitser syndrome (NCBRS)	BAFopathy	ARID1B; ARID1A; SMARCB1; SMARCA4; SMARCA2	135900; 614607; 614608; 614609; 601358
Coffin–Siris syndrome-4 (CSS4)	CSS_c.2656	SMARCA4	614609
Coffin–Siris syndrome-9 (CSS9)	CSS9	SOX11	615866
Cohen–Gibson syndrome; Weaver syndrome	PRC2	EED; EZH2	617561; 277590
Cornelia de Lange syndromes 1–4	CdLS	NIPBL; SMC1A; SMC3; RAD21	122470; 300590; 610759; 614701
Down syndrome	Down	Chr21 trisomy	190685
Dystonia-28, childhood onset	DYT28	KMT2B	617284
Epileptic encephalopathy, childhood onset	EEOC	CHD2	615369
Floating-Harbour syndrome	FLHS	SRCAP	136140
Fragile X syndrome	FXS	FMR1	300624
Gabriele de Vries syndrome	GADEVS	YY1	617557
Genitopatellar syndrome (see also Ohdo syndrome, SBBYSS variant)	GTPTS	KAT6B	606170
Helsmoortel–Van der Aa syndrome (ADNP syndrome (Central))	HVDAS_C	ADNP	615873

Table 1. Cont.

Syndrome	Episignature Abbreviation	Underlying Gene(s) or Region	OMIM
Helsmoortel–Van der Aa syndrome (ADNP syndrome (Terminal))	HVDAS_T	ADNP	615873
Hunter–McAlpine craniosynostosis syndrome	HMA	Chr5q35-qter duplication	601379
Immunodeficiency, centromeric instability, facial anomalies syndrome 1 (ICF1)	ICF_1	DNMT3B	242860
Immunodeficiency, centromeric instability, facial anomalies syndrome 2,3,4 (ICF2,3,4)	ICF_2_3_4	ZBTB24; CDCA7; HELLS	614069; 616910; 616911
Intellectual developmental disorder-65	KDM4B	KDM4B	619320
Intellectual developmental disorder with seizures and language delay	IDDSELD	SETD1B	619000
Intellectual developmental disorder, X-linked 93	MRX93	BRWD3	300659
Intellectual developmental disorder, X-linked 97	MRX97	ZNF711	300803
Intellectual developmental disorder, X-linked, Snyder–Robinson type	MRXSSR	SMS	309583
Intellectual developmental disorder, X-linked, syndromic, Armfield type	MRXSA	FAM50A	300261
Intellectual developmental disorder, X-linked, syndromic, Claes-Jensen type	MRXSCJ	KDM5C	300534
Intellectual developmental disorder, X-linked syndromic, Nascimento-type	MRXSN	UBE2A	300860
Kabuki syndromes 1, 2	Kabuki	KMT2D; KDM6A	147920; 300867
Kagami–Ogatta syndrome	KOS	Chr14q32	608149
KDM2B-related syndrome	KDM2B	KDM2B	unofficial
Kleefstra syndrome 1	Kleefstra	EHMT1	610253
Koolen de Vries syndrome	KDVS	KANSL1	610443
Luscan–Lumish syndrome	LLS	SETD2	616831
Menke–Hennekam syndrome-1, 2	MKHK_ID4	CREBBP; EP300	618332; 618333
Mental retardation, autosomal dominant 23	MRD23	SETD5	615761
Mental retardation, autosomal dominant 51	MRD51	KMT5B	617788
Mental retardation, FRA12A type	DIP2B	DIP2B	136630
Myopathy, lactic acidosis, and sideroblastic anemia-2	MLASA2	YARS2	613561

Table 1. Cont.

Syndrome	Episignature Abbreviation	Underlying Gene(s) or Region	OMIM
Ohdo syndrome, SBBYSS variant	SBBYSS	KAT6B	603736
Phelan–McDermid syndrome	PHMDS	Chr22q13.3 deletion	606232
Prader–Willi syndrome	PWS	Chr15q11 (SNRPN, NDN)	176270
Rahman syndrome	RMNS	HIST1H1E	617537
Renpenning syndrome	RENS1	PQBP1	309500
Rubinstein–Taybi syndrome 1	RSTS1	CREBBP	180849
Rubinstein–Taybi syndrome-1, 2	RSTS	CREBBP; EP300	180849; 613684
Rubinstein–Taybi syndrome-2	RSTS2	EP300	613684
Silver–Russell syndrome 1	SRS1	Chr11p15.5	180860
Silver–Russell syndrome 2	SRS2	Chr7p11.2	618905
Sotos syndrome 1	Sotos	NSD1	117550
Tatton–Brown–Rahman syndrome	TBRS	DNMT3A	615879
Temple syndrome	Temple	Chr14q32	616222
Velocardiofacial syndrome	VCFS	Chr22q11.2 deletion	192430
Wiedemann–Steiner syndrome	WDSTS	KMT2A	605130
Williams–Beuren deletion syndrome (Chr7q11.23 deletion syndrome)	Williams	Chr7q11.23 deletion	194050
Williams–Beuren duplication syndrome (Chr7q11.23 duplication syndrome)	Dup7	Chr7q11.23 duplication	609757
Wolf-Hirschhorn syndrome	WHS	Chr4p16.13 deletion	194190

In parallel with screening for episignatures, EpiSign also permits concurrent detection of FRX in males [37] and common imprinting disorders [76], thereby consolidating tests and reducing the need for additional reflexive testing [45]. In addition, its clinical utility in the assessment and reclassification of VUSs in genes with existing episignatures was recently reported in multiple studies [45,72,77,78]. EpiSign is the first and currently the only genome-wide DNAm clinical test offered for screening individuals with NDDs, and can be used as part of the diagnostic work up or for reclassification of VUSs. The reference EpiSign Knowledge Database (EKD) [44] utilized by the EpiSign assay contains thousands of peripheral blood DNAm profiles from both reference controls and NDD.

The cost of completing a methylation array is comparable to the cost of most CMAs, and the results are highly reproducible. The assay uses peripheral blood, similar to current CMA platforms, allowing streamlined adaption in the clinical setting given the overlap in equipment and laboratory techniques.

The ability to detect episignatures in patients with NDDs has been shown to increase the diagnostic yield, helping to resolve the diagnostic odyssey. A recent study assessing the clinical impact of EpiSign for patients with rare Mendelian disorders demonstrated a 27.6% diagnostic yield among patients with previous ambiguous/inconclusive genetic findings including genetic VUSs [45]. As episignature discovery expands and more disorders are added to the test repertoire, the diagnostic yield is likely to increase significantly, ultimately benefiting patients, their families and the related health care systems. This expansion in episignatures, however, may bring with it challenges, as it is likely to uncover syndromes with overlapping episignatures which may require the implementation of novel computational methods in order to classify these disorders.

7. Episignature Development in CNV-Associated Genomic Disorders Provides Insight into Pathological Mechanism

Changes in DNAm profiles, or episignatures, in patients with large CNV defects associated with genomic disorders have not been systematically studied, and it is plausible that large CNVs, much like gene specific variants, may exhibit unique diagnostic methylation signatures in patients with NDDs.

Our group recently published findings describing episignature discovery in patients with PHMDS [46], highlighting the novel insights DNA methylation analysis can contribute to the pathogenesis of CNV disorders. PHMDS is a genomic disorder associated with deletions of chromosome 22, involving partial or whole-gene disruption of the SH3 and multiple ankyrin repeat domains 3 gene (*SHANK3*). Intragenic variants in *SHANK3* alone are responsible for a broad range of the phenotypic features observed in PHMDS [79]. However, this gene does not explain the entire phenotype in many patients, particularly speech and motor deficits, as well as renal abnormalities. The phenotypic variability and potential involvement of additional genes within the region has been previously assessed by multiple groups [80,81]. We demonstrated an episignature in patients with large deletions that was not observed in those with small deletions or *SHANK3* gene level variants (Figure 1a–c). The minimal region of difference between these two deletion types, large versus small, included the bromodomain-containing protein 1 gene (*BRD1*), a gene involved in epigenetic mechanisms and a likely candidate gene for the methylation signature observed in these patients (Figure 1d). *BRD1* is a component of a histone acetyltransferase complex that interacts with chromatin remodeling proteins and, before now, there was limited genotype–phenotype association reported in this gene. In addition, metabolic studies confirmed that these patients also exhibited very different metabolic profiles [46], further providing functional evidence for disease pathogenesis, as well as indicating targets for future therapies.

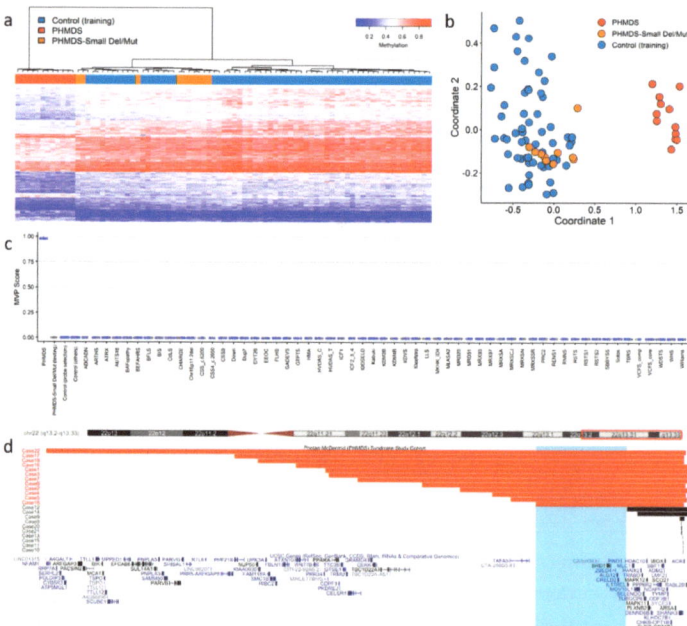

Figure 1. Phelan–McDermid syndrome (PHMDS) episignature demonstrating the critical *BRD1* region: (**a**) Euclidean hierarchical clustering (heatmap); each column represents a single PHMDS case or control, each row represents one of the CpG probes selected for the episignature. This heatmap

shows clear separation between large deletion (2–6 Mb in size) PHMDS cases (red) from controls (blue). Smaller deletions (0.01–1 Mb) and intragenic *SHANK3* gene variants (Small Del/Mut) (orange) are shown to segregate with controls. (**b**) Multidimensional scaling (MDS) plot shows segregation of large deletion PHMDS cases from both controls and Small Del/Mut cases. (**c**) Support vector machine (SVM) classifier model. Model was trained using the selected probes for the PHMDS episignature, 75% of controls and 75% of other neurodevelopmental disorder samples (blue). The remaining 25% of controls and 25% of other disorder samples were used for testing (grey). Plot shows the large deletion PHMDS cases with a methylation variant pathogenicity (MVP) score close to 1 compared with all other samples, showing the specificity of the classifier and episignature. (**d**) PHMDS deletions illustrating the critical region of interest associated with DNA methylation episignature. The horizontal red bars represent large deletion PHMDS cases associated with the presence of a distinct episignature. The horizontal black bars represent Small Del/Mut cases that do not have a distinct DNA methylation episignature. Highlighted in light blue is the common critical region of interest (Chr22:49,228,863–50,429,645) of deletions associated with the episignature. The common region of interest contains the candidate *BRD1* gene. Cytogenetic bands and known genes are presented in this figure using the UCSC genome browser [82] 2009 (GRCh37/hg19) genome build. Figure adapted with permission from Schenkel et al. [46].

8. Defined Episignatures in Other CNV-Associated Genomic Disorders Provide Rationale to Further Expand Episignature Discovery

Symmetrical dose-dependent DNAm profiles have been reported in individuals with deletion of the 7q11.23 region (Williams syndrome; WS) or duplication of the same region (7q11.23 duplication syndrome) [83], highlighting the importance of DNAm in the pathogenesis of these disorders. This region contains a number of genes associated with epigenetic mechanisms, and a study by Aref-Eshghi et al. later showed that these methylation changes resulted in unique episignatures that could differentiate WS and 7q11.23 duplication syndrome from 40 other NDDs and congenital anomaly disorders [44]. In the same study, Aref-Eshghi et al. demonstrated another example of symmetrical DNAm pattern, this time when comparing Hunter–McAlpine syndrome (HMS) and Sotos syndrome. A distinct hypermethylation episignature is observed in HMS patients with duplications involving the 5q35 region containing the *NSD1* gene, a direct contrast to the robust hypomethylation episignature seen in patients with Sotos syndrome, which is the result of loss of function variants in the same *NSD1* gene [44].

A DNAm signature was reported in a cohort with the genomic disorder 16p11.2 deletion syndrome (16p11.2DS) [84]—a disorder associated with a variable phenotype that includes increased susceptibility to ASD. Several genes within this region play a role in histone or chromatin function; however, to date, no single candidate gene has been identified to be causative of this disorder or its resultant episignature. Moreover, 16p11.2DS shows reduced penetrance and variable expressivity, and although most deletions are de novo, many are inherited from apparently unaffected parents. These so-called "susceptibility CNVs" present challenges for clinicians in counselling families [41]. Due to the presence of a cluster of LCRs in this region that mediate CNVs through NAHR, there is a reciprocal duplication disorder (16p11.2 duplication syndrome) with similar diagnostic challenges. Studying methylation changes in patients with these susceptibility CNVs and their carrier parents could potentially unlock novel insights into the role of aberrant DNAm in reduced penetrance CNV disorders.

Our group recently described an aberrant DNAm pattern in patients with deletions of 12q24.31 encompassing the known histone modifier gene SET domain-containing protein 1B (*SETD1B*), and demonstrated that patients who harbored point mutations within *SETD1B* shared the same methylation episignature [78]. This study highlights that larger CNVs may exhibit the same methylation affects as gene specific variants within these regions.

The most common genomic disorder is a 22q11.2 deletion syndrome and is the result of a 1.5–3 Mb deletion also mediated by NAHR at a cluster of LCRs. Clinical manifestations of this disorder include DiGeorge and Velocardiofacial syndromes, and, to date, the phenotype–genotype relationship has not been fully elucidated. Through analysis of a cohort of individuals with 22q11.2 deletions, we identified an episignature that can differentiate 22q11.2 deletion syndrome from other NDDs on the clinical EpiSign test, including those considered in the differential diagnosis of this syndrome [85]. Among other findings, assessment of DMRs showed overlap with loci for orofacial clefting, a key phenotypic feature of this disorder. Through further analysis of atypical deletions and gene level variants, it may be possible to determine the gene, or genes, that play a role in the aberrant DNAm pattern observed, as well as insight into the mechanisms contributing to this disorder.

Only a few of the most prevalent genomic disorders have a candidate gene considered responsible for the entire phenotypic spectrum. Interestingly, where these candidate genes have been identified, they are predominantly involved in epigenetic regulation including chromatin remodeling or histone modification, e.g., *CREBBP* in Rubinstein–Taybi syndrome [86] and *NSD1* in Sotos syndrome [87] (Table 2). Variants in most of these genes have already been assessed for genome-wide DNAm changes, and have been shown to exhibit unique and specific episignatures [43]. Overall, the majority of CNV disorders do not have a known or suspected candidate gene of interest. However, almost all of these regions contain one or more genes with epigenetic function (Table 2), e.g., chromodomain helicase DNA-binding protein 1-like (*CHD1L*) gene in 1q21.1 deletions and duplications, a gene that has a role in chromatin remodeling following DNA damage [88].

Table 2. Common CNV disorders including the candidate genes involved in the clinical phenotype (where applicable), and genes contained within with reported epigenetic machinery roles.

Syndrome	Chromosome Region	Candidate Gene	Genes in Region with Epigenetic Function
1p36 Deletion/Duplication	1p36	-	ICMT, CHD5, TP73, PMRD16, SKI, NOC2L
1q21.1 Deletion/Duplication	1q21.1	-	CHD1L
1q43q44 Deletion	1q43q44	-	HNRNPU, DESI2, ZBTB18, AKT3
2q11.2 Deletion/Duplication	2q11.2	-	KANSL3, ARID5A
2q13 Deletion/Duplication	2q13	-	MIR4435-2HG
2q37 Deletion	2q37	-	HDAC4, D2HGDH, ING5, HDLBP, PASK
3q29 Deletion/Duplication	3q29	-	PAK2, RNF168
4p16.3 Deletion (Wolf–Hirschhorn)/4p16.3 Duplication	4p16.3	NSD2	NSD2, CTBP1, SLBP, CTBP1, PCGF3
5p15 Deletion (Cri du Chat)/5p15 Duplication	5p15	-	ATPSCKMT, MTRR, NSUN2, LPCAT1, BRD9
5q35 Deletion (Sotos)/5q35 Duplication (Hunter–McAlpine)	5q35	NSD1	NSD1, UIMC1
7q11.23 Deletion (Williams–Beuren)/7q11.23 Duplication	7q11.23	-	METTL27, BUD23, BCL7B, BAZ1B
8p23.1 Deletion/Duplication	8p23.1	-	TNKS
9q34 Deletion (Kleefstra)/9q34 Duplication	9q34	EHMT1	EHMT1
10q22.3q23.2 Deletion/Duplication	10q22.3q23.2	-	WAPL, DYDC1, MAT1A

Table 2. Cont.

Syndrome	Chromosome Region	Candidate Gene	Genes in Region with Epigenetic Function
11p11.2 Deletion (Potocki–Shaffer)/11p11.2 Duplication	11p11.2	-	PHF21A, CD82, ALKBH3
11q13.2q13.4 Deletion	11q13.2q13.4	-	KMT5B
15q11.2 Deletion (non-imprinting region)	15q11.2	-	-
15q11q13 Deletion (Prader–Willi/Angelman)/15q11q13 Duplication	15q11q13	-	HERC2
15q13.3 Deletion/Duplication	15q13.3	-	OTUD7A, KLF13
15q24 (BP0-BP1) Deletion/Duplication	15q24	-	-
15q24 (BP2-BP3) Deletion	15q24	-	SIN3A, COMMD4
15q25.2 Deletion	15q25.2	-	HDGFL3, BNC1
16p13.3 Deletion (Rubinstein–Taybi)/16p13.3 Duplication	16p13.3	CREBBP	CREBBP
16p13.11 Deletion/16p13.11 Duplication	16p13.11	-	NDE1
16p11.2 Distal Deletion/Duplication	16p11.2	-	SH2B1
16p11.2 Deletion/Duplication	16p11.2	-	PPP4C, HIRIP3, PAGR1, INO80E
17p13.3 Deletion (Miller–Dieker)/17p13.3 Duplication	17p13.3	-	HIC1, SMYD4, MYO1C
17p11.2 Deletion (Smith–Magenis)/17p11.2 Duplication (Potocki–Lupski)	17p11.2	RAI1	ALKBH5, RAI1, PEMT
17q11.2 Deletion/Duplication	17q11.2	-	SUZ12
17q12 Deletion/Duplication	17q12	-	HNF1B, TADA2A, AATF, PIGW
17q21.31 Deletion (Koolen–de Vries)/17q21.31 Duplication	17q21.31	KANSL1	KANSL1
22q11.2 Tetrasomy/Triplication (Cat eye syndrome)	22q11.2	-	CECR2, ADA2
22q11.2 Deletion (DiGeorge/Velocardiofacial)/22q11.2 Duplication	22q11.2	-	THAP7, TRMT2A, COMT, HIRA
22q11.2 recurrent region distal type I (D-E/F) Deletion/Duplication	22q11.2	-	TOP3B, PPM1F
22q13.3 Deletion (Phelan–McDermid)	22q13.3	SHANK3	BRD1
Xp11.22 Duplication (MRX17)	Xp11.22	-	HUWE1, HSD17B10, SMC1A

Taken together, the evidence suggests that CNV-associated genomic disorders may exhibit aberrant DNAm as the result of genes affected in their underlying deletions and duplications, especially when those regions include genes with epigenetic regulatory roles. CNV-associated genomic disorders are therefore strong candidates for episignature discovery. Investigating these syndromes further, including atypical CNVs and gene level variants within the same regions for possible sub-signatures, may uncover novel insights into the pathogenesis of these disorders. These studies may also identify new candidate genes responsible for some of the phenotypic presentation—should sub-signatures be uncovered for specific deleted or duplicated regions—and potentially unlock novel targets for more personalized treatment approaches.

9. Combined Detection of CNVs and DNA Methylation Episignatures in a Single Assay

Recent studies have shown it is possible to detect CNVs by applying computational methods to data obtained from DNAm arrays, such as the Illumina 450K and EPIC Bead Chip arrays [89–91]. Many of these pipelines are publicly available in Bioconductor, e.g., ChAMP [91,92], CopyNumber450k [93] and EpiCopy [89] (https://bioconductor.org/packages/, accessed on 19 May 2022). The ability to integrate the detection of genetic and epigenetic findings can provide a more complete view of underlying pathogenic mechanisms.

We applied a similar computational approach using the DNAcopy package (Bioconductor.org) to our PHMDS cohort, and confirmed we could detect breakpoint coordinates similar to those obtained from conventional clinical CMA at the time of original diagnosis [46]; these findings are in line with previous studies [89–93].

Combining these detection methods is not without challenges, most notably in coverage of the genome, as CpG sites are not uniformly distributed throughout the genome and therefore methylation arrays lack the "backbone coverage" observed in high-density SNP arrays. However, it is plausible that, with modifications, a combined array could be developed containing a combination of copy number and CpG targeted probes to produce a clinically targeted array enabling accurate episignature and CNV analysis on a single platform. This has the potential to impact healthcare resource utilization by reducing concurrent testing in NDD patients, and decreasing the need for reflexive testing for disorders such as those associated with imprinting. There would continue to be limitations in the ability to detect low level mosaicism, as seen with existing CNV platforms; however, studies have shown the ability to detect mosaicism from methylation arrays in Kabuki syndrome 1 [94], imprinting disorders [76] and FRX [37].

Additional benefits of a combined testing platform include those to the patient; a combined array would permit screening for more disorders in a single assay, thereby potentially increasing diagnostic yield over that of the current first-tier clinical test (chromosome microarray), and shortening the time spent in the diagnostic odyssey. This approach could concurrently reduce the burden on clinical services and genetic counselling by providing results for CMA, FRX, imprinting and methylation in a single report, leading to a reduction in requisitions and clinic visits. A combined platform would also benefit oncology studies, where limitations in tumor sample availability can often impact research and diagnosis; this would permit the detection of CNVs and methylation status from the same volume of tissue as traditional testing.

10. Conclusions

The identification of episignatures in genomic disorders associated with CNVs could facilitate the expansion of screening capabilities for patients with NDDs, improving the diagnostic yield of clinical testing. This work may also provide novel insights into the pathogenesis of genomic disorders and provide targets for future therapies. The ability to combine CNV and episignature detection into a single assay would reduce the overall cost of testing, increase the number of disorders being screened for, and contribute to the reduction in alternative reflexive and concurrent genetic tests ordered. The benefit to patients and families in reducing wait times and increasing screened disorders, as well as reducing clinician and laboratory burden via fewer clinic visits and fewer genetic tests ordered, would have significant impacts on healthcare resource utilization and the costs associated with the diagnosis of NDDs.

Author Contributions: K.R. and B.S. conceived, performed the literature review and wrote the manuscript. All authors have read and agreed to the published version of the manuscript.

Funding: This work was funded by the Government of Canada through Genome Canada and the Ontario Genomics Institute (OGI-188).

Data Availability Statement: Not applicable.

Acknowledgments: The authors would like to thank Haley McConkey for administrative support.

Conflicts of Interest: The authors declare no conflict of interest.

Abbreviations

aCGH, array-based comparative genomic hybridization; ADHD, attention deficit hyperactivity disorder; ASD, autism spectrum disorder; CMA, chromosomal microarray analysis; CNV, copy number variant; DD, developmental delay; DNAm, DNA methylation; DNMT, DNA methyltransferases; FRX, fragile X syndrome; HMS, Hunter–McAlpine syndrome; ID, intellectual disability; LCR, low copy repeats; MLM, machine learning models; NAHR, non-allelic homologous recombination; NCBRS, Nicolaides–Baraitser syndromes; NDD, neurodevelopmental disorder; PHMDS, Phelan–McDermid syndrome; SAM, S-adenosylmethionine; SNV, single nucleotide variants; TBRS, Tatton–Brown–Rahman syndrome; VUS, variant of uncertain significance; WES, whole exome sequencing; WGS, whole genome sequencing; WS, Williams syndrome.

References

1. López-Rivera, J.A.; Pérez-Palma, E.; Symonds, J.; Lindy, A.S.; McKnight, D.A.; Leu, C.; Zuberi, S.; Brunklaus, A.; Møller, R.; Lal, D. A catalogue of new incidence estimates of monogenic neurodevelopmental disorders caused by de novo variants. *Brain* **2020**, *143*, 1099–1105. [CrossRef] [PubMed]
2. Institute of Medicine (US) Committee on Nervous System Disorders in Developing Countries. *Neurological, Psychiatric, and Developmental Disorders: Meeting the Challenge in the Developing World*; National Academies Press: Washington, DC, USA, 2001.
3. Morris-Rosendahl, D.J.; Crocq, M.-A. Neurodevelopmental disorders—The history and future of a diagnostic concept. *Dialogues Clin. Neurosci.* **2020**, *22*, 65–72. [CrossRef] [PubMed]
4. Parenti, I.; Rabaneda, L.G.; Schoen, H.; Novarino, G. Neurodevelopmental Disorders: From Genetics to Functional Pathways. *Trends Neurosci.* **2020**, *43*, 608–621. [CrossRef] [PubMed]
5. Sheridan, E.; Wright, J.; Small, N.; Corry, P.C.; Oddie, S.; Whibley, C.; Petherick, E.S.; Malik, T.; Pawson, N.; McKinney, P.A.; et al. Risk factors for congenital anomaly in a multiethnic birth cohort: An analysis of the Born in Bradford study. *Lancet* **2013**, *382*, 1350–1359. [CrossRef]
6. Pinto, D.; Delaby, E.; Merico, D.; Barbosa, M.; Merikangas, A.; Klei, L.; Thiruvahindrapuram, B.; Xu, X.; Ziman, R.; Wang, Z.; et al. Convergence of Genes and Cellular Pathways Dysregulated in Autism Spectrum Disorders. *Am. J. Hum. Genet.* **2014**, *94*, 677–694. [CrossRef]
7. Miller, D.T.; Adam, M.P.; Aradhya, S.; Biesecker, L.G.; Brothman, A.R.; Carter, N.P.; Church, D.M.; Crolla, J.A.; Eichler, E.E.; Epstein, C.J.; et al. Consensus Statement: Chromosomal Microarray Is a First-Tier Clinical Diagnostic Test for Individuals with Developmental Disabilities or Congenital Anomalies. *Am. J. Hum. Genet.* **2010**, *86*, 749–764. [CrossRef]
8. Silva, M.; De Leeuw, N.; Mann, K.; Schuring-Blom, H.; Morgan, S.; Giardino, D.; Rack, K.; Hastings, R. European guidelines for constitutional cytogenomic analysis. *Eur. J. Hum. Genet.* **2019**, *27*, 1–16. [CrossRef]
9. Shaw-Smith, C.; Redon, R.; Rickman, L.; Rio, M.; Willatt, L.; Fiegler, H.; Firth, H.; Sanlaville, D.; Winter, R.; Colleaux, L.; et al. Microarray based comparative genomic hybridisation (array-CGH) detects submicroscopic chromosomal deletions and duplications in patients with learning disability/mental retardation and dysmorphic features. *J. Med. Genet.* **2004**, *41*, 241–248. [CrossRef]
10. Vissers, L.E.; de Vries, B.B.; Osoegawa, K.; Janssen, I.M.; Feuth, T.; Choy, C.O.; Straatman, H.; van der Vliet, W.; Huys, E.H.; van Rijk, A.; et al. Array-Based Comparative Genomic Hybridization for the Genomewide Detection of Submicroscopic Chromosomal Abnormalities. *Am. J. Hum. Genet.* **2003**, *73*, 1261–1270. [CrossRef]
11. Haraksingh, R.R.; Abyzov, A.; Urban, A.E. Comprehensive performance comparison of high-resolution array platforms for genome-wide Copy Number Variation (CNV) analysis in humans. *BMC Genom.* **2017**, *18*, 321. [CrossRef]

12. McCarroll, S.; Kuruvilla, F.G.; Korn, J.M.; Cawley, S.; Nemesh, J.; Wysoker, A.; Shapero, M.H.; Bakker, P.I.W.D.; Maller, J.; Kirby, A.; et al. Integrated detection and population-genetic analysis of SNPs and copy number variation. *Nat. Genet.* **2008**, *40*, 1166–1174. [CrossRef] [PubMed]
13. Feuk, L.; Carson, A.R.; Scherer, S. Structural variation in the human genome. *Nat. Rev. Genet.* **2006**, *7*, 85–97. [CrossRef] [PubMed]
14. Levy, B.; Burnside, R.D. Are all chromosome microarrays the same? What clinicians need to know. *Prenat. Diagn.* **2019**, *39*, 157–164. [CrossRef] [PubMed]
15. D'Amours, G.; Langlois, M.; Mathonnet, G.; Fetni, R.; Nizard, S.; Srour, M.; Tihy, F.; Phillips, M.S.; Michaud, J.L.; Lemyre, E. SNP arrays: Comparing diagnostic yields for four platforms in children with developmental delay. *BMC Med. Genom.* **2014**, *7*, 70. [CrossRef]
16. Zhang, Y.; Haraksingh, R.; Grubert, F.; Abyzov, A.; Gerstein, M.; Weissman, S.; Urban, A.E. Child Development and Structural Variation in the Human Genome. *Child Dev.* **2013**, *84*, 34–48. [CrossRef] [PubMed]
17. Tuzun, E.; Sharp, A.J.; Bailey, J.A.; Kaul, R.; Morrison, V.A.; Pertz, L.M.; Haugen, E.; Hayden, H.S.; Albertson, D.G.; Pinkel, D.; et al. Fine-scale structural variation of the human genome. *Nat. Genet.* **2005**, *37*, 727–732. [CrossRef]
18. Liu, J.; Zhou, Y.; Liu, S.; Song, X.; Yang, X.Z.; Fan, Y.; Chen, W.; Akdemir, Z.C.; Yan, Z.; Zuo, Y.; et al. The coexistence of copy number variations (CNVs) and single nucleotide polymorphisms (SNPs) at a locus can result in distorted calculations of the significance in associating SNPs to disease. *Hum. Genet.* **2018**, *137*, 553–567. [CrossRef]
19. Akhtar, M.S.; Ashino, R.; Oota, H.; Ishida, H.; Niimura, Y.; Touhara, K.; Melin, A.D.; Kawamura, S. Genetic variation of olfactory receptor gene family in a Japanese population. *Anthr. Sci.* **2022**, 211024. [CrossRef]
20. Lee, J.A.; Lupski, J.R. Genomic Rearrangements and Gene Copy-Number Alterations as a Cause of Nervous System Disorders. *Neuron* **2006**, *52*, 103–121. [CrossRef]
21. Cooper, G.M.; Coe, B.P.; Girirajan, S.; Rosenfeld, J.A.; Vu, T.H.; Baker, C.; Williams, C.; Stalker, H.; Hamid, R.; Hannig, V.; et al. A Copy Number Variation Morbidity Map of Developmental Delay. *Nat. Genet.* **2011**, *43*, 838–846. [CrossRef]
22. Le Gouard, N.R.; Jacquinet, A.; Ruaud, L.; Deleersnyder, H.; Ageorges, F.; Gallard, J.; Lacombe, D.; Odent, S.; Mikaty, M.; Manouvrier-Hanu, S.; et al. Smith-Magenis syndrome: Clinical and behavioral characteristics in a large retrospective cohort. *Clin. Genet.* **2021**, *99*, 519–528. [CrossRef] [PubMed]
23. Eichler, E.E. Recent duplication, domain accretion and the dynamic mutation of the human genome. *Trends Genet.* **2001**, *17*, 661–669. [CrossRef]
24. Sharp, A.J.; Cheng, Z.; Eichler, E.E. Structural Variation of the Human Genome. *Annu. Rev. Genom. Hum. Genet.* **2006**, *7*, 407–442. [CrossRef] [PubMed]
25. Liu, P.; Lacaria, M.; Zhang, F.; Withers, M.; Hastings, P.; Lupski, J.R. Frequency of Nonallelic Homologous Recombination Is Correlated with Length of Homology: Evidence that Ectopic Synapsis Precedes Ectopic Crossing-Over. *Am. J. Hum. Genet.* **2011**, *89*, 580–588. [CrossRef] [PubMed]
26. Smajlagić, D.; Lavrichenko, K.; Berland, S.; Helgeland, Ø.; Knudsen, G.P.; Vaudel, M.; Haavik, J.; Knappskog, P.M.; Njølstad, P.R.; Houge, G.; et al. Population prevalence and inheritance pattern of recurrent CNVs associated with neurodevelopmental disorders in 12,252 newborns and their parents. *Eur. J. Hum. Genet.* **2021**, *29*, 205–215. [CrossRef]
27. Tatton-Brown, K.; Douglas, J.; Coleman, K.; Baujat, G.; Chandler, K.; Clarke, A.; Collins, A.; Davies, S.; Faravelli, F.; Firth, H.; et al. Multiple mechanisms are implicated in the generation of 5q35 microdeletions in Sotos syndrome. *J. Med. Genet.* **2005**, *42*, 307–313. [CrossRef]
28. Goldenberg, P. An Update on Common Chromosome Microdeletion and Microduplication Syndromes. *Pediatr. Ann.* **2018**, *47*, e198–e203. [CrossRef]
29. Bernardini, L.; Alesi, V.; Loddo, S.; Novelli, A.; Bottillo, I.; Battaglia, A.; Digilio, M.C.; Zampino, G.; Ertel, A.; Fortina, P.; et al. High-resolution SNP arrays in mental retardation diagnostics: How much do we gain? *Eur. J. Hum. Genet.* **2010**, *18*, 178–185. [CrossRef]
30. De Ligt, J.; Willemsen, M.H.; Van Bon, B.W.; Kleefstra, T.; Yntema, H.G.; Kroes, T.; Vulto-van Silfhout, A.T.; Koolen, D.A.; De Vries, P.; Gilissen, C.; et al. Diagnostic Exome Sequencing in Persons with Severe Intellectual Disability. *N. Engl. J. Med.* **2012**, *367*, 1921–1929. [CrossRef]
31. Lemke, J.R.; Riesch, E.; Scheurenbrand, T.; Schubach, M.; Wilhelm, C.; Steiner, I.; Hansen, J.; Courage, C.; Gallati, S.; Bürki, S.; et al. Targeted next generation sequencing as a diagnostic tool in epileptic disorders. *Epilepsia* **2012**, *53*, 1387–1398. [CrossRef]
32. Schwarze, K.; Buchanan, J.; Taylor, J.C.; Wordsworth, S. Are whole-exome and whole-genome sequencing approaches cost-effective? A systematic review of the literature. *Genet. Med.* **2018**, *20*, 1122–1130. [CrossRef] [PubMed]
33. Sikkema-Raddatz, B.; Johansson, L.F.; de Boer, E.N.; Almomani, R.; Boven, L.G.; van den Berg, M.P.; van Spaendonck-Zwarts, K.Y.; van Tintelen, J.P.; Sijmons, R.H.; Jongbloed, J.D.H.; et al. Targeted Next-Generation Sequencing can Replace Sanger Sequencing in Clinical Diagnostics. *Hum. Mutat.* **2013**, *34*, 1035–1042. [CrossRef] [PubMed]
34. Fraiman, Y.S.; Wojcik, M.H. The influence of social determinants of health on the genetic diagnostic odyssey: Who remains undiagnosed, why, and to what effect? *Pediatr. Res.* **2021**, *89*, 295–300. [CrossRef]
35. Michaels-Igbokwe, C.; McInnes, B.; MacDonald, K.V.; Currie, G.R.; Omar, F.; Shewchuk, B.; Bernier, F.P.; Marshall, D.A. (Un)standardized testing: The diagnostic odyssey of children with rare genetic disorders in Alberta, Canada. *Genet. Med.* **2021**, *23*, 272–279. [CrossRef] [PubMed]

36. Thevenon, J.; Duffourd, Y.; Masurel-Paulet, A.; Lefebvre, M.; Feillet, F.; El Chehadeh-Djebbar, S.; St-Onge, J.; Steinmetz, A.; Huet, F.; Chouchane, M.; et al. Diagnostic odyssey in severe neurodevelopmental disorders: Toward clinical whole-exome sequencing as a first-line diagnostic test. *Clin. Genet.* **2016**, *89*, 700–707. [CrossRef]
37. Schenkel, L.C.; Schwartz, C.; Skinner, C.; Rodenhiser, D.I.; Ainsworth, P.J.; Pare, G.; Sadikovic, B. Clinical Validation of Fragile X Syndrome Screening by DNA Methylation Array. *J. Mol. Diagn.* **2016**, *18*, 834–841. [CrossRef]
38. Coffee, B.; Ikeda, M.; Budimirovic, D.B.; Hjelm, L.N.; Kaufmann, W.E.; Warren, S.T. Mosaic *FMR1* Deletion Causes Fragile X Syndrome and Can Lead to Molecular Misdiagnosis. *Am. J. Med. Genet. Part A* **2008**, *146A*, 1358–1367. [CrossRef] [PubMed]
39. van Nimwegen, K.; Schieving, J.; Willemsen, M.; Veltman, J.; van der Burg, S.; van der Wilt, G.; Grutters, J. The diagnostic pathway in complex paediatric neurology: A cost analysis. *Eur. J. Paediatr. Neurol.* **2015**, *19*, 233–239. [CrossRef]
40. Copeland, H.; Kivuva, E.; Firth, H.V.; Wright, C.F. Systematic assessment of outcomes following a genetic diagnosis identified through a large-scale research study into developmental disorders. *Genet. Med.* **2021**, *23*, 1058–1064. [CrossRef]
41. Kleinendorst, L.; Heuvel, L.M.V.D.; Henneman, L.; Van Haelst, M.M. Who ever heard of 16p11.2 deletion syndrome? Parents' perspectives on a susceptibility copy number variation syndrome. *Eur. J. Hum. Genet.* **2020**, *28*, 1196–1204. [CrossRef]
42. Savatt, J.M.; Myers, S.M. Genetic Testing in Neurodevelopmental Disorders. *Front. Pediatr.* **2021**, *9*, 526779. [CrossRef] [PubMed]
43. Levy, M.A.; McConkey, H.; Kerkhof, J.; Barat-Houari, M.; Bargiacchi, S.; Biamino, E.; Bralo, M.P.; Cappuccio, G.; Ciolfi, A.; Clarke, A.; et al. Novel diagnostic DNA methylation episignatures expand and refine the epigenetic landscapes of Mendelian disorders. *Hum. Genet. Genom. Adv.* **2021**, *3*, 100075. [CrossRef] [PubMed]
44. Aref-Eshghi, E.; Kerkhof, J.; Pedro, V.P.; Barat-Houari, M.; Ruiz-Pallares, N.; Andrau, J.-C.; Lacombe, D.; Van-Gils, J.; Fergelot, P.; Dubourg, C.; et al. Evaluation of DNA Methylation Episignatures for Diagnosis and Phenotype Correlations in 42 Mendelian Neurodevelopmental Disorders. *Am. J. Hum. Genet.* **2020**, *106*, 356–370. [CrossRef]
45. Sadikovic, B.; Levy, M.A.; Kerkhof, J.; Aref-Eshghi, E.; Schenkel, L.; Stuart, A.; McConkey, H.; Henneman, P.; Venema, A.; Schwartz, C.E.; et al. Clinical epigenomics: Genome-wide DNA methylation analysis for the diagnosis of Mendelian disorders. *Genet. Med.* **2021**, *23*, 1065–1074. [CrossRef] [PubMed]
46. Schenkel, L.C.; Aref-Eshghi, E.; Rooney, K.; Kerkhof, J.; Levy, M.A.; McConkey, H.; Rogers, R.C.; Phelan, K.; Sarasua, S.M.; Jain, L.; et al. DNA methylation epi-signature is associated with two molecularly and phenotypically distinct clinical subtypes of Phelan-McDermid syndrome. *Clin. Epigenetics* **2021**, *13*, 2. [CrossRef]
47. Berger, S.L.; Kouzarides, T.; Shiekhattar, R.; Shilatifard, A. An operational definition of epigenetics. *Genes Dev.* **2009**, *23*, 781–783. [CrossRef] [PubMed]
48. Deans, C.; Maggert, K.A. What Do You Mean, "Epigenetic"? *Genetics* **2015**, *199*, 887–896. [CrossRef]
49. Gibney, E.R.; Nolan, C.M. Epigenetics and gene expression. *Heredity* **2010**, *105*, 4–13. [CrossRef]
50. Li, E.; Zhang, Y. DNA Methylation in Mammals. *Cold Spring Harb. Perspect. Biol.* **2014**, *6*, a019133. [CrossRef]
51. Miller, J.L.; Grant, P.A. The Role of DNA Methylation and Histone Modifications in Transcriptional Regulation in Humans. In *Epigenetics: Development and Disease*; Kundu, T.K., Ed.; Springer: Dordrecht, The Netherlands, 2013; pp. 289–317. [CrossRef]
52. Jones, P.A. Functions of DNA methylation: Islands, start sites, gene bodies and beyond. *Nat. Rev. Genet.* **2012**, *13*, 484–492. [CrossRef]
53. Aref-Eshghi, E.; Schenkel, L.C.; Lin, H.; Skinner, C.; Ainsworth, P.; Paré, G.; Rodenhiser, D.; Schwartz, C.; Sadikovic, B. The defining DNA methylation signature of Kabuki syndrome enables functional assessment of genetic variants of unknown clinical significance. *Epigenetics* **2017**, *12*, 923–933. [CrossRef] [PubMed]
54. Schenkel, L.C.; Aref-Eshghi, E.; Skinner, C.; Ainsworth, P.; Lin, H.; Paré, G.; Rodenhiser, D.I.; Schwartz, C.; Sadikovic, B. Peripheral blood epi-signature of Claes-Jensen syndrome enables sensitive and specific identification of patients and healthy carriers with pathogenic mutations in KDM5C. *Clin. Epigenetics* **2018**, *10*, 21. [CrossRef] [PubMed]
55. Kernohan, K.D.; Schenkel, L.C.; Huang, L.; Smith, A.; Pare, G.; Ainsworth, P.; Care4Rare Canada Consortium; Boycott, K.M.; Warman-Chardon, J.; Sadikovic, B. Identification of a methylation profile for DNMT1-associated autosomal dominant cerebellar ataxia, deafness, and narcolepsy. *Clin. Epigenetics* **2016**, *8*, 91. [CrossRef] [PubMed]
56. Klein, C.J.; Bird, T.; Ertekin-Taner, N.; Lincoln, S.; Hjorth, R.; Wu, Y.; Kwok, J.; Mer, G.; Dyck, P.J.; Nicholson, G.A. DNMT1 mutation hot spot causes varied phenotypes of HSAN1 with dementia and hearing loss Background: Mutations in DNA methyltransferase 1 (DNMT1) have been identified in 2 autosomal. *Neurology* **2013**, *80*, 824–828. [CrossRef]
57. Klein, C.J.; Botuyan, M.; Wu, Y.; Ward, C.J.; Nicholson, G.A.; Hammans, S.; Hojo, K.; Yamanishi, H.; Adam, R.; Wallace, D.C.; et al. Mutations in *DNMT1* cause hereditary sensory neuropathy with dementia and hearing loss. *Nat. Genet.* **2011**, *43*, 595–600. [CrossRef]
58. Tatton-Brown, K.; Childhood Overgrowth Consortium; Seal, S.; Ruark, E.; Harmer, J.; Ramsay, E.; Duarte, S.D.V.; Zachariou, A.; Hanks, S.; O'Brien, E.; et al. Mutations in the DNA methyltransferase gene DNMT3A cause an overgrowth syndrome with intellectual disability. *Nat. Genet.* **2014**, *46*, 385–388. [CrossRef]
59. Jin, B.; Tao, Q.; Peng, J.; Soo, H.M.; Wu, W.; Ying, J.; Fields, C.R.; Delmas, A.I.; Liu, X.; Qiu, J.; et al. DNA methyltransferase 3B (DNMT3B) mutations in ICF syndrome lead to altered epigenetic modifications and aberrant expression of genes regulating development, neurogenesis and immune function. *Hum. Mol. Genet.* **2008**, *17*, 690–709. [CrossRef]
60. Levy, M.A.; Beck, D.B.; Metcalfe, K.; Douzgou, S.; Sithambaram, S.; Cottrell, T.; Ansar, M.; Kerkhof, J.; Mignot, C.; Nougues, M.-C.; et al. Deficiency of TET3 leads to a genome-wide DNA hypermethylation episignature in human whole blood. *NPJ Genom. Med.* **2021**, *6*, 92. [CrossRef]

61. Beck, D.B.; Petracovici, A.; He, C.; Moore, H.W.; Louie, R.J.; Ansar, M.; Douzgou, S.; Sithambaram, S.; Cottrell, T.; Santos-Cortez, R.L.P.; et al. Delineation of a Human Mendelian Disorder of the DNA Demethylation Machinery: TET3 Deficiency. *Am. J. Hum. Genet.* **2020**, *106*, 234–245. [CrossRef]
62. Hood, R.L.; Schenkel, L.C.; Nikkel, S.M.; Ainsworth, P.J.; Pare, G.; Boycott, K.M.; Bulman, D.E.; Sadikovic, B. The defining DNA methylation signature of Floating-Harbor Syndrome. *Sci. Rep.* **2016**, *6*, 38803. [CrossRef]
63. Schenkel, L.C.; Kernohan, K.D.; McBride, A.; Reina, D.; Hodge, A.; Ainsworth, P.J.; Rodenhiser, D.I.; Pare, G.; Bérubé, N.G.; Skinner, C.; et al. Identification of epigenetic signature associated with alpha thalassemia/mental retardation X-linked syndrome. *Epigenet. Chromatin* **2017**, *10*, 10. [CrossRef] [PubMed]
64. Aref-Eshghi, E.; Bend, E.G.; Hood, R.L.; Schenkel, L.C.; Carere, D.A.; Chakrabarti, R.; Nagamani, S.C.S.; Cheung, S.W.; Campeau, P.M.; Prasad, C.; et al. BAFopathies' DNA methylation epi-signatures demonstrate diagnostic utility and functional continuum of Coffin–Siris and Nicolaides–Baraitser syndromes. *Nat. Commun.* **2018**, *9*, 4885. [CrossRef] [PubMed]
65. Wieczorek, D.; Bögershausen, N.; Beleggia, F.; Steiner-Haldenstätt, S.; Pohl, E.; Li, Y.; Milz, E.; Martin, M.; Thiele, H.; Altmüller, J.; et al. A comprehensive molecular study on Coffin–Siris and Nicolaides–Baraitser syndromes identifies a broad molecular and clinical spectrum converging on altered chromatin remodeling. *Hum. Mol. Genet.* **2013**, *22*, 5121–5135. [CrossRef] [PubMed]
66. Cappuccio, G.; Sayou, C.; Tanno, P.L.; Tisserant, E.; Bruel, A.L.; Kennani, S.E.; Sá, J.; Low, K.J.; Dias, C.; Havlovicová, M.; et al. De novo SMARCA2 variants clustered outside the helicase domain cause a new recognizable syndrome with intellectual disability and blepharophimosis distinct from Nicolaides–Baraitser syndrome. *Genet. Med.* **2020**, *22*, 1838–1850. [CrossRef]
67. Bend, E.G.; Aref-Eshghi, E.; Everman, D.B.; Rogers, R.C.; Cathey, S.S.; Prijoles, E.J.; Lyons, M.J.; Davis, H.; Clarkson, K.; Gripp, K.W.; et al. Gene domain-specific DNA methylation episignatures highlight distinct molecular entities of ADNP syndrome. *Clin. Epigenet.* **2019**, *11*, 64. [CrossRef]
68. Breen, M.S.; Garg, P.; Tang, L.; Mendonca, D.; Levy, T.; Barbosa, M.; Arnett, A.B.; Kurtz-Nelson, E.; Agolini, E.; Battaglia, A.; et al. Episignatures Stratifying Helsmoortel-Van Der Aa Syndrome Show Modest Correlation with Phenotype. *Am. J. Hum. Genet.* **2020**, *107*, 555–563. [CrossRef]
69. Tolmacheva, E.N.; Kashevarova, A.A.; Nazarenko, L.P.; Minaycheva, L.I.; Skryabin, N.A.; Lopatkina, M.E.; Nikitina, T.V.; Sazhenova, E.A.; Belyaeva, E.O.; Fonova, E.A.; et al. Delineation of Clinical Manifestations of the Inherited Xq24 Microdeletion Segregating with sXCI in Mothers: Two Novel Cases with Distinct Phenotypes Ranging from UBE2A Deficiency Syndrome to Recurrent Pregnancy Loss. *Cytogenet. Genome Res.* **2020**, *160*, 245–254. [CrossRef]
70. Wojcik, F.; Dann, G.P.; Beh, L.Y.; Debelouchina, G.T.; Hofmann, R.; Muir, T.W. Functional crosstalk between histone H2B ubiquitylation and H2A modifications and variants. *Nat. Commun.* **2018**, *9*, 1394. [CrossRef]
71. Selmi, C.; Feghali-Bostwick, C.A.; Lleo, A.; Lombardi, S.A.; De Santis, M.; Cavaciocchi, F.; Zammataro, L.; Mitchell, M.M.; LaSalle, J.M.; Medsger, T.; et al. X chromosome gene methylation in peripheral lymphocytes from monozygotic twins discordant for scleroderma. *Clin. Exp. Immunol.* **2012**, *169*, 253–262. [CrossRef]
72. Aref-Eshghi, E.; Bend, E.G.; Colaiacovo, S.; Caudle, M.; Chakrabarti, R.; Napier, M.; Brick, L.; Brady, L.; Carere, D.A.; Levy, M.A.; et al. Diagnostic Utility of Genome-wide DNA Methylation Testing in Genetically Unsolved Individuals with Suspected Hereditary Conditions. *Am. J. Hum. Genet.* **2019**, *104*, 685–700. [CrossRef]
73. Alisch, R.S.; Barwick, B.G.; Chopra, P.; Myrick, L.K.; Satten, G.A.; Conneely, K.N.; Warren, S.T. Age-associated DNA methylation in pediatric populations. *Genome Res.* **2012**, *22*, 623–632. [CrossRef] [PubMed]
74. Houseman, E.A.; Accomando, W.P.; Koestler, D.C.; Christensen, B.C.; Marsit, C.J.; Nelson, H.H.; Wiencke, J.K.; Kelsey, K.T. DNA methylation arrays as surrogate measures of cell mixture distribution. *BMC Bioinform.* **2012**, *13*, 86. [CrossRef] [PubMed]
75. Jaffe, A.; Murakami, P.; Lee, H.; Leek, J.; Fallin, M.D.; Feinberg, A.; Irizarry, R.A. Bump hunting to identify differentially methylated regions in epigenetic epidemiology studies. *Int. J. Epidemiol.* **2012**, *41*, 200–209. [CrossRef] [PubMed]
76. Aref-Eshghi, E.; Schenkel, L.C.; Lin, H.; Skinner, C.; Ainsworth, P.; Paré, G.; Siu, V.; Rodenhiser, D.; Schwartz, C.; Sadikovic, B. Clinical Validation of a Genome-Wide DNA Methylation Assay for Molecular Diagnosis of Imprinting Disorders. *J. Mol. Diagn.* **2017**, *19*, 848–856. [CrossRef]
77. Aref-Eshghi, E.; Rodenhiser, D.I.; Schenkel, L.C.; Lin, H.; Skinner, C.; Ainsworth, P.; Paré, G.; Hood, R.L.; Bulman, D.E.; Kernohan, K.D.; et al. Genomic DNA Methylation Signatures Enable Concurrent Diagnosis and Clinical Genetic Variant Classification in Neurodevelopmental Syndromes. *Am. J. Hum. Genet.* **2018**, *102*, 156–174. [CrossRef]
78. Krzyzewska, I.M.; Maas, S.M.; Henneman, P.; Lip, K.V.D.; Venema, A.; Baranano, K.; Chassevent, A.; Aref-Eshghi, E.; Van Essen, A.J.; Fukuda, T.; et al. A genome-wide DNA methylation signature for SETD1B-related syndrome. *Clin. Epigenet.* **2019**, *11*, 156. [CrossRef]
79. De Rubeis, S.; Siper, P.M.; Durkin, A.; Weissman, J.; Muratet, F.; Halpern, D.; Trelles, M.D.P.; Frank, Y.; Lozano, R.; Wang, A.T.; et al. Delineation of the genetic and clinical spectrum of Phelan-McDermid syndrome caused by SHANK3 point mutations. *Mol. Autism* **2018**, *9*, 31. [CrossRef]
80. Sarasua, S.M.; Dwivedi, A.; Boccuto, L.; Chen, C.-F.; Sharp, J.L.; Rollins, J.D.; Collins, J.S.; Rogers, R.C.; Phelan, K.; DuPont, B.R. 22q13.2q13.32 genomic regions associated with severity of speech delay, developmental delay, and physical features in Phelan–McDermid syndrome. *Genet. Med.* **2014**, *16*, 318–328. [CrossRef]
81. Wilson, H.L.; Crolla, J.A.; Walker, D.; Artifoni, L.; Dallapiccola, B.; Takano, T.; Vasudevan, P.; Huang, S.; Maloney, V.; Yobb, T.; et al. Interstitial 22q13 deletions: Genes other than SHANK3 have major effects on cognitive and language development. *Eur. J. Hum. Genet.* **2008**, *16*, 1301–1310. [CrossRef]

82. Kent, W.J.; Sugnet, C.W.; Furey, T.S.; Roskin, K.M.; Pringle, T.H.; Zahler, A.M.; Haussler, D. The Human Genome Browser at UCSC. *Genome Res.* **2002**, *12*, 996–1006. [CrossRef]
83. Strong, E.; Butcher, D.T.; Singhania, R.; Mervis, C.B.; Morris, C.A.; De Carvalho, D.; Weksberg, R.; Osborne, L.R. Symmetrical Dose-Dependent DNA-Methylation Profiles in Children with Deletion or Duplication of 7q11.23. *Am. J. Hum. Genet.* **2015**, *97*, 216–227. [CrossRef] [PubMed]
84. Siu, M.T.; Butcher, D.T.; Turinsky, A.L.; Cytrynbaum, C.; Stavropoulos, D.J.; Walker, S.; Caluseriu, O.; Carter, M.; Lou, Y.; Nicolson, R.; et al. Functional DNA methylation signatures for autism spectrum disorder genomic risk loci: 16p11.2 deletions and CHD8 variants. *Clin. Epigenetics* **2019**, *11*, 103. [CrossRef] [PubMed]
85. Rooney, K.; Levy, M.A.; Haghshenas, S.; Kerkhof, J.; Rogaia, D.; Tedesco, M.G.; Imperatore, V.; Mencarelli, A.; Squeo, G.M.; Di Venere, E.; et al. Identification of a DNA Methylation Episignature in the 22q11.2 Deletion Syndrome. *Int. J. Mol. Sci.* **2021**, *22*, 8611. [CrossRef] [PubMed]
86. Van Gils, J.; Magdinier, F.; Fergelot, P.; Lacombe, D. Rubinstein-Taybi Syndrome: A Model of Epigenetic Disorder. *Genes* **2021**, *12*, 968. [CrossRef] [PubMed]
87. Choufani, S.; Cytrynbaum, C.; Chung, B.H.Y.; Turinsky, A.L.; Grafodatskaya, D.; Chen, Y.A.; Cohen, A.S.A.; Dupuis, L.; Butcher, D.T.; Siu, M.T.; et al. NSD1 mutations generate a genome-wide DNA methylation signature. *Nat. Commun.* **2015**, *6*, 10207. [CrossRef]
88. Singh, H.R.; Nardozza, A.P.; Möller, I.R.; Knobloch, G.; Kistemaker, H.A.V.; Hassler, M.; Harrer, N.; Blessing, C.; Eustermann, S.; Kotthoff, C.; et al. A Poly-ADP-Ribose Trigger Releases the Auto-Inhibition of a Chromatin Remodeling Oncogene. *Mol. Cell* **2017**, *68*, 860–871. [CrossRef]
89. Cho, S.; Kim, H.-S.; Zeiger, M.A.; Umbricht, C.B.; Cope, L.M. Measuring DNA Copy Number Variation Using High-Density Methylation Microarrays. *J. Comput. Biol.* **2019**, *26*, 295–304. [CrossRef]
90. Feber, A.; Guilhamon, P.; Lechner, M.; Fenton, T.; Wilson, G.A.; Thirlwell, C.; Morris, T.J.; Flanagan, A.M.; Teschendorff, A.E.; Kelly, J.D.; et al. Using high-density DNA methylation arrays to profile copy number alterations. *Genome Biol.* **2014**, *15*, R30. [CrossRef]
91. Tian, Y.; Morris, T.J.; Webster, A.P.; Yang, Z.; Beck, S.; Feber, A.; Teschendorff, A.E. ChAMP: Updated methylation analysis pipeline for Illumina BeadChips. *Bioinformatics* **2017**, *33*, 3982–3984. [CrossRef]
92. Morris, T.J.; Butcher, L.M.; Feber, A.; Teschendorff, A.E.; Chakravarthy, A.R.; Wojdacz, T.K.; Beck, S. ChAMP: 450k Chip Analysis Methylation Pipeline. *Bioinformatics* **2014**, *30*, 428–430. [CrossRef]
93. Papillon-Cavanagh, S.; Fortin, J.-P.; De Jay, N. CopyNumber 450k: An R Package for CNV Inference Using Illumina 450k DNA Methylation Assay. 2013. Available online: http://rdrr.io/github/spapillon/CopyNumber450k/ (accessed on 15 May 2022).
94. Montano, C.; Britton, J.F.; Harris, J.R.; Kerkhof, J.; Barnes, B.T.; Lee, J.A.; Sadikovic, B.; Sobreira, N.; Fahrner, J.A. Genome-wide DNA methylation profiling confirms a case of low-level mosaic Kabuki syndrome 1. *Am. J. Med. Genet. Part A* **2022**, *188*, 2217–2225. [CrossRef] [PubMed]

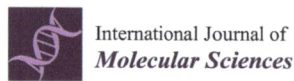
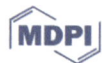

Case Report

A Complex Genomic Rearrangement Resulting in Loss of Function of *SCN1A* and *SCN2A* in a Patient with Severe Developmental and Epileptic Encephalopathy

Valeria Orlando [1,*,†], Silvia Di Tommaso [1,*,†], Viola Alesi [1], Sara Loddo [1], Silvia Genovese [1], Giorgia Catino [1], Licia Martucci [1], Maria Cristina Roberti [1], Marina Trivisano [2], Maria Lisa Dentici [3,4], Nicola Specchio [2], Bruno Dallapiccola [4], Alessandro Ferretti [2] and Antonio Novelli [1]

1. Laboratory of Medical Genetics, Translational Cytogenomics Research Unit, Bambino Gesù Children Hospital, IRCCS, 00146 Rome, Italy
2. Rare and Complex Epilepsy Unit, Department of Neuroscience, Bambino Gesù Children Hospital, IRCCS, 00146 Rome, Italy
3. Medical Genetics Unit, Bambino Gesù Children Hospital, IRCCS, 00146 Rome, Italy
4. Genetics and Rare Disease Research Division, Bambino Gesù Children Hospital, IRCCS, 00146 Rome, Italy
* Correspondence: valeria.orlando@opbg.net (V.O.); silvia.ditommaso@opbg.net (S.D.T.)
† These authors contributed equally to this work.

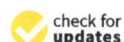

Citation: Orlando, V.; Di Tommaso, S.; Alesi, V.; Loddo, S.; Genovese, S.; Catino, G.; Martucci, L.; Roberti, M.C.; Trivisano, M.; Dentici, M.L.; et al. A Complex Genomic Rearrangement Resulting in Loss of Function of *SCN1A* and *SCN2A* in a Patient with Severe Developmental and Epileptic Encephalopathy. *Int. J. Mol. Sci.* **2022**, *23*, 12900. https://doi.org/10.3390/ijms232112900

Academic Editors: David E. Godler and Olivia J. Veatch

Received: 1 September 2022
Accepted: 17 October 2022
Published: 26 October 2022

Publisher's Note: MDPI stays neutral with regard to jurisdictional claims in published maps and institutional affiliations.

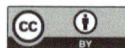

Copyright: © 2022 by the authors. Licensee MDPI, Basel, Switzerland. This article is an open access article distributed under the terms and conditions of the Creative Commons Attribution (CC BY) license (https://creativecommons.org/licenses/by/4.0/).

Abstract: Complex genomic rearrangements (CGRs) are structural variants arising from two or more chromosomal breaks, which are challenging to characterize by conventional or molecular cytogenetic analysis (karyotype and FISH). The integrated approach of standard and genomic techniques, including optical genome mapping (OGM) and genome sequencing, is crucial for disclosing and characterizing cryptic chromosomal rearrangements at high resolutions. We report on a patient with a complex developmental and epileptic encephalopathy in which karyotype analysis showed a de novo balanced translocation involving the long arms of chromosomes 2 and 18. Microarray analysis detected a 194 Kb microdeletion at 2q24.3 involving the *SCN2A* gene, which was considered the likely translocation breakpoint on chromosome 2. However, OGM redefined the translocation breakpoints by disclosing a paracentric inversion at 2q24.3 disrupting *SCN1A*. This combined genomic high-resolution approach allowed a fine characterization of the CGR, which involves two different chromosomes with four breakpoints. The patient's phenotype resulted from the concomitant loss of function of *SCN1A* and *SCN2A*.

Keywords: array CGH; CGR; complex genomic rearrangements; chromothripsis; cryptic rearrangement; OGM; optical genome mapping; genome sequencing; DEE; developmental and epileptic encephalopathy; *SCN1A*; *SCN2A*

1. Introduction

Complex genomic rearrangements (CGRs) include structural variants with two or more breakpoints that are not fully characterized by conventional G-banded karyotyping and FISH. CGRs are non-recurrent rearrangements mostly caused by microhomology-mediated recombination processes [1]. Recently, a new phenomenon, chromothripsis, was defined as the shattering and reshuffling of one or a few chromosome segments during a one-step catastrophic event, associated with the incomplete repair of double-strand breaks (DSBs) through non-homologous end-joining (NHEJ) [2]. Initially, this phenomenon was reported in cancer cells, in which tens to hundreds of genomic rearrangements have been acquired in a single catastrophic event [3], while other studies suggest a similar mechanism of NHEJ in both CGRs and cancer [4]. However, recent evidence argues that chromothripsis could occur in the germline and in the early stage of embryonic development, leading to stable and heritable CGRs [5,6].

A fine characterization of CGRs is crucial for the identification of gene disruption at breakpoints and for evaluating the clinical outcome. Karyotype and FISH analysis can provide important genomic information but are unable to provide a fine characterization of the rearrangements. A combined approach of genomic high-resolution methods overcomes these limits and provides clues to a deeper genotype–phenotype analysis.

Genome sequencing and optical genome mapping (OGM) analysis, a non-sequencing genome imaging tool, are innovative approaches providing high-resolution information about numerical and structural rearrangements.

We report on a female patient affected by developmental and epileptic encephalopathy (DEE) [7] in which OGM and genome sequencing detected a de novo complex genomic rearrangement, not fully resolved by standard techniques, explaining the clinical phenotype.

Clinical Description

We describe an 8-year-old girl with an unremarkable perinatal history, born at term from non-consanguineous parents. Family history was negative. Her 6-year-old brother is healthy. The patient had a normal development up to the age of 16 months, when neurodevelopmental regression was noticed with worsening of vigilance, feeding difficulties, and asthenic body habitus, following a first episode of seizures, occurring in conjunction with fever. A cranial TC scan and electroencephalogram (EEG) were considered normal. Afterwards, she developed afebrile generalized tonic–clonic, focal to bilateral tonic–clonic and myoclonic seizures, associated with resistance to anti-seizure medications (ASMs), including valproate, clonazepam, levetiracetam, phenobarbital, clobazam, sulthiame, rufinamide, lacosamide, carbamazepine, ketogenic diet, vigabatrin, topiramate, cannabidiol, and phenytoine, which did not result in a significant benefit or worsening of epilepsy and development. She also experienced several episodes of status epilepticus.

The patient was firstly evaluated by us at the age of 5 years, when she manifested severe cognitive and intellectual disability with limited social interaction, poor eye contact, absent speech, behavior disturbances and moderate axial hypotonia and hyporeflexia. She experienced drug-resistant focal–tonic seizures with secondary bilateral clonic-tonic diffusion and myoclonic seizures, with multiple clusters per day. Video-EEG recording revealed a severe disruption of background activity with recurrent high voltage slow waves intermingled with epileptiform abnormalities, predominantly over the bilateral frontal and temporal regions. Ictal discharge showed a diffuse low-voltage fast activity, increasing in amplitude and decreasing in frequency, bilateral and symmetrical, associated with a massive and diffuse tonic contraction, with flushing of the face and trunk, perioral cyanosis, and sialorrhea, followed by tonic–clonic contraction of upper and lower limbs lasting 90 s (Figure S1). A clinical diagnosis of developmental and epileptic encephalopathy (DEE) was made.

2. Results

NGS analysis was performed on the patient's blood as a first-line test, focusing on genes associated with epileptic encephalopathies, but no pathogenic variants were detected. Cytogenetic analysis revealed a female karyotype with a de novo balanced translocation involving the long arms of chromosomes 2 and 18 (Figure 1). Array-CGH analysis disclosed a de novo microdeletion at 2q24.3, spanning 194 Kb of genomic DNA (arr[GRCh37]2q24.3(166,079,043_166,273,000) × 1 dn), including the entire *SCN2A* gene (Figure 2), which was considered the likely translocation breakpoint on chromosome 2.

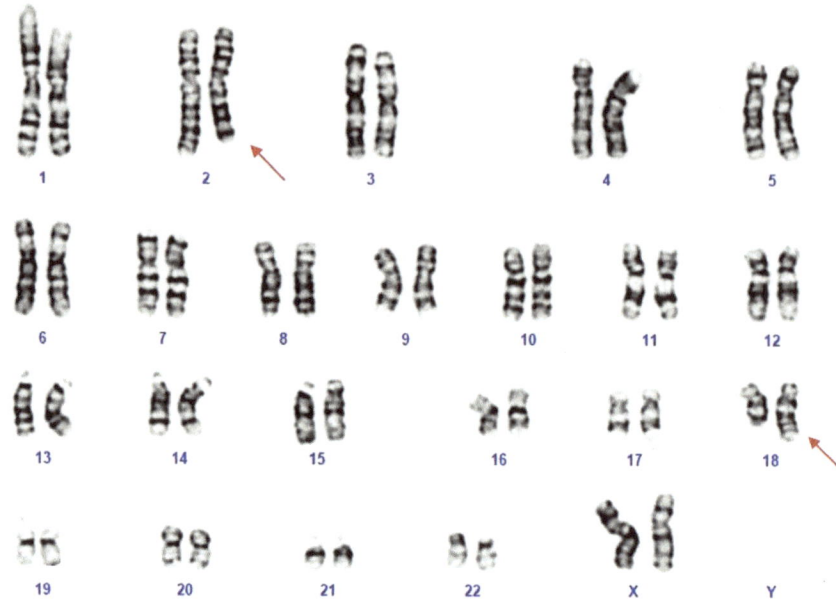

Figure 1. The patient's karyotype showing a reciprocal translocation between the long arm of chromosomes 2 and 18.

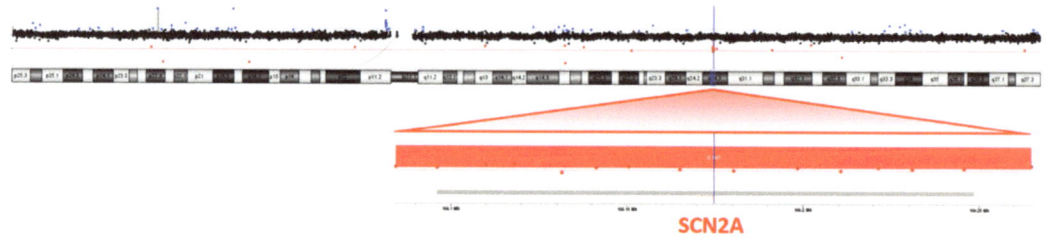

Figure 2. Array-CGH (4 × 180K platform) showing a microdeletion at 2q24.3, spanning 194 Kb of genomic DNA including the entire *SCN2A* gene.

Genome sequencing and OGM confirmed the 2q24.3 deletion and the reciprocal 2q;18q translocation, but ruled out the association between the two rearrangements. In fact, the translocation breakpoint was found to map several Mb downstream in a gene "desert" region at 2q32.1. A paracentric inversion was detected within this region, with the distal breakpoint at 2q32.1, overlapping the translocation breakpoint and the proximal breakpoint at 2q24.3, 655 Kb downstream the deletion disclosed by CMA. Interestingly, the 2q24.3 proximal breakpoint disrupted the first intron of the *SCN1A* gene, probably causing its functional inactivation (Figure 3). The translocation breakpoint on chromosome 18, at 18q21.32, disrupted the *ALPK2* gene, whose haploinsufficiency is not associated with clinical outcome to date.

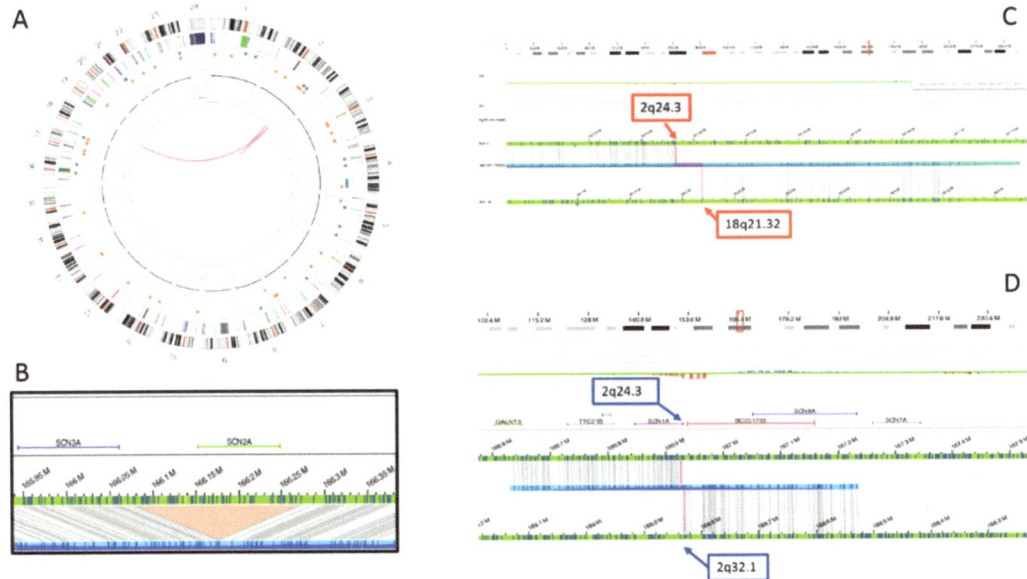

Figure 3. Complex genomic rearrangements (CGR) disclosed by optical genome mapping. Graphic visualizations of the rearrangement include the circle plot (**A**), the *SCN2A* gene deletion (**B**), the 2;18 translocation with breakpoints at 2q24.3 and 18q21.32 (**C**) and paracentric inversion involving 2q24.3 and 2q32.1 breakpoints (**D**).

3. Discussion

The integrated use of high-resolution platform (CMA) and new technologies, including OMG and genome sequencing, proves to be helpful in the fine characterization of CGRs, which is mandatory in establishing accurate genotype–phenotype correlation. The present patient showed a complex phenotype of developmental and epileptic encephalopathy (DEE) with neurodevelopmental regression since 16 months of age, when the epilepsy started, with different seizures semiology and a strong resistance to ASMs.

Cytogenetic analysis revealed a balanced translocation involving the long arm of chromosomes 2 and 18, and CMA detected a small de novo 2q24.3 microdeletion, including the *SCN2A* gene. These results did not seem per se capable of explaining the rapid evolution and the complexity of clinical outcome, since recent studies report loss-of function variations of the *SCN2A* gene in association to intellectual disability (ID) without seizures [8].

Thus, OGM and genome sequencing were used for a deeper characterization of the rearrangement, with the aim of refining the correlation between the 2q24.3 microdeletion and the translocation breakpoints. Genome sequencing and OGM highlighted a CGR involving the 2q24.3 region, characterized by four breakpoints, two delimiting the known *SCN2A* gene deletion and two more distal, delimiting a paracentric inversion, including one overlapping the translocation breakpoint and one into the first intron of the *SCN1A* gene. The inversion causes the displacement of the 5′ UTR region and the first exon of the *SCN1A* gene from 2q24.3 to 2q32.1, leading to probable inactivation of the gene (Figure 4). To our knowledge, this is the first patient in which the concomitant inactivation of both the *SCN1A* and *SCN2A* genes has been documented.

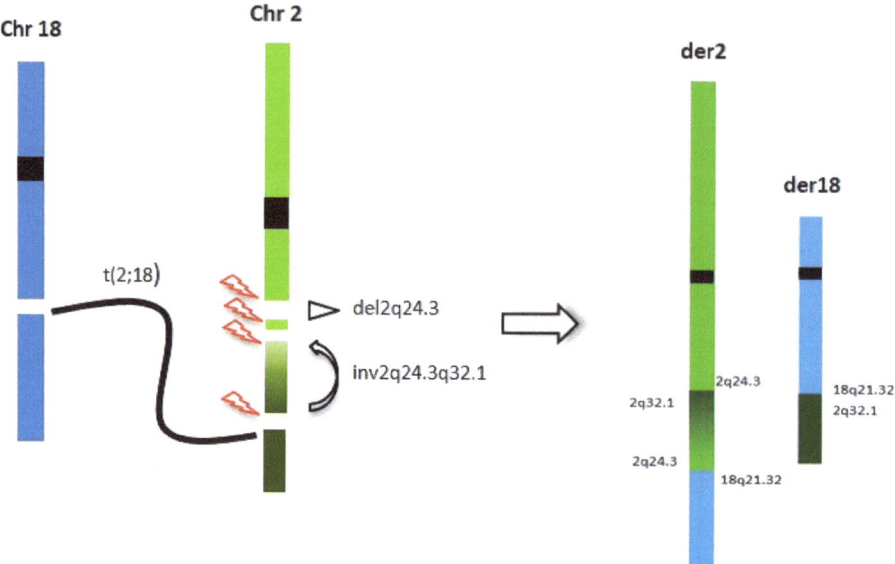

Figure 4. Chromotripsis event underlying the CGR identified in our patient: breakpoints are reported and chromosome segments reshuffling is represented.

SCN1A and SCN2A encode Nav1.1 and Nav1.2, respectively, two of nine α-subunits of the channel pore of voltage-gated sodium (Nav) channels, together with more β-subunits modulating function [9]. Nav channels have an essential role in correcting the neurological functions involved in the initiation and propagation of action potentials across the central nervous system [10]. SCN1A and SCN2A are the most commonly mutated epilepsy-associated genes, with different pathogenic variants leading to a wide range of phenotypes with variable disease severity [11]. More than 140 variants in SCN1A and more than 200 in SCN2A have been described [12].

Pathogenic variants in SCN2A are associated with a wide spectrum of neurodevelopmental disorders and four different phenotypes have been delineated, including benign familiar neonatal-infantile seizures (BFIS3) (OMIM # 607745), episodic ataxia type 9 (EA9) (OMIM #618924), developmental and epileptic encephalopathy-11 (DEE11) (OMIM #613721), autism spectrum disorder and intellectual disability (ASD/ID) [13,14].

Causative variants in SCN1A were identified in patients with an age-dependent epileptic encephalopathy, known as Dravet syndrome (DS) (OMIM # 607208), and in patients showing a spectrum of seizure disorders, ranging from early-onset isolated febrile seizures to generalized epilepsy with febrile seizures plus, type 2 (GEFSP2) (OMIM # 604403). Missense variants of SCN2A are the most common variants in epileptic encephalopathies and they typically have a gain-of-function effect (GOF), resulting in patients which usually benefit from sodium channel blockers (SCBs), whereas de novo loss of function variants inducing SCN1A haploinsufficiency are usually associated with DS [13].

The clinical characteristics of our patient do not exactly match with any specific phenotype classified in association with SCN1A or SCN2A gene variations. In the present patient, the epilepsy onset was after the first year of life, while in Dravet syndrome the onset of seizures typically is around 6 months of age, although a minority of cases manifest seizures in the second year of life. On the other hand, in the present case the first seizure was associated with a fever, and she experienced different seizure semiology (focal and generalized tonic–clonic and myoclonic seizures) as reported in Dravet syndrome, as well as psychomotor regression and behavior disorder [15].

Interstitial deletions of 2q24.3 are very rare. In 2015, Lim et al. [16] reviewed the literature of 2q24.3 deletions with variable extensions and, thus, differently involving the various sodium channel gene clusters (*SCN3A*, *SCN2A*, *SCN1A*, *SCN9A*, and *SCN7A*). *SCN1A* is considered the major contributor to the epileptic phenotype, although the role of other sodium channel genes that map within this cluster is less delineated. Patients with deletion of the entire sodium channel gene cluster exhibited a complex epilepsy phenotype characterized by migrating partial seizures of infancy with neonatal seizure onset, severe developmental delay and acquired microcephaly. Individuals with partial deletion of *SCN1A* and *SCN9A* and whole *SCN1A* deletion present with an epileptic phenotype of Dravet syndrome. Our patient presented a neurodevelopmental regression in conjunction with multiple drug-resistant afebrile generalized tonic–clonic and myoclonic seizures, followed by developmental and epileptic encephalopathy (DEE). The loss of function of *SCN1A* and the concurrent *SCN2A* gene deletion, due to cryptic CGRs likely arising from a chromotripsis event at germinal level or in the very early mitotic divisions, might explain her complex phenotype as result of a double hit. These results support the hypothesis that these events occur during an "all in one" chromosomal catastrophe rather than through the progressive acquirement of mutations or rearrangements.

In conclusion, the application of a combined genomic high-resolution approach allows the fine characterization of CGRs, and improves the molecular diagnosis leading to precise treatments and better clinical outcome.

4. Materials and Methods

4.1. Sample Collection and Consent

EDTA and Na-Heparin peripheral blood samples of the patient and her parents were collected and used for molecular and cytogenetic testing. DNA was isolated by means of a Qiagen blood kit (Qiagen, Hilden, Germany) according to the manufacturer's instructions. The patient's parents signed an informed consent for genetic analysis and publication purpose. The study was approved by the Ethics Committee of OPBG Hospital in compliance with the Helsinki Declaration.

4.2. Mutation Analysis

A custom gene panel including genes associated with epileptic encephalopathy was analyzed by next-generation sequencing (NGS) on genomic DNA. The patient's library preparation and targeted resequencing were performed using the NimbleGen SeqCap Target Enrichment kit (Roche, Basilea, Switzerland) on a NextSeq550 (Illumina, San Diego, CA, USA) platform, according to the manufacture's protocol. The BaseSpace pipeline (Illumina, San Diego, CA, USA) and the Geneyx Analysis software (Geneyx, Genomex Ltd., Herzliya, Israel) were used for the variant calling and annotating variants, respectively. Sequencing data were aligned to the hg19 human reference genome.

4.3. Cytogenetics Analysis

Karyotype analysis was performed on metaphases from lymphocyte cultures according to standard G-banding techniques.

4.4. Array

CMA (chromosomal microarray analysis) was performed on an array-CGH 4×180K platform (Agilent Technologies, Santa Clara, CA, USA) using standard procedures. Images were obtained using an Agilent DNA Microarray Scanner and analyses were performed by Agilent CytoGenomics (v 5.1.2.1). Confirmation and segregation tests on the patient's and parents' DNA were performed by Sybr Green qPCR [17] on the *SCN2A* gene with the *TERT* gene as internal control.

4.5. Optical Genome Mapping (OGM)

A fresh blood sample was collected in EDTA and stored at −80 °C just after sampling. Ultra-high molecular weight (UHMW) DNA was extracted according to manufacturer's instructions (SP Frozen Human Blood DNA Isolation Protocol, Bionano Genomics, San Diego, CA, USA) and enzymatically labeled (Bionano Prep Direct Label and Stain Protocol). Labeled DNA was uploaded on nanochannel chips and scanned on a Saphyr instrument (Bionano Genomics). An effective genome coverage >100× was achieved. Images were analyzed by Access software v3.6, using Bionano De novo genome assembly pipeline. Genome maps obtained were aligned with Human Genome Reference Consortium GRCh38/hg38 assembly for structural variant detection.

4.6. Genome Sequencing

Library preparation was carried out according to the manufacturer's protocol from DNA PCR-Free Library Prep (Illumina), and sequenced on a NovaSeq6000 (Illumina) platform. The obtained NGS assay presented a mean coverage of 35×, with Q30 bases around 87%. The TruSight Software Suite (Illumina) and the integrated DRAGEN platform and IGV software were used for alignment, variant calling and breakpoint data visualization. Sequencing data were aligned to the hg38 human reference genome.

Supplementary Materials: The following supporting information can be downloaded at: https://www.mdpi.com/article/10.3390/ijms232112900/s1. Figure S1: Ictal video-polygraphic recording of patient at the age of 5 years. The ictal discharge starts with a diffuse low-voltage fast activity, increasing in amplitude and decreasing in frequency, bilateral and symmetrical. Seizure ends after 90 s with intravenous midazolam administration and is followed by a post-ictal suppression of brain electrical activity (Post-Ictal Generalized EEG, PGES). Clinically: abrupt and massive tonic contraction with flushing of the face and trunk, followed by bilateral tonic-clonic contraction of upper and lower limbs 50 s after its beginning.

Author Contributions: Case report writing, V.O. and S.D.T.; patient clinical evaluation, A.F., M.T., N.S. and M.L.D.; review and editing, V.A., S.L., M.C.R., B.D. and A.N.; data analysis, V.O. and S.G.; technical support, L.M. and G.C. All authors have read and agreed to the published version of the manuscript.

Funding: This research was funded by Ministero della Salute, grant number RC2021, to A.N.

Institutional Review Board Statement: The study was conducted according to the guidelines of the Declaration of Helsinki, and approved by the Institutional Review Board of Bambino Gesù Children's Hospital (protocol code RC2021).

Informed Consent Statement: Informed consent was obtained from all subjects involved in the study.

Data Availability Statement: The data that support the findings of this study are available on request from the corresponding author. The data are not publicly available due to privacy or ethical restrictions.

Conflicts of Interest: The authors declare they have no conflicts of interest. The data that support the findings of t his study are available on request from the corresponding author. The data are not publicly available due to privacy or ethical restrictions.

References

1. Zhang, F.; Carvalho, C.M.; Lupski, J.R. Complex human chromosomal and genomic rearrangements. *Trends Genet.* **2009**, *25*, 298–307. [CrossRef]
2. Pellestor, F.; Gatinois, V. Chromoanagenesis: A piece of the macroevolution scenario. *Mol. Cytogenet.* **2020**, *13*, 3. [CrossRef] [PubMed]
3. Stephens, P.J.; Greenman, C.D.; Fu, B.; Yang, F.; Bignell, G.R.; Mudie, L.J.; Pleasance, E.D.; Lau, K.W.; Beare, D.; Stebbings, L.A.; et al. Massive genomic rearrangement acquired in a single catastrophic event during cancer development. *Cell* **2011**, *144*, 27–40. [CrossRef] [PubMed]
4. Liu, P.; Erez, A.; Nagamani, S.C.; Dhar, S.U.; Kołodziejska, K.E.; Dharmadhikari, A.V.; Cooper, M.L.; Wiszniewska, J.; Zhang, F.; Withers, M.A.; et al. Chromosome catastrophes involve replication mechanisms generating complex genomic rearrangements. *Cell* **2011**, *146*, 889–903. [CrossRef]

5. Kloosterman, W.P.; Guryev, V.; van Roosmalen, M.; Duran, K.J.; de Bruijn, E.; Bakker, S.C.; Letteboer, T.; van Nesselrooij, B.; Hochstenbach, R.; Poot, M.; et al. Chromothripsis as a mechanism driving complex de novo structural rearrangements in the germline. *Hum. Mol. Genet.* **2011**, *20*, 1916–1924. [CrossRef] [PubMed]
6. Chiang, C.; Jacobsen, J.C.; Ernst, C.; Hanscom, C.; Heilbut, A.; Blumenthal, I.; Mills, R.E.; Kirby, A.; Lindgren, A.M.; Rudiger, S.R.; et al. Complex reorganization and predominant non-homologous repair following chromosomal breakage in karyotypically balanced germline rearrangements and transgenic integration. *Nat. Genet.* **2012**, *44*, 390–397. [CrossRef] [PubMed]
7. Raga, S.; Specchio, N.; Rheims, S.; Wilmshurst, J.M. Developmental and epileptic encephalopathies: Recognition and approaches to care. *Epileptic Disord.* **2021**, *23*, 40–52. [CrossRef] [PubMed]
8. Begemann, A.; Acuña, M.A.; Zweier, M.; Vincent, M.; Steindl, K.; Bachmann-Gagescu, R.; Hackenberg, A.; Abela, L.; Plecko, B.; Kroell-Seger, J.; et al. Further corroboration of distinct functional features in *SCN2A* variants causing intellectual disability or epileptic phenotypes. *Mol. Med.* **2019**, *25*, 6. [CrossRef] [PubMed]
9. Meisler, M.H.; Kearney, J.A. Sodium channel mutations in epilepsy and other neurological disorders. *J. Clin. Investig.* **2005**, *115*, 2010–2017. [CrossRef] [PubMed]
10. Brunklaus, A.; Ellis, R.; Reavey, E.; Semsarian, C.; Zuberi, S.M. Genotype phenotype associations across the voltage-gated sodium channel family. *J. Med. Genet.* **2014**, *51*, 650–658. [CrossRef] [PubMed]
11. Oliva, M.; Berkovic, S.F.; Petrou, S. Sodium channels and the neurobiology of epilepsy. *Epilepsia* **2012**, *53*, 1849–1859. [CrossRef] [PubMed]
12. Kong, Y.; Yan, K.; Hu, L.; Wang, M.; Dong, X.; Lu, Y.; Wu, B.; Wang, H.; Yang, L.; Zhou, W. Data on mutations and Clinical features in *SCN1A* or *SCN2A* gene. *Data Brief* **2018**, *22*, 492–501. [CrossRef] [PubMed]
13. Wolff, M.; Johannesen, K.M.; Hedrich, U.B.S. Genetic and phenotypic heterogeneity suggest therapeutic implications in *SCN2A*-related disorders. *Brain* **2017**, *140*, 1316–1336. [CrossRef] [PubMed]
14. Reynolds, C.; King, M.D.; Gorman, K.M. The phenotypic spectrum of *SCN2A*-related epilepsy. *Eur. J. Paediatr. Neurol.* **2020**, *24*, 117–122. [CrossRef] [PubMed]
15. Lagae, L. Dravet syndrome. *Curr. Opin. Neurol.* **2021**, *34*, 213–218. [CrossRef] [PubMed]
16. Lim, B.C.; Hwang, H.; Kim, H.; Chae, J.H.; Choi, J.; Kim, K.J.; Hwang, Y.S.; Yum, M.S.; Ko, T.S. Epilepsy phenotype associated with a chromosome 2q24.3 deletion involving SCN1A: Migrating partial seizures of infancy or atypical Dravet syndrome? *Epilepsy Res.* **2015**, *109*, 34–39. [CrossRef] [PubMed]
17. Livak, K.J.; Schmittgen, T.D. Analysis of relative gene expression data using real-time quantitative PCR and the 2(-Delta Delta C(T)) Method. *Methods* **2001**, *25*, 402–408. [CrossRef] [PubMed]

MDPI AG
Grosspeteranlage 5
4052 Basel
Switzerland
Tel.: +41 61 683 77 34

International Journal of Molecular Sciences Editorial Office
E-mail: ijms@mdpi.com
www.mdpi.com/journal/ijms

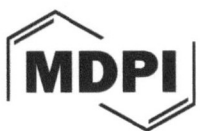

Disclaimer/Publisher's Note: The title and front matter of this reprint are at the discretion of the Guest Editors. The publisher is not responsible for their content or any associated concerns. The statements, opinions and data contained in all individual articles are solely those of the individual Editors and contributors and not of MDPI. MDPI disclaims responsibility for any injury to people or property resulting from any ideas, methods, instructions or products referred to in the content.

www.ingramcontent.com/pod-product-compliance
Lightning Source LLC
LaVergne TN
LVHW072344090526
838202LV00019B/2480